INTERPERSONAL RECONSTRUCTIVE THERAPY

Interpersonal Reconstructive Therapy
Promoting Change in Nonresponders

LORNA SMITH BENJAMIN

THE GUILFORD PRESS
New York   London

© 2003 The Guilford Press
A Division of Guilford Publications, Inc.
72 Spring Street, New York, NY 10012
www.guilford.com

Printed in the United States of America

Last digit is print number: 9   8   7   6   5   4   3   2   1

Library of Congress Cataloging-in-Publication Data

Benjamin, Lorna Smith.
   Interpersonal reconstructive therapy : promoting change in
nonresponders / Lorna Smith Benjamin.
        p.   cm.
Includes bibliographical references and index.
   ISBN 1-57230-538-X (hardcover : alk. paper)
   1. Personality disorders—Treatment.   2. Psychotherapy.   3. Impasse.
(Psychotherapy) 4. Resistance (Psychoanalysis) I. Title.
RC554 .B453 2003
616.89′14—dc21

                                                    2002014668

About the Author

Born and raised in Rochester, New York, **Lorna Smith Benjamin** graduated from Oberlin College and subsequently obtained a PhD in Psychology from the University of Wisconsin in 1960. Because her long-range goal was to try to make clinical practice more amenable to scientific standards, she chose to emphasize acquisition of technical skills in graduate school. There, her specialties were learning theory and neurophysiology, with an outside department minor in mathematical statistics. Four years of post-doctoral clinical training in the University of Wisconsin Department of Psychiatry were followed by several years of part-time work as a research consultant, while she put most of her energy into caring for her two young children. Starting in 1971, she taught principles of human development to medical students, and instructed psychiatry residents and psychology interns in interviewing, assessment, and psychotherapy for adults. She maintained a large clinical practice, as she simultaneously developed the concepts and technology for the Structural Analysis of Social Behavior, her method for objectifying social perceptions and internalized representations. In 1987, Dr. Benjamin left a position as Full Professor of Psychiatry at the University of Wisconsin to become Full Professor in the Department of Psychology and Adjunct Full Professor of Psychiatry at the University of Utah. Presently, she is Co-Director of the Interpersonal Reconstructive Therapy Clinic at the University of Utah Neuropsychiatric Institute. In addition to providing effective service, research tests of efficacy, and training in IRT to students and staff, the hope is that the clinic will soon become able to offer continuing education training in IRT to practicing clinicians.

Preface

This book is for clinicians who work with difficult cases that have not shown adequate improvement, no matter what approach is taken. Many, but not all, individuals with apparently treatment-refractory conditions— the so-called nonresponder population—meet criteria for one or more personality disorders. These patients typically have been tried on many different combinations of medications, and have had one or more extended courses of treatment with psychotherapy. They suffer significantly and are greatly impaired in functioning. The time and money invested by them and by their care providers in trying to find effective relief is likely to have been substantial.

Readers may think that an approach claiming to be useful for nonresponders must be efficacious for Borderline Personality Disorder (BPD). Clinical experience suggests that it is. Interpersonal Reconstructive Therapy (IRT) that is supported by the promise of a long-term working relationship is usually rapidly effective in stopping chronic suicidal and self-mutilating behaviors, as well as other system-rattling characteristics of BPD. However, as suggested by the examples in this book, IRT can be equally useful for the other personality disorders, and for selected other chronic presentations from Axis I. Although no treatment is 100% successful, IRT's success rate does represent an improvement over the baseline rate for this difficult group. Let it be clear that IRT is rarely brief. Few treatments are completed in less than a year, and most are multiyear.

On the basis of IRT theory and practice, which are illustrated by four cases in Chapter 1 and explained in more detail in Chapter 2, IRT provides a sensible, attachment-based explanation for why nonresponders have remained symptomatic. The fundamental idea of IRT is that treatment-refractory patients are responding to internalizations of important persons more than they are to persons in their present-day real world. IRT addresses their relationship with those internalizations. After old expectations and hopes in relation to the internalizations are given up, usual and customary treatment procedures (e.g., medications, cognitive-behavioral or psychodynamic therapy) have a better chance to work. This fundamental idea is applied as follows.

In the IRT case formulation and treatment method, problem patterns are linked to learning with important early loved ones via one or more of three copy processes: (1) Be like him or her; (2) Act as if he or she is still there and in control; and (3) Treat yourself as he or she treated you. For example, if a female child lives with a relentlessly critical parent, the child is very likely to become critical of and displeased with herself. The copying is maintained by fantasies that Important Persons and their Internalized Representations (IPIRs) ultimately will provide the desired love if the patient's living testimony to the IPIR's rules and values is good enough. This illustrative patient, who morbidly criticizes and disapproves of herself, is treating herself as an important loved one treated her. In an often unrecognized way, applying that old view to herself represents incorporation of the perceived parental rules and values. Such intense devotion to relentless self-criticism suggests a continuing wish to please that parent.

Since the relationship with the internalization is immensely powerful, treatment must focus sharply on grieving and letting go of these fantasy residues of early attachments. In IRT, there are flow charts that guide the clinician in using the theory to develop the individual case formulation, and to choose optimal treatment interventions on a moment-to-moment basis. The core algorithm details the required domains of focus. There are five steps in IRT, each requiring activities that facilitate self-discovery (psychodynamic) and self-management (behavioral). All steps address a basic conflict between the Regressive Loyalist (Red; the part that seeks the approval of the IPIRs) and the Growth Collaborator (Green; the part that comes to therapy for constructive change). The five steps are as follows: (1) collaboration (the therapy relationship); (2) about patterns, where they are from, and what they are for (insight); (3) blocking problem patterns (crisis and stalemate management); (4) enabling the will to change (in steps that compare to Prochaska's transtheoretical stages of change); and (5) learning new patterns (via standard behavioral technology).

The effectiveness of IRT has not yet been demonstrated by a formal clinical trials protocol. A small pilot study (mentioned in Chapter 10) has shown significant reduction in symptomatology, as well as marked reduction in suicide attempts and frequency of hospitalizations. Perhaps of greater interest to clinicians are the reports from many experienced practitioners that IRT ideas are immediately useful in the treatments of their difficult cases. Beginning therapists find IRT to be helpful, too. For example, a number of psychology graduate students trained in IRT have said that they found its concepts to be helpful in preparing them for the challenges of internship, while their peers declared that when confronted with difficult cases, they had little idea of what to do.

Useful background readings for skills frequently used in implementing IRT include Rogers's (1951) revolutionary presentation of client-centered therapy, Goldfried and Davison's (1994) authoritative and clinically informed summary of behavior therapy, and Thoma and Kachele's (1987) very readable account of psychoanalytic treatment. An understanding of Structural Analysis of Social Behavior (SASB; Benjamin, 1996d) usually enhances the clinician's ability to recognize patterns and their links to IPIRs. Familiarity with SASB is recommended, but not required, for the practice of IRT. On the other hand, SASB is essential to the research tests of the validity of IRT case formulations, of adherence, and of links between therapy process and outcome.

Writing this book involved challenge, patience, and repetitive toil similar to that asked of patients and therapists using IRT to modify intractable patterns. At first, my self-imposed task of summarizing wisdom cumulated over three decades of practice, teaching, and research seemed insurmountable. The biggest breakthrough came when I was supervising yet another good student in how to handle a suicidal patient, and realized I was repeating things I had said many times before. There was an underlying logic to my recommendations for handling this problem, even though the details varied a lot from patient to patient. At the time, I happened to have a new "toy"—a computer program that makes flow charts. It seemed that the "system" for handling crisis could be organized by the flow chart program. The result was an early version of Figure 7.1 in this book. The idea of using flow charts was then applied to other problems, and made it possible to organize the material in this book sensibly.

Now that the basic ideas are summarized in this book, a future step with a high priority is to develop workbooks illustrating the varieties of ways in which the core algorithm and flow charts can be implemented. Such workbooks will focus primarily on enhancing clinicians' ability to adhere to IRT procedures. The most common form of adherence failure is to forget to consider the case formulation and the Red–Green conflict with every intervention.

One barrier to learning to focus on the underlying IPIRs is the fact that many younger therapists' training emphasizes giving priority to symptom management. According to IRT, focus on symptoms can be helpful, but it can also be iatrogenic. The case formulation helps predict response to a focus on symptoms. For example, suppose a man with Passive–Aggressive Personality Disorder (PAG) is very slow in getting ready in the morning, and is about to lose his job because of chronic lateness. Focus on the steps of getting ready and meeting the arrival time deadline is highly likely to escalate rather than diminish symptoms. The reason is that, for this particular patient, the therapist is repeating parts of his earlier experiences that led to his oppositional and self-destructive method of self-definition via PAG. Such severely disordered individuals are responding to internalizations of earlier relationships rather than to "contingencies" in their present lives. Under the IRT protocol, symptom-focused therapists would learn to conduct their functional analyses in relation to attachments to underlying IPIRs that have been identified by the case formulation. Interventions would then target the relationship with the particular IPIR associated with the symptom, rather than the symptom itself.

Whereas younger therapists tend to be preoccupied with symptoms, older therapists are likely to suffer from a lack of interest in developing any sharp focus at all. They have been trained that a clinician who has a preconceived notion of what is important will inappropriately impose his or her prejudices, and get in the patient's way of true understanding. Clinicians with this perspective are more likely to concentrate on generic facilitative processes, such as empathy, remembering, and "getting it out." These facilitative methods and many other procedures are also important in IRT, but not *ad libitum*, and not for every patient or situation.

Learning IRT is a complex task. Like other forms of learning, it requires substantial patience and effort. Learning is faster for therapists who already have the component skills. For example, consider therapists who encourage experiencing distinct parts of the self, as in emotion-focused therapy (Greenberg, Rice, & Elliott, 1993). Using different language, these experientially oriented therapists are experts in helping patients develop compassion for what is called Green in IRT, and let go of Red wishes and hurts. Although they are ahead of the curve in facilitating such self-discovery, these therapists might need coaching in drawing upon behavioral techniques to enhance self-management. Under the IRT protocol, they would follow the core algorithm and use the flow charts selectively to become more directive. Their new therapist behaviors would have the purpose of helping patients build more adaptive ways of being, once they have discovered and begun to let go of their problem wishes.

A second future step is to conduct formal clinical trials to test whether IRT is as effective with nonresponders as it has seemed to be. The University of Utah Neuropsychiatric Institute (UNI) believes that it is, and is sponsoring an IRT specialty clinic that provides teaching, research, and service to the nonresponder population.

There are many who deserve thanks for their valuable contributions to IRT and to this book. First, I want to thank Tom Woolf and Ross VanVranken of UNI for their willingness to bring the IRT specialty clinic to life. Next, I gratefully acknowledge Seymour Weingarten, editor-in-chief of The Guilford Press, who has been very patient and supportive. If he had made me stick to the original time line, this book would never have happened. Jim Nageotte, my editor, has been diligent and challenging in help-ful and much-appreciated ways. Many of the notes and clarifying examples are the result of his good work.

Deep gratitude is also extended to the patients who have participated in some or all steps of IRT and have agreed to help others by granting per-mission to share their stories with others. In addition to these patients (who cannot be named), students and former students have greatly shaped the development and description of IRT concepts. Some, but not all, who deserve thanks include Tracey Smith, David Moore, Kok Mun Soo-Tho, JuHui Park, Wilson Butz-Whittaker, Arlin Hatch, and Melissa Hawkins.

Likewise, many clinical and research collaborators are due thanks and acknowledgments. Kathleen Levenick is at the top of that list. For many years, Kathleen has been teaching SASB and various versions of IRT to practicing clinicians. Her commentary on this book has been particularly valuable, because she knows what kinds of questions are most likely to come from practicing clinician learners. She also, of course, has good an-swers to them! Paul Pilkonis, an expert in formulating clinical concepts in ways that are amenable to research, was helpful. Thanks also go to Jennifer Skeem, whose energy and intelligence mobilized an IRT study group at Western Psychiatric Institute. For their continuing support and encouragement over many years, I thank Marjorie and Norman Green-field, Allen Frances, Ted Millon, Robert Carson, Marvin Goldfried, Robert Spitzer, and Pio Scilligo. I am grateful, too, to more recent colleagues who have contributed to IRT as well as to applications of SASB. These include Aaron Pincus, Steffan Sohlberg, Wolfgang Tress, Gherardo Amadei, and Karla Moras. Finally, I owe much to Harry F. Harlow, my major advisor, for modeling how to sift wheat from the chaff, and for his compelling dem-onstrations of the impact of attachment on social development.

To all of these good people, and to my loving children and grandchil-dren, I offer my heartfelt thanks for being who you are and for letting me be with you.

LORNA SMITH BENJAMIN

Contents

CHAPTER 1.   Introduction and Overview   1

CHAPTER 2.   Case Formulation   31

CHAPTER 3.   Choosing Interventions   72

CHAPTER 4.   Structural Analysis of Social Behavior: 120
              The Clarifying Lens

CHAPTER 5.   Step 1: Collaboration   154

CHAPTER 6.   Step 2: Learning about Patterns, Where   193
              They Are From, and What They Are For

CHAPTER 7.   Step 3: Blocking Maladaptive Patterns   226

CHAPTER 8.   Step 4: Enabling the Will to Change   262

CHAPTER 9.   Step 5: Learning New Patterns   299

CHAPTER 10.   Interpersonal Reconstructive Therapy   325
              in Clinical and Research Contexts

References   352

Index   364

1

Introduction and Overview

PROLOGUE: FOUR NONRESPONDERS

Case 1. Marie: Scared to Death

Marie, a 56-year-old school teacher, was brought to the hospital for treatment of her long-standing anxiety and depression. She had been given antidepressants throughout her illness. About 4 years ago, anxiolytics had been added, and they had successfully contained the anxiety until the 3 months preceding this hospitalization. It then intensified to a level that Marie called "ultimate fear." She declared, "Anxiety is the major feeling of my whole life." Marie's primary diagnosis was Major Depressive Disorder, according to the prevalent practice of letting depression preempt anxiety. She was also suffering from a significant medical condition. The patient summarized her understanding of the basis of the problem: "They believe my father began incesting when I was 3 months old." She had been in psychotherapy for 15 years.

Case 2. Kenneth: Wrong-Patient Syndrome

Kenneth was a 42-year-old man who came to the hospital for treatment of suicidal thoughts associated with his belief that his wife had been "stepping out on him." He was extremely angry, vaguely threatening his wife and her alleged lover; he declared he was so upset that he did not want to be alive. Along with agitation, there were many vegetative signs. Kenneth was diagnosed with Major Depressive Disorder. A few months before this hospitalization, Kenneth had started psychotherapy, but had "fired" three counselors so far. He continued to take his Prozac. Other than taking medication, Kenneth refused to participate in the psychosocial treatment programs offered by the hospital. Rather, he was devoted to repetitive description of all the evidence of his wife's infidelity.

1

Case 3. Jessica: "It Is Only a Question of When and How to Die

Jessica, a 39-year-old woman, had recently separated from her husband of 20 years. A valued customer service representative for a well-known hotel chain, she had been on medical leave for 4 months because of her severe depression. She had recurrent severe Major Depressive Disorder, and for the past 21 years had been given all classes of antidepressants, as well as an antipsychotic. Jessica had also had a variety of psychotherapies. The current hospitalization was for evaluation of suicidality, because she had recently been "researching" suicide, declaring that she did not want to choose a method that would fail. About a year previous to this hospitalization, symptoms of anxiety and panic had appeared, particularly when Jessica was shopping for groceries or for clothing. The fear of shopping was a mystery to her and to all of the family, because, she explained, "everybody knows I love to shop." Although Jessica's narratives were quite logical, and her behavior and appearance were well socialized, the patient disclosed that she had heard "voices" for many years. One voice was "reasonable and good"; another was "bad." When Jessica found herself in difficult situations, these voices would start talking simultaneously and were very confusing.

Case 4. Patsy: "I Can't Deal with Life"

Patsy was a 40-year-old woman who had suffered from severe and recurrent Major Depressive Disorder for 6 years. Recently, her suicidal ideation had escalated. Patsy had taken Prozac at first, but later was switched to Zoloft. During all of this time, she had been trying to separate from her physically abusive, alcohol-dependent husband. Patsy frequently asked him to leave, but much to the consternation of family and friends, invited him back shortly afterward. Patsy provided the sole support for the family, while the husband spent large sums on his own personal interests—motorcycles, boats, and related paraphernalia. She was "getting tired." On more than one occasion in the past, Patsy had assaulted her oldest child to the point that medical care was required; however, she had been in cognitive therapy and said she had learned skills in anger management. Although Patsy believed she would never again attack one of her children, her impulses to do so were now beginning to return.

HOW CAN RESULTS FOR NONRESPONDERS BE IMPROVED?

Such cases as the ones just described are not unusual in today's hospital practices. These four were referred for consultation for evaluation of potential complications from personality disorders. Such referrals for evaluation of "possible Axis II involvement" (defined in the *Diagnostic and Statistical Manual of Mental Disorders*, fourth edition [DSM-IV]; American Psychiatric Association, 1994) are typically brought about by apparent unresponsiveness to state-of-the-art treatments. Marie had been in psychotherapy for 15 years, and felt she must continue her work on the residual effects of sexual abuse. She had had good treatment with psychoactive drugs, but her depression, anxiety, and medical condition had made it difficult to function in her job as a filing clerk. Luckily, her employer was highly tolerant of her many absences. Kenneth was depressed, suicidal, and perhaps homicidal. As far as he was concerned, the whole problem was his wife. Except for taking Prozac, he was completely unwilling to accept anything from health care providers except empathic listening to his legalistic logic about the crimes of his wife. His depression had yet to remit. Jessica was experiencing chronic and severe depression; she had been tried on every possible antidepressant plus an antipsychotic. At the time of hospitalization, she was lethally suicidal—scaring everyone with her cool, systematic search for a good method, backed up by her recent preparation of a will. Patsy was greatly stressed by her abusive husband, but could not leave him for more than a few days. Although she had been helped to manage her temper in important ways, her urges to attack her children were returning, and her depression was escalating out of control.

Clinical facts suggest that a substantial number of mentally disordered individuals, like these four, do not respond well either to medications or to psychotherapy. Like most such patients, they have been tried on several classes of drugs and often have had repeated hospitalizations. They also have had psychotherapy, sometimes for many years. Despite such efforts, they continue to suffer. In studies of DSM-IV Axis I clinical syndromes, such individuals are called nonresponders, or are said to have treatment-refractory or treatment-resistant disorders. For example, the problems of treatment-refractory depression (Bonner & Howard, 1995) and schizophrenia (Buckley, Wiggins, Sebastian, & Singer, 2001) are well documented. Personality disorders themselves have long been recognized as treatment-refractory (Reich, 1949; Shea, 1993), and this may be a reason why Axis II disorders come to mind as a possible explanation for nonresponsiveness of some patients with Axis I disorders. In this volume, these individuals are called nonresponders. The term can apply to disorders, individuals, populations and more. It simply describes a history of minimal responsiveness.

Most researchers and clinicians agree that the presence of personality disorders significantly worsens the prognosis for treatment of clinical syndromes (Perry, Bannon, & Ianni, 1999; Johnson, Rabkin, Williams, Reiman, & Gorman, 2000). Indeed, the boundary between Axis I (clinical syndromes) and Axis II (personality disorders) is beginning to fade, as major researchers/clinicians directly address the interface between Axis I and

Axis II when dealing with treatment-refractory conditions. For example, Thase, Friedman, and Howland (2001) report (p. 18): "The impact of prior pharmacologic interventions may have been adversely affected by a poor therapeutic alliance, low social support, life stress, or chronic adversity and cognitive or personality factors such as neuroticism or pessimism."

This book pursues in depth the question of how to work with psychosocial factors (including but not limited to Axis II complications) to improve results with nonresponders or patients with treatment-refractory disorders. The method, called Interpersonal Reconstructive Therapy (IRT), is primarily psychosocial, but does recommend medications for specific situations. IRT does not offer any new treatment techniques per se, such as a new drug or a new way of relating to patients. Rather, IRT offers a way of thinking about patients that helps clinicians more effectively choose interventions from the array of possibilities available within any and all frequently used methods of intervention, called treatment as usual (TAU). The therapy, divided into five steps or stages, draws techniques from TAU according to highly specific algorithms (flow charts). After successful negotiation of the fourth of five therapy steps, so-called nonresponders become more amenable to TAU. The IRT perspective on how Marie, Kenneth, Jessica, and Patsy could be moved from nonresponder to responder subgroups of their respective DSM categories is presented at the end of this chapter. But first there is a discussion of TAU in general, and as it had previously been applied to these patients[1] in particular.

THE STATE OF THE ART

The TAU plans in place for these four patients were typical of most modern-day inpatient and outpatient systems. Practitioners draw from a number of interventions to address each specific symptom or problem. Examples include medications targeted toward symptoms or group of symptoms, such as depression, anxiety, or thought disorder; and cognitive-behavioral therapy (CBT) for specific problems, such as phobia, failure to perform, angry outbursts, depressive self-talk, and the like.[2] Usually, there is no particular theory or perspective that convincingly explains the patient's total predicament. Rather, the person is characterized by a list of symptoms and problems, and these are targeted and treated, one by one. The goal is reduction of the symptoms that characterize the disorders listed in the DSM-IV.

Increasingly, insurance plans and research-funding agencies demand not only that treatment be targeted toward symptoms appearing within a particular DSM-IV category, but also that an acceptable treatment be documented by a clinical-trials research protocol. An intervention (e.g., an antidepressant) must significantly reduce a symptom or group of symptoms (e.g., depression) within a brief period of time (e.g., 6 weeks), relative to a control condition (in this case, placebo). The intervention must be well operationalized (a drug with a specific chemical structure must be given in a specific dose for a specific duration to address a specific group of symptoms). Subjects from a relevant population (depressed individuals) are selected on a random basis, and they must respond significantly better than subjects assigned to a control condition. In research protocols, it is also acceptable to use an extant validated treatment as a control condition.

This standard, exemplified by the typical clinical-trials drug protocol, has been applied to interventions based on psychotherapy (Task Force on Promotion and Dissemination of Psychological Procedures, 1995). Like the validation studies for drugs, some psychotherapies have been "operationalized" (in manuals); they are targeted toward specific populations; they have demonstrated that randomly chosen subjects show significant improvement, relative to subjects receiving a control condition; their effects have been demonstrated within a relatively brief period of time. A list of interventions that have met this standard, both pharmacological and psychological, was named the "empirically validated therapies" (EVTs). Not surprisingly, the initial list of EVTs included the major classes of psychoactive medications, electroconvulsive therapy, and CBT for depression, anxiety, phobias, smoking, and chronic pain. Klerman and Weissman's interpersonal psychotherapy (IPT) for depression, recently updated by Weissman, Markowitz, and Klerman (2000), has also been well validated in large clinical trials studies (Elkin et al., 1989; Frank, Kupfer, Wagner, McEachran, & Cornes, 1991).

Counterarguments against requiring validation of the effectiveness of (especially longer-term) psychotherapy by the clinical-trials design have been vigorous (e.g., Seligman, 1995).[3] An illustrative group of papers that presented arguments and counterarguments appeared in the *American Psychologist* in 1996 (see the introduction to these papers by VandenBos, 1996).

In response to these and other criticisms about the narrowness of the EVT standards, Chambless and Hollon (1998) subsequently presented the results of a task force effort that introduced a new nomenclature, the "empirically supported therapies" (ESTs). These standards addressed some of the previous criticisms (e.g., Seligman, 1995), and added two new categories to the original EVT description. One includes therapies that have practical value in less "purified" settings; the other focuses strictly on savings in cost of treatment. The resulting three EST categories respectively describe studies that seek to answer three questions, phrased by Chambless and Hollon (1998, p. 7) as follows:

(a) Has the treatment been shown to be beneficial in controlled research?
(b) Is the treatment useful in applied clinical settings and, if so, with what

patients and under what circumstances? (c) Is the treatment efficient in the sense of being cost-effective relative to other alternative interventions? These questions respectively are addressed by studies on efficacy (including clinical significance), effectiveness (or clinical utility), and efficiency (or cost-effectiveness).

Thus the word efficacious now indicates that the approach has been validated by EVT standards; effective means that it has been validated by the softer second category, marking clinical utility; and efficient means that the treatment is validated by the cost-effectiveness standard.

The slightly relaxed standards associated with the new EST categories added some treatment approaches to the previous EVT list, but psychopharmacological and behavioral therapies or CBT still dominate. In general, ESTs remain the most likely to receive reimbursement from insurance companies. Moreover, insurance companies frequently authorize payment on the basis of a policy of "stepped care." This refers to the practice of starting with the least expensive and least intrusive intervention possible, and moving on to more expensive and/or more intrusive interventions only if necessary to achieve a specific therapeutic goal.

The problem of how to establish that therapy is efficacious, effective, or efficient without compromising needed (if not yet "validated") care is yet to be resolved (Davison, 2000). With nonresponders, who are often severely disabled, this issue is particularly acute by definition.[4]

Remarks on Overstated Effectiveness and Problematic Side Effects

Few could doubt that there have been stunning advances in understanding of the mechanisms of psychopharmacology and neurochemistry (e.g., Julien, 1995). Nonetheless, the gap between descriptions of psychopharmacological mechanisms and our understanding of the causes of mental disorder remains large. Optimal medical practice uses treatments that directly address cause more than symptoms. For example, pneumonia is treated primarily with a drug (e.g., penicillin) that kills the causal bacterium. Treatments that only address symptoms (e.g., aspirin for fever in a case of pneumonia) are helpful, but less definitive. So far, psychiatry is better at treating symptoms than in identifying and directly addressing causal agents.[5] The discipline awaits further theory-based research on the origins of the chemical imbalances and structural abnormalities presently treated by psychoactive drugs. Even if, as some would argue (e.g., Soloff, 1997), such theory is not necessary, others have suggested that the state of the art of treating chemical imbalances does have room for improvement.[6]

Also under pressure to demonstrate effectiveness with the EST protocol, advocates of psychotherapy have marshaled evidence to show that it is effective, even when applied to treatment of personality disorders (Perry et al., 1999). In contrast to the literature on psychopharmacological treatments, problematic side effects of psychotherapy have been largely ignored except for the work of Bergin and Lambert (1978), who described "deterioration effects."[7] About a decade and a half after they first described deterioration, the same authors (Lambert & Bergin, 1994) summarized their earlier observations and noted that the problem continues:

> . . . it was concluded that the occurrence of therapy- or therapist-induced worsening was widespread, occurring across a variety of treatment modalities including group and family therapies. Further, we implied that there was a causal link between negative outcomes and therapeutic activities, particularly for some specific clients. . . . Many more recent studies continue to document rates of deterioration in patients, even in those who participate in carefully controlled research protocols. . . . Those studies that use controls usually show that *deterioration is lower in controls than in treated samples.* (p. 176, emphasis added)[8]

It would make sense that the EST standards, as well as the research upon which they are based, should more specifically address the problem of deterioration along with concern about improvement. Sometimes publications include a footnote to the Subjects section reporting the number of cases that had to be taken off a protocol for various reasons, including dangerous deterioration (e.g., escalating suicidality).[9] If not excluded from the research protocol in the first place, dangerous cases dropped from a protocol are frequently not included in analyses and discussions of treatment effectiveness.[10] Davison (2000) has called for consideration of deterioration in response to psychosocial treatments, while Lunnen and Ogles (1998) have explored related methodological issues (e.g., how does one define clinically significant deterioration and distinguish it from simple failure to improve?).

A Need for Sound Theory That Accounts for the Totality of a Patient's Symptoms

The record of efficacy, effectiveness, or efficiency for any approach should be enhanced by use of a valid theory of psychopathology and treatment. Such a theory would offer clear, testable, and refutable hypotheses about etiology that have direct treatment implications. It would link mechanisms to cause and to treatment response. It would provide a means to account for all of a patient's psychological symptoms simultaneously, in a logical and clinically coherent manner. It would be able to account for why the observed symptoms in an individual are currently in exacerbation. It would be consistent with all available empirical observations. It would be able to make a diagnosis independently[11] of response to treatment. It would be able to define normality as well as pathology. It would have powerful preventative implications. Such a theory has yet to appear for mental disorders.

Psychoanalysts continue to strive to meet these illustrative standards for ideal theory (e.g., OPD Task Force, 2001),[12] as do advocates of the idea that mental disorder is a brain disease (e.g., Janicak, Davis, Preskorn, & Ayd, 1997). However, in addition to conceptual challenge to these claims, the continued problem of nonresponders suggests that there is room for improvement, no matter what the approach or ideology of the clinician.

THE IRT PERSPECTIVE

The IRT Approach to Questions about Nature, Nurture, and the Will

The theory of psychopathology that forms the basis of IRT also strives to meet the standards of testable, refutable theory just discussed. It is firmly rooted in Darwin's (1871/1952) theory of evolution. The IRT approach assumes that humans, placed at the peak[13] of the primate branch of the phylogenetic continuum, are greatly affected by learning.[14] The fact that learning deeply affects humans is both a blessing and a curse. It is a blessing, because human development is characterized by great flexibility and hence adaptability to a large number of conditions. It is a curse, because there is more opportunity for the process of ontogeny to stray from the genetic plan within a single generation than there is in species less affected by the vicissitudes of experience.

Kagan's (1994) suggestion that heritability provides an "envelope" of potentials for each individual offers a useful way to think about the interaction between heritable and acquired traits in humans. Kagan has shown that temperamental differences destined to persist for a lifetime can be detected in newborns.[15] Experience locates the person within a given envelope (not just for temperament, but for musical ability, athletic ability, intelligence, etc.). Temperament and these other inherited abilities or disabilities will interact with social experience to shape the personality. For now, it is reasonable to agree with those who suggest that approximately half the available variance in personality belongs to the genes, and half to environmental factors (Reiss, Plomin, & Hetherington, 1991; Rose, 1995).

Although the concepts of personal agency, will, or choice are not typically studied by biologists, the developmental theory invoked by IRT assumes for practical reasons that these factors are also important determinants of human behavior.

In sum, the IRT perspective presented in this book assumes that individual, familial, and societal learning join inherited chemistry and structure as important factors to consider when one is addressing questions of cause, mechanisms, and treatment of mental disorder in general, and patients in the office in particular. It is also assumed that the behavior of a human being is affected by will or agency. It is probably not possible to know the degree to which will is independent of heritage or experience. The treatment approach does attempt to modify the will in specific ways for specific reasons. In sum, IRT is a psychosocial approach that focuses mostly on the impact of learning, current situation, and the consequences of choice. However, there is due respect for the inherited envelope of potential. Medications are used under specific conditions.

The Theory of Psychopathology That Forms the Basis of IRT

Developmental Learning and Loving (DLL) theory is the key to developing a case formulation in IRT. The case formulation is the focal point for every treatment intervention, because it attempts to identify the causes[16] that need to be addressed. DLL theory is introduced in this chapter by showing how it applies to Marie, Kenneth, Jessica, and Patsy. Its background and rationale are presented in detail in Chapter 2. The treatment method that rationally follows from the DLL assumptions about how a disorder is shaped and maintained is presented in Chapters 3–10.

A thumbnail sketch of the case formulation method[17] and its treatment implications is as follows: Each of the presenting problems must be related in an empirically informed manner to perceived rules and values expressed by one or more key attachment figures. The resulting case formulation should be a coherent, integrated, data-based, testable, and refutable, and should reasonably account for the total presentation. The case formulation has clear treatment implications and is used to guide the choice of interventions.

This challenge is approached by assuming, as proposed by Bowlby (1977), that important early relationships provide "internal working models" for a child. According to DLL theory, the connection between presenting maladaptive patterns in the adult and internalizations of specific early relationships (working models) occurs via one or more of three "copy processes" (Benjamin, 1993, 1994b, 1996a, 1996b). These are (1) "Be like him or her," (2) "Act as if he or she is still there and in control," and (3) "Treat yourself as he or she treated you." It follows that if presenting behaviors and associated thoughts and affects are organized by internalized representations, then an effective intervention must somehow affect these organizing templates—these acquired habitual instructions[18] concerning rules and values.

Once copy processes that link problem behaviors to an attachment figure have been identified, it is necessary to identify and target whatever sustains these processes. The working hypothesis is that copy processes are maintained by the wish that the internalized representations of early figures will forgive, forget, apologize, wake up, make restitution, relent—or otherwise make it possible for there to be rapprochement and unfettered love. In other words, while manifesting the problem behaviors, affects, and cognitions, the patient has assumed that the key to reconciliation is to live by and provide testimony to the perceived rules and values of the internalized figures. These key figures are called Important Persons and their Internalized Representations (IPIRs). The implied motivation for maintaining the problem behaviors is that the patient will persist in these ways of being until the message is "heard" by the IPIRs and rapprochement can be realized. The patient is therefore said to seek psychic proximity to the IPIRs. If that plan is what sustains the disorder, then the treatment must target these wishes so that they can be either realized more constructively or let go and grieved. IRT focuses relentlessly on releasing the patient from the need to meet the identified wishes underlying the problem behaviors. After the organizing wishes are transformed or given up, the patient can leave the nonresponder category. He or she can benefit more from assistance, because response is less likely to be sabotaged by the need to maintain problem behaviors and their associated affects and cognitions. Both learning technology and medications can become more effective, because the patient is no longer so (unconsciously) determined to maintain old patterns.

DLL CASE FORMULATIONS
FOR THE FOUR NONRESPONDERS

Marie: Scared to Death

Review of the Presenting Problems

Recall that Marie suffered from chronic depression and anxiety that she described as "ultimate fear." Her own explanation for her problem was this: "They believe my father began incesting when I was 3 months old." She had been in psychotherapy for 15 years. Following her long-term separation from a severely abusive man, she became focused on helping her adult children, who returned to live with her whenever they had difficulties. At the time of her hospitalization, her youngest daughter was leaving to marry a kind man, and everyone else also was doing well. Marie suddenly became nonfunctional and dependent.

Relation of the History to the Presenting Problems

Marie's history provided some insight into why being alone with nobody to take care of was so frightening. Her father was reportedly alcoholic and abusive—physically, emotionally, and sexually. Marie provided details of severe and chronic physical abuse (beatings, punchouts, being dragged by the hair, being slammed against walls) that were compellingly specific. Not only did Marie's mother fail to protect Marie and her siblings, but her mother used Marie to deal with the father. "She felt I had all the strength. He would be raging, and she sent me out to deal with it. I was always the go-between. They would send me here, there—'Do this, do that.' " In addition to her assigned role of protecting her mother and siblings from her father's rages, Marie was subjected to a sexual relationship with him. The sexual abuse[19] was not violent: "When I was a teen, he made me lie on the bed while he sexually touched me." As is the case for many victims of childhood abuse, in addition to the helplessness, fear, and pain inherent in physical and verbal abuse, there was pleasurable sexual activity. Once the pleasure can be acknowledged, it can be easier for a patient like Marie to understand and give up the ensuing attachment to violent men.

Marie recalled a particularly traumatic moment in her early teens that was central to her disorder. After her parents divorced, she was sitting in the car with her younger brother and sister at the start of a long visitation with her father. Marie and her siblings were terrified of what lay in store for them. They watched their mother wave goodbye, seemingly happy to be rid of them. "All there is, is endless black. I knew I was completely and utterly alone. No one or nothing would ever save me. To take away the horror, I decided I should take as good care of my sister and brother as I could. It was all left to me. At that moment, I was totally abandoned." In a context of terror before spending an extended period alone with her violent father, Marie seized on her assigned, well-practiced role as mediator. She became a dedicated protector of others. She would be doing what she was supposed to do, and her brother and sister would at least have what she could not. This sense of choice and control calmed her.

Marie retained this role through adulthood. While others in the family did battle with each other, "I was the head of the world. They went through me. I was the one to whom everybody came. The one who would finally do something was me." In addition to a vision of herself as rescuer, there were two other safe havens. The first was that when Marie was ill, her mother did take care of her. She noted, "I always loved hospitals and doctors and shots." The second safe haven was the bathroom: "You could lock the door and it was really safe. It was socially unacceptable to walk in on anybody in the bathroom." It was probably relevant that her unyielding medical disorder frequently took her to a safe place (hospitals and doctors) and also happened to force her to spend thousands of hours in another safe place, the bathroom. (Consider also that a natural response to terror is digestive upset and diarrhea.)

As an adult, Marie was psychologically trapped in a world wherein her (by then deceased) father might attack at any minute, and there would be no mother to protect her. Her defense had been to take care of others who were in trouble. When her last daughter decided to leave home to marry well, Marie's nameless fear, her anxiety began to escalate. Unable any longer to implement the caregiver's identity, Marie experienced "ultimate fear." When she was not allowed to be a rescuer and a coper, she next tried being demandingly dependent, like her mother. Nobody in her present family supported that solution. Marie was defeated—left alone without her defense of caring for others, and frightened by her loss of identity with its accompanying sense of control.

If correct, this formulation would, among other things, explain why 15 years of therapy that attempted to get Marie to confront her father for sexual abuse had not achieved the desired effect. His physical abuse, and the mother's long-standing demands that she be the one to cope with it, would be better explanations for her anxiety. Marie was quite attached to her father, and to her identity as the one who could manage him and protect the others. This sense of closeness and of the ability to influence him was surely intensified by the sexuality in their relationship. Talking in therapy about her sexual relationship as if it were "the" dreadful experience that accounted for her anxiety may have been beside the point. Rather, the sexual abuse, albeit highly inappropriate, was a complicating feature of a much larger picture. Marie agreed with the interviewer's suggestion that talking so long and so much about her father in a sense kept her closer to him (psychic proximity). Marie was startled by, but agreed to, the thought that her difficulties in sexual relations with her husband[20] reflected continuing loyalty to her father. This reframing of her abuse history seemed to strengthen her resolve to separate from these old patterns and to find new and better ones.

Marie's Reaction to the Case Formulation

Marie and I discussed the thesis that Marie had been trained to be a rescuer and now was "out of work." I noted that it is natural to be very anxious when one's whole identity has suddenly been taken away. I suggested that she needed "a birthday,"[21] to which Marie responded, "For heaven's sake." Then I discussed her present opportunity to find new ways of relating to others.

MARIE: How interesting. How should I go about doing that?

THERAPIST: Be careful about asking questions like that. Somebody might answer them. What if I suggested something stupid?

Marie laughed heartily. Then she talked quite a bit about the incest with her father. She mentioned how painful the thought of it was and how she never wanted to think about it again.

THERAPIST: I hear your anger about that, and I like it. But if you are not having pleasure sexually, you are giving your father a lot of control in your life now.

MARIE: Wow. (*Long silence*) Will I have a copy of this later? I don't want to forget what you are saying to me.

Kenneth: Wrong-Patient Syndrome

Review of the Presenting Problems

Recall that Kenneth came to the hospital for treatment of suicidal thoughts associated with his belief that his wife had been "stepping out on him." Kenneth was vaguely threatening her and her alleged lover. He was so upset that he did not want to be alive. Other than taking medication, Kenneth refused to participate in the psychosocial treatment programs offered by the hospital. Rather, he was devoted to repetitive description of all the evidence of his wife's infidelity.

Relation of the History to the Presenting Problems

Kenneth's developmental history helped explain his current behavior. His father was rarely home, and his mother "ruled the house." She was very loving, affectionate, and a good friend. In her grief about the father's absence, she would come to Kenneth's bedroom and ask for a back rub. Very often they would "talk and discuss everything." Sometimes Kenneth felt that she commanded affection; in this and other ways, she was "dictatorial." A "stickler for cleanliness," she often punished him with a willow switch for failure to get things spotless. Kenneth was invited to "pick the willow that I wanted."

After years of marriage, Kenneth's father "had an affair on my mother." There were many long nights of fighting about the infidelity. His mother would yell and scream at his father, "How could you?" As this went on and on, Kenneth's excellent grades deteriorated. Eventually his father confessed, his mother forgave, and they reconciled.

Kenneth's treatment plan might be called "courtroom therapy" and he learned it at his mother's side. He wanted therapists to agree his wife was wrong. Acting like his mother (his main IPIR) and being loyal to his parents' ways of doing things, Kenneth sabotaged his chances to reconcile with his wife. Until Kenneth decided to abandon his loyalty (psychic proximity) to his mother's beliefs and her method of relentless blaming for marital infidelity, few therapy interventions could succeed.

Kenneth's Response to the Case Formulation

At the end of the interview, I explained to Kenneth that I thought he was being like his mother as he confronted his wife with evidence for infidelity. It seemed that he was hoping for the same result he saw her get—namely, confession and reconciliation. Kenneth took notes, but said nothing. A few hours after the interview, he left a long, somewhat tearful message on my answering machine, providing examples of that connection and of other ways he was like his mother. Kenneth asked to talk more about this with me. I did not get the message then, and by the next day, the hospital staff said he had forgotten the interview entirely. Without strong and specific support, he was unable to sustain this profoundly altered view of what he was doing and why.

Jessica: "It Is Only a Question of When and How to Die"

Review of the Presenting Problems

Recall that Jessica had been on medical leave because her recurrent severe Major Depressive Disorder from the past 21 years had failed to respond to any class of antidepressant, to an antipsychotic, or to a variety of psychotherapies. She was admitted for evaluation of suicidality, since she had recently been "researching" suicide. In the hospital she was interested in treatment programs only to the extent that they might inform her on better ways to commit suicide. Anxiety and panic had appeared in the past year, particularly when she was shopping for groceries or for clothing. Despite Jessica's logical narratives and her well-socialized behavior and appearance, she disclosed that she had heard "voices" for many years—both "reasonable and good" and "bad" ones. When Jessica was in difficult situations, these voices would start talking simultaneously and confusingly.

Jessica had recently filed for divorce from her husband of 20 years; there had been chronic marital rape. Moreover, at work new corporate rules had recently been introduced to assure efficiency. Jessica was a valued customer service representative, and she felt that the rules interfered with her ability to be truly responsive to customers. Nonetheless, she kept her job because the family needed the money, which until the separation she had turned over to her husband. He had given her back less than she needed when she went shopping for groceries, clothing, and other household items. He'd denied her requests occasionally to go to a movie or out to a restaurant with him, explaining they could not afford it. Recently, however, she had learned that over the years he had accumulated $100,000 in a secret investment that was in his name only. Moreover, he was now stalking her every move during the day. Despite all these undeniably difficult challenges, Jessica believed that the precipitating event for this hospitalization was the disapproval of a certain brother over her handling of a recent family reunion.

Relation of the History to the Presenting Problems

Jessica's developmental history helped explain her long-standing tolerance of extreme sexual, financial, and personal exploitation, as well as her immutable devotion to suicide in response to a family fight at a reunion. Jessica was the youngest of nine children and said the family was very close. Positive highlights of her childhood were the occasions when her mother would take her shopping. Otherwise, her stories from childhood were painful. Jessica felt sorry for her parents because when she was an infant, they would often have to take her with them to restaurants, movies, evenings at friends' houses, and so on. Jessica also felt like a burden to her siblings, because they had to watch her at home or take her along with them. They expressed their displeasure freely and often. Jessica's response was to "apologize and try to make things right so they would be happy with me again." When she realized there was nothing she could do about the situation, Jessica "would go sit in front of the TV but not watch it. I would be crying in front of cartoons. I would wish I was not around. I wanted them to be able to do what they wanted to do."

Later, Jessica attempted to justify her existence by serving others. She did a lot of the cooking and cleaning because her mother worked. She often did her siblings' share to protect them from her father's discipline for their failures to perform. Up to the time of her current hospitalization, some adult siblings still called her to ask that she clean their houses. She did.

Jessica declined to discuss childhood relations with the brother who had just refused to pay his share of the costs of the recent family reunion. Asked to rate their relationship on a scale of 0–10, which would reflect the seriousness of the danger he posed to her, she quickly replied, "10." She said that throughout childhood, this particular brother would "do something to her, and afterwards put his hands around my throat and threaten to kill me if I told anybody." She said she had tried to be "real nice and good" around him, so he would not get mad. Also, she believed he would have been "beaten to death" if she had told their father. Jessica compellingly described her own beatings with the father's belt or being kicked repeatedly for small crimes.

Jessica's Panic Disorder was characterized by feeling closed in and trapped by any high aisles encountered when shopping. As noted above, she had an impossibly small allowance for groceries and other needed items for herself and the children. Shopping for household necessities probably intensified her (unacceptable) resentment about her husband's inordinate control of the money. Providing basic care for her children was very important to her. It probably also was important that being allowed to go shopping with her mother had been a very positive experience in her childhood, which was otherwise painfully lonely. In other words, her husband forced Jessica to take responsibility for basic household items, while he withheld for his own use the needed resources that she herself had provided. Moreover, his habit of coercing sexual activity was likely to have reactivated feelings of fear, helplessness, and hopelessness in relation to suspected sexual abuse by her brother. In short, she had married a replica of her severely abusive and exploitative brother. She had long endured the requirement that she work while she had to hand all her earnings over to her husband and the chronic marital rape. But she had only recently learned about his very large, sequestered bank account. Simultaneously, she happened to have been confronted with a concrete reminder of the origins of this pattern: The terrifying brother whom she had always labored to please refused even to respond to the simple request that he pay his share of the costs of the family reunion.

Detailed inquiry about the voices revealed that the "good" one told Jessica to perform as others (employer, husband, siblings) asked. The "bad" voice seemed to express what Jessica might understandably wish to say and do, but did not. It supported assertiveness and self-protection. It was also inclined to swear—a serious transgression within the family. The voices concretely reflected her intrapsychic conflict. The "good" voice usually won, but tension was mounting. In a family that was supposed to be close, with no dissent allowed, it would make sense that Jessica could not have internal dissent either. The voices that directly reflected her conflicts with her loved ones were not "her."

The suicidality related most directly to Jessica's long-standing belief, based on her experience with her siblings, that she simply should not exist. Her presence was a burden to her parents and her siblings (her IPIRs). Until her hospitalization, Jessica had reacted to this by working very hard to please and to avoid displeasing others. With the fight about the payment for the family reunion, she felt she was failing at pleasing her siblings. The gravity of this failure can be understood only if one bears in mind that she spent years appeasing first her brother, and then her husband. It followed, according to her logic, that Jessica should kill herself. If she could not please and appease important family members by performing well, she could please them by getting out of their way. Jessica calmly acknowledged that her lethal suicidality was "for them." Her wish for psychic proximity to her siblings was leading her inexorably to suicide, and she was quite peaceful about her decision to kill herself. After death, Jessica believed, she would be reunited with a kind figure from early adulthood. Until her will to present her death as a gift to her siblings was transformed, all therapy interventions were likely to fail. Jessica was at extremely high risk for successful suicide.

Jessica's Response to the Case Formulation

At the end of the interview, I summarized the idea that Jessica believed she was "in the way" with her parents, her siblings, and now her children.

JESSICA: (*Nods*) Hum hum.

THERAPIST: Does that sound right?

JESSICA: Definitely. Yeah.

THERAPIST: So when you attack yourself, you treat yourself as your family did. If you die, you stop bothering them. You are out of here and you take care of them. You are smiling.

JESSICA: (*Laughs outright*)

THERAPIST: Why are you laughing?

JESSICA: (*Loudly*) Because that is *true*.

The laugh was alarming because it suggested that Jessica was enjoying the thought of removing herself. This indicated that a great priority needed to be placed on exploring her perception that her siblings thought she was perpetually "in the way." Her self-destructive attachment to them needed major revision—and soon.

Patsy: "I Can't Deal with Life"

Review of the Presenting Problems

Recall that Patsy had had severe Major Depressive Disorder for years, and recently had attempted to separate from her severely abusive husband. Much to the consternation of family and friends, she invited him back shortly after she'd finally managed to get him to leave. Patsy said that she wanted to be loved and not to have to continue to be the breadwinner. She did not like her job working for a woman who was very controlling and unappreciative. Her husband was dependent on alcohol, had lost many jobs, and showed little interest in work. Patsy had tried a range of ways of trying to keep him from drinking, but with little success. He had also recently incensed her by rather blatantly having an affair. Patsy said, "I was forced into filing for divorce by friends and coworkers, but I wasn't ready." There was some moving in and out. As Patsy explained the most recent change, "I asked him back because I need somebody to love me. After another beating last week, my therapist told me to tell him to get his stuff out of the house. I was visiting my mother for the weekend and decided to kill myself on the way back. I don't want to live with him, and I don't want to live without him. Everybody thinks I am a fool."

Patsy said that in the past, she would hit her children "way too hard."

She sometimes broke a wooden spoon on them as she administered the blows. Other times, she would hurl them across the room. Stitches were needed on occasion. Usually her rages were due to the fact she was "a clean fanatic. I'd walk in the house and see the mess and yell and ask, 'What is the matter with you?' " Patsy explained that her husband kept her "mellow." Last week, without him, she had a sudden urge to attack one of her grown-up daughters. She did not, but the close call upset her. Interestingly, she had rarely attacked one of her children, a son. Patsy said that when she got angry at this son, "he would say, 'Don't be mad. I love you, Mom.' And then he would leave. I would laugh at how scared he was. It would calm me." The child who got the most severe beatings, a daughter, was strong-willed and would not cry. "I wanted her to cry. I don't remember why. I got mad at her defiance."

Relation of the History to the Presenting Problems

Patsy's developmental history helped clarify her problem patterns. When Patsy's mother disapproved of her appearance, she would tear off the offending item of clothing. Patsy did the same thing to her children, for the same reason. The mother was extremely clean, and the house was absolutely "sterile." Everything had to be just so.

Patsy said her that father was "crazy" and very abusive to her mother. Patsy had once seen him tie up the mother and then whip her. "When he hurts someone, his eyes sparkle." The father would corner his boys and slug them, and seemed to delight in torturing the children's pets to the point of death. Patsy's own punishment involved being thrown in the closet and being punched by her father. This went on from infancy to age 10. Patsy said that she remembered her mother yelling at him, "Don't hit her." She added that "I would always pee in my pants" at these times. Nonetheless, she also remembered her father hugging her and being loving.

All six of the children had inherited their father's temper, Patsy said. She described her own rages: "It is a problem of my control. A thing goes off in my head. It gets hot. I want to lash out at whatever is nearest. I want to tear something."

The psychosocial analysis suggested that Patsy had identified with both her mother and her father. Her devotion to cleanliness and her penchant for tearing things were rather direct imitations of her mother. During the times that she became violent with her children, Patsy was identifying more directly with her abusive father. She recognized the connections, but said she did not think she got the same pleasure out of hurting a child that her father did. Patsy's report that she was harsher if there was no crying, and lenient if the child showed fear and love, suggests that her motive was to be in control, feared, and loved. That was exactly what Patsy had provided her father: She'd obeyed, feared, and loved him. Her imitation of him was her attempt at psychic proximity. The strength of her attachment to him was further manifested by the fact that she was the one in the family who looked after him in his declining years.

Patsy's Response to the Case Formulation

Patsy's husband's abuse was what she was used to. She agreed with several comparisons, including the idea that staying with her husband was being like her mother. Moreover, the husband was an exact replacement for her father. Patsy's husband hugged and held her and told her he loved her. When he was around, she was less inclined to be violent with her children. It was as if he were a "stand-in " for the father. When her husband was not there, then Patsy got closer to her father by becoming just like him and having urges to beat the children.

THERAPIST: It seems that you are acting like your father at times.

PATSY: That's terrible. But my husband tells me that too. He says, "OK, [father's name]." That is a button.

THERAPIST: What do you do when your husband says that?

PATSY: It upsets me. That [my father] is one person I do not want to be like.

THERAPIST: But do you see the connection?

PATSY: Well, I have seen the connection to my father more in the past. I haven't done that [abuse children] lately. But the "having things just so" part. That is new. Well, that is just like Mom too. It is like both of them. My mother is a wonderful grandmother now, but I don't really want to be like her.

The interview continued along these lines, and then I said:

THERAPIST: We have this way of being like them. In your case, it is really dramatic. The part of you that is like your father is locked up, but now and then comes out.

PATSY: I wish I could lock it out forever. (*Sigh*) This is probably true.

I then suggested that staying with an abusive husband was another way she was being like her mother. The two of us worked on further examples of this point. Then Patsy spontaneously said, "You are pretty much right on."

Summary of the Findings about Links between Early History and Presenting Problems

Marie, Kenneth, Jessica, and Patsy were devoted to rules and values that had been created long ago in relation to loved ones. They were repeating interpersonal and intrapsychic habits that were generated within important childhood relationships. Their maladaptive patterns were sustained by wishes and fears that made sense in childhood. The connections between current patterns and the earlier ones were traced by the three simple "copy processes": "Be like him or her," "Act as if he or she is still there and in control," and "Treat yourself as he or she did." According to DLL theory, these three copy processes link problem patterns to perceived rules and values held by early loved ones, called IPIRs. Copy processes are sustained by the wish for psychic proximity to the IPIRs. The hope is that demonstrating loyalty to the views of the IPIRs will cause them to forgive, forget, apologize, wake up, make restitution, relent—or otherwise make rapprochement and unfettered love possible.

These "explanations" of presenting problems demonstrate how DLL theory attempts to account for seemingly unrelated lists of presenting symptoms in a systematic, organized way. As indicated before, further details are provided in Chapter 2.

Relation of the Case Formulations to Treatment Planning

When these patients' psychoactive treatments failed to address the underlying rules and values that organized the pathology, little change was observed. This was what defined them as nonresponders. IRT holds that if those underlying organizing wishes are directly addressed, such patients can become accessible to treatment. Aids for case formulation and treatment planning are offered in Chapter 2, and methods for carrying out the planned treatment are the topic of Chapters 3–10.

STRUCTURAL ANALYSIS OF SOCIAL BEHAVIOR: THE LENS THAT CLARIFIES THE PATTERNS AND LINKS

Most readers will intuitively understand the connections between the problem patterns described in the four cases and the patients' early learning. There is also a formal method that can guide the interviewer's intuition and operationalize the connections. The method involves formal (in research) or informal (in clinical practice) coding of patient narratives and therapy processes with a model called Structural Analysis of Social Behavior (SASB; Benjamin, 1996b), presented in detail in Chapter 4. The SASB model is generic in its ability to describe interpersonal and intrapsychic interactions. Each relationship is dissected in terms of these three underlying dimensions:

1. Focus ("You focus on me; I react to your focus on me; I focus on myself").
2. Affiliation (love vs. hate).

3. Interdependence—that is, enmeshment (control/submit) versus differentiation (emancipate/separate).

One can understand and practice IRT without learning how to use the SASB model. The uses of SASB, for those who choose to learn it, are illustrated by presenting SASB-coded descriptions of therapy narrative and process in footnotes throughout this book. The words are everyday, so readers unfamiliar with the model can nonetheless get the "feel" of how it works. If the reader then chooses to read about the SASB model in Chapter 4 and Appendix 4.1 to Chapter 4, he or she will then be able to understand the precision and rigor that support the use of its everyday words to clarify patterns; understand developmental roots; and plan, implement, and assess the effects of treatment interventions.

A BRIEF OVERVIEW OF IRT

The Five Steps of Therapy

IRT seeks to guide the practitioner in choosing interventions from TAU to more directly and consistently address the underlying organizing wishes for the presenting problem—that is, its interpersonal and intrapsychic patterns. The IRT treatment approach is summarized for patients quite simply in a prototypic learning speech:

> "Therapy starts with learning to recognize your patterns, where they came from and what they are for. Once you see that clearly, you can make a decision about whether to change and begin learning new and better patterns."

There are five approximately sequential steps in this therapy learning:

1. *Collaboration.* For example, a therapist and Marie would work together to help her implement self-care activities and enjoy being with others even if she was not helping them with trouble.
2. *Learning what the patterns are, where they are from, and what they are for.* For example, Marie would need to learn at many levels that her only sense of control and meaning came when she was able to master a terrifying situation on behalf of others. She had been loyal to the self-definition that emerged in relation to her father, her mother, and her siblings. Now that her family did not need her to mediate and rescue any more, she felt as terrified and alone as she did when she first assumed this role. Her rescuer identity made great sense then, but now it was no longer necessary or possible.
3. *Blocking maladaptive patterns.* For example, Marie would need to learn behaviorally to resist the call to rescue, except when truly appropri-

ate. Rather than plunging into the midst of others' troubles, she would need to "reframe" her "ultimate fear" as an undesired residual effect of her relationship with her father.

4. *Enabling the will to change.* For example, Marie would need to decide that her father could no longer be so central to her psyche and life. She would need to stop giving him control of her phenomenology, now that he was no longer a threat to her and others. If she could "let go" of her wish to remain psychically engaged with him, she could find better ways to live and love.

5. *Learning new patterns.* For example, Marie would need to learn ways of soothing herself when she became anxious about being alone, as well as alternative ways of relating to family members and others. She might be able to engage in new activities that had long interested her, but that she could not develop because of her overwhelming anxiety. At this final stage of IRT, Marie could begin to reconstruct herself. The IRT therapist would support this goal actively by encouraging constructive new activities, whether they were social, cognitive, or affective.

The five steps are simple, but not simplistic. They draw upon all schools of psychoactive treatment. Experienced clinicians may recognize that these five steps are "easier said than done." They are described so simply here because IRT attempts to embrace all available knowledge about constructive change in therapy via TAU and "boil it down" to basics that seek to change underlying motivation, followed by new learning.

The Core Algorithm: "Rules of Engagement" in IRT

There are six guidelines that the skilled IRT therapist tries to implement with each intervention. These constitute the core algorithm, reviewed in more detail in Chapter 3.

- *Rule 1: Work from a baseline of accurate empathy.* Empathy is to IRT as breathing is to the living person. A therapist's ability to focus on the patient in a friendly way that is profoundly supportive of the patient's own strength and well-being is essential to IRT. It is so omnipresent and so fundamental that it is hardly noticed until it is no longer there. When it is missing, the therapy process is no longer viable.
- *Rule 2: Support the Growth Collaborator (Green) more than the Regressive Loyalist (Red).* At each of the five steps of therapy, but especially at step 4, the therapist is aware of a fundamental conflict between two parts of the patient. One part presents for treatment and wishes to become better adjusted, while the other wants to continue to demonstrate the problem behaviors, affects, and cognitions consistent with the perceived rules and values of the IPIRs. Focus on this conflict is so central to the

treatment that it is represented in relation to the five steps in Figure 1.1. The part of the patient that wishes to become better adjusted is shown as the Growth Collaborator (GC in Figure 1.1, or Green). The part that wishes to remain loyal to the old ways is named the Regressive Loyalist (RL in Figure 1.1, or Red). Because the figure represents the early period of therapy, Red is much larger than Green. The terms "Red" and "Green" are explained in greater detail in Chapter 3.

In Figure 1.1, the Red is very large relative to the Green, since that is the case with the nonresponder population. A diagram of the "worried well" population would, of course, reverse the magnitudes of the circles representing the Red and the Green. In Figure 1.1, the conflict between the Red and the Green is represented by the arrow connecting them. Again, this conflict is at the center of step 4 (enabling the will to change), but it is also present at each of the other steps. Patients quickly grasp the meaning of Figure 1.1 and appreciate the simplicity and symbolism of the words

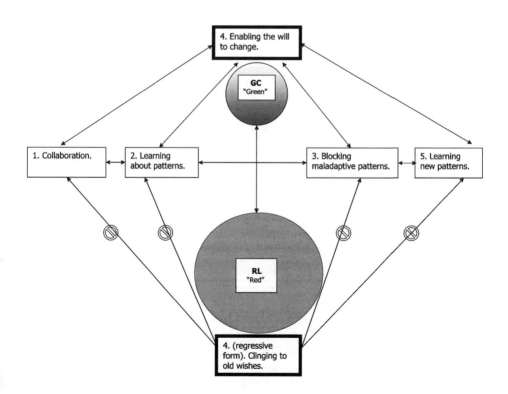

FIGURE 1.1. The five steps early in therapy, with emphasis on the conflict between the Growth Collaborator (GC) and the Regressive Loyalist (RL) at step 4.

Red (Stop) and Green (Go). They also, as illustrated by the responses of Marie, Kenneth, Jessica, and Patsy to the IRT interview, understand that the symptoms arise from a wish to cling to the rules and values formed in relation to key figures.

Ideally, the therapist's reflections will be phrased in a way that supports Green more than Red parts of the patient. However, it is not always possible or even wise to do that. Sometimes the Regressive Loyalist is too powerful and must be allowed to prevail. In that case, the clinician supports the Red and looks for a chance to amplify the Green as soon as possible.

- *Rule 3: Relate every intervention to the case formulation.* Suppose a paranoid patient becomes angry that her boss asked her whether she had a nice weekend, but she feels it is none of her boss's business. "What does the boss mean, anyway?" the patient wonders. Encouraging the patient to express her anger at her boss is not going to help her change the paranoid orientation. It may not help her position at work, either. On the other hand, suppose this anger is reminiscent of her anger about the severe abuse she suffered at the hands of her stepmother. Recognizing and exploring expression of this anger in therapy could be helpful if it helps her distance from the internalization of her stepmother, and does not merely exchange the "blamer" role with the stepmother. The meaning of expression of anger in therapy, then, is contingent on the specific details of how it relates to the case formulation.

- *Rule 4: Seek concrete illustrative details about input, response, and impact on self.* This rule assures that the treatment approach will be primarily interpersonal. Sullivan (1953) is responsible for the very useful interpersonal emphasis found in modern psychodynamic therapies (Greenberg & Mitchell, 1983). In IRT, every story that potentially relates to presenting problems and key figures is amplified in terms of three elements: input, response, and impact on self. Important episodes need to be discussed until the patient and therapist share understanding of what set this off, how the patient reacted, and how this affected the patient's self-concept. It is extremely important that the answers to these questions be phrased in very concrete terms. Specificity is the key to the "white heat of relevance" (Benjamin, 1996a, p. 89).

- *Rule 5: Explore in terms of the ABCs.* Every episode of input, response and impact on self also needs to be explored in three domains: affect (A), behavior (B), and cognition (C). Merely understanding the case formulation is not enough. There has to be affective as well as cognitive learning that will deepen appreciation of what organizes the problem interpersonal and intrapsychic behaviors. Interviewer questions that facilitate exploration with the ABCs include "What do you feel now [or what did you feel]?" "What do you want to do now [or what did you do]?" What do you think about this now [or what did you think about it]?" The IRT therapist gives equal priority to affective experiencing, intellectual understanding, and behavioral manifestations.[22]

• *Rule 6: Relate the intervention drawn from TAU to one or more of the five steps described above.* The five steps are so central to IRT that a separate chapter of this book is devoted to each of them.

How Can a Therapist Do Six Things at Once?

Beginning IRT therapists are frequently overwhelmed with the idea of having to think about six rules when deciding on an intervention. This is a natural reaction that can be observed when undertaking any complex learning task. The learner needs to scale back expectations at first, and proceed with patience and willingness to practice. As each skill is mastered, it drops into the preconscious and then happens more or less automatically. This is normal in any kind of learning.

Consider the process of learning to type. When the typist begins, he or she must be aware of where each letter is on the keyboard. Typing is difficult, laden with errors, and slow. As the learner practices more, accuracy and speed improve, and soon the accomplished typist is hardly aware of where the keys are. The same principles apply when one is learning IRT.

Consider the process of showing accurate empathy—the first rule described above, and a most important initial skill. Without empathy, there is unlikely to be collaboration in the therapy process. Beginning therapists have to work hard to remember to listen carefully and reflect compassionately and accurately. After some practice, therapist empathy happens naturally and usually outside of awareness, like breathing.

Experienced therapists already have many of the core skills embodied in the six rules of the core algorithm, and need only to learn how to focus them around the case formulation. Consider empathy, for example. The therapist already skilled in accurate reflection can begin to work on adding further core skills to the way empathic reflections are phrased. To the extent that an empathic reflection keeps the therapy narrative focused on the case formulation, for example, it shows greater IRT adherence, and presumably better outcome.

Many examples of how to implement each element of the core algorithm appear throughout this book. In Chapter 10, there are further suggestions for how to learn the IRT approach. Despite the risk of reader overload, the six rules have been listed here and elsewhere to help the reader focus on critical components of this difficult task. The core algorithm also provides a clear template for assessment of adherence.

ILLUSTRATIVE RESULTS OF IRT

Here are examples of successful reconstructions that followed from application of DLL theory and the IRT core algorithm.

A housewife and mother had been "depressed all of her life" and was, by her own description, hard to live with.

> "We had some friends over for dinner this weekend. I can't believe what I was doing before. It is *so* different now. Usually I ruin it. This time I approached it altogether differently. I was able to enjoy what was happening right then, not feeling could I do something else with this time. I was much more enjoyable, too. Something has broken loose in me. Definitely. It feels as dramatic as birth. A bag of waters has burst after a very long process of building."

Another example comes from a nonresponder who had been chronically suicidal and implacably depressed for over a decade. She had been unmoved by years of TAU, including pharmacological as well as psychological approaches. She brought up the idea of terminating her course of IRT, which had lasted 2 years. "Several people have told me how good I look. They say I look younger, that I even walk different. As I think about leaving, my mood is not happy. I do feel like crying. And I have these anxiety attacks. But overall, I think I am hopeful and positive." Later, she came back from a business trip and said, "I can't remember when I was so happy at a meeting. I enjoyed myself. I did not do things because I felt I had to. I spoke up when I felt like it and I was comfortable with myself."

A gifted woman who had dropped out of a college program in engineering kept her giant talent totally out of view, and devoted herself to "making myself as unattractive as possible." This alienated and withdrawn person, who had relations with imaginary figures that more or less directed her life, eventually went back to school and finished her degree. After some years, she put those fantasy figures to rest, came out of her social withdrawal, and subsequently characterized herself very well when she hesitantly described herself as "a diamond in the sand." Her way of seeing the world was fascinating, and watching her realize her talents in very concrete and public terms was marvelous.

A woman who had been withdrawn and crippled by paranoia for years noticed herself one day beginning to suspect that coworkers were talking about her. She reported that she said to herself, "I know that I might be seeing them as I see my sisters. But even if they are saying bad things about me, I don't have to react to it. They can not like me, and I can deal with it. I can choose."

These people have met the goals of IRT, which are clearly detailed in Chapters 4, 5, and 9. Basically, they have learned to function from a baseline of friendliness, with moderate degrees of enmeshment and differentiation. The affects and cognitions that parallel these ways of relating are pleasant and functional.[23]

IRT: A LONGER-TERM TREATMENT

The recommendations made in this book are most effective in the context of a longer-term psychotherapy. Nonetheless, IRT does also offer a framework that allows the clinician to determine when a particular intervention might be helpful on a short-term basis. If outcome can be measured in terms of stages, short-term impact can be assessed. For example, a brief inpatient hospitalization would be a success if it were associated with any of the five steps in IRT. Recognition of patterns as problems or making a conscious decision to try to give up old wishes would represent significant progress. Experienced clinicians will know that declaration of intent is, at best, only the beginning. The Green part of the person may plan to change things, but the Red will delay that process with frustrating regularity. The difficulty in letting go of the underlying wishes assures that for a full reconstruction[24] of personality to take place, it is appropriate to expect to invest 1–3 years, or even more.

I have argued (Benjamin, 1997, 2000c) that longer-term therapies might be seen as equal or superior to current ESTs in effectiveness if assessed in terms of longer remission of symptoms, fewer rehospitalizations, reductions in other medical problems, fewer lost days of work, and so on. Within this broader perspective, the slower, "more expensive," longer-term therapies—like the one being described in this book—are expected ultimately to prove more cost-effective. A review of research from 1984 to 1994 (Gabbard, Lazar, Hornberger, & Spiegel, 1997) supports that expectation. Their survey showed that psychotherapy "appears to have a beneficial impact on a variety of costs when used in the treatment of the most severe psychiatric disorders, including schizophrenia, bipolar affective disorder, and borderline personality disorder. Much of that impact accrues from reductions in inpatient treatment and decreases in work impairment" (p. 147). If IRT were to be used with more nonresponders, it is suggested that these numbers could be even better.

OVERVIEW OF THE CHAPTERS THAT FOLLOW

Following this introductory summary, a more complete rationale for IRT, along with detailed instructions for making a case formulation, appears in Chapter 2. Chapter 3 follows with a detailed description of the core algorithm in IRT. It includes a wealth of therapy aids, including flow charts, speeches, recommendations for enhancing adherence, methods of tracking progress, and more. Chapter 4 presents a brief description of the SASB model, which helps the clinician see the quintessence of patterns and provides predictive principles that link presenting problems to key figures more clearly. Clinicians interested in learning more about the SASB model might read Appendix 4.1 to Chapter 4, which provides more detail. Chapters 5–9 discuss the five steps of IRT. Chapter 10 reviews the approach; compares it to a few other major therapy approaches (e.g., psychodynamic, behavioral, family, group); assesses its status as a testable, refutable theory; and provides suggestions for how the reader can begin to practice IRT.

NOTES

1. In this book, individuals who present for treatment are called patients. They could also be called clients. There are varying perspectives on whether one term is preferable to another. As I said in Benjamin (1996a, p. 6), the list of "synonyms" for the word patient (as an adjective) "better characterizes what we need from those we seek to help."

2. In this book, the terms behavioral and cognitive-behavioral are used indiscriminately. Sometimes a technique involves working with mental events (cognitive-behavioral) and sometimes not. Quite often, the clinician does well to attend to both mental events and to behavior. Trying to make a clear distinction does not seem useful for present purposes.

3. Here is Seligman's (1995, p. 965) abstract of his widely cited position:

    > Consumer Reports (1995, November) published an article which concluded that patients benefited very substantially from psychotherapy, that long-term treatment did considerably better than short-term treatment, and that psychotherapy alone did not differ in effectiveness from medication plus psychotherapy. Furthermore, no specific modality of psychotherapy did better than any other for any disorder; psychologists, psychiatrists, and social workers did not differ in their effectiveness as treaters; and all did better than marriage counselors and long-term family doctors. Patients whose length of therapy or choice of therapist was limited by insurance or managed care did worse. The methodological virtues and drawbacks of this large-scale survey are examined and contrasted with the more traditional efficacy study, in which patients are randomized into a manualized, fixed duration treatment or into control groups. I conclude that the Consumer Reports survey complements the efficacy method, and that the best features of these two methods can be combined into a more ideal method that will best provide empirical validation of psychotherapy.

4. Recall that a nonresponder is defined by failure to respond to TAU, including the EST approaches. Such patients do not fall into any single diagnostic category, but into subsets of standard diagnostic categories (Axis I and/or Axis II). IRT's claim to move nonresponders to a responder subset can be validated by showing that such patients improve during IRT, compared to their previous year or more of multiple treatments. Alternatively, nonresponder patients in IRT can be compared to a group of such patients receiving TAU that is not informed by IRT procedures.

5. Interestingly, the EST standards also focus exclusively on symptom relief.

6. Breggin (1994) published a passionate indictment of overuse of psychoactive medications on the grounds that statements about effectiveness are inflated, while descriptions of destructive side effects are minimized. A comparatively balanced review of the weaknesses as well as strengths of contemporary brain disorder theory and practice appears in Valenstein (1998).

7. "Deterioration" was defined as negative change, meaning some individual's outcome scores were worse, compared to their starting scores.

8. References within quotations are not included in my reference list unless I refer to them in an independent context.

9. Zimmerman, Mattia, and Posternak (2002) surveyed patients presenting in routine clinical practice, and formally assessed them for eligibility in the efficacy protocols. From their sample of 346 patients presenting for outpatient treatment, 29 would have been admissible to those studies that form the basis of EST treatment recommendations. Exclusion criteria were gathered from treatment efficacy studies published from 1994 to 1998 in five psychiatric journals, including the *Archives of General Psychiatry* and the *American Journal of Psychiatry*. Not incidentally, exclusion criteria for some efficacy studies included suicidality—a feature of great concern to clinicians, and common in treatment-resistant disorders.

10. A colleague and I (Benjamin & Karpiac, 2001) recommend that assessment of effectiveness of treatments should include consideration of subjects who drop out because of deterioration. For example, if it is reported that $X\%$ of a sample showed clinically significant improvement, the denominator should be the original number of subjects, not just the number of subjects that completed the protocol. Adjustments for dropout for reasons unrelated to the presenting problems and treatment would be permissible.

11. A very clear exposition of the logical problems inherent in the practice of making a diagnosis on the basis of response to treatment (e.g., a particular medication) is offered by Valenstein (1998, pp. 132–147).

12. The OPD Task Force's approach draws heavily on an adaptation of the Structural Analysis of Social Behavior (SASB) model, shown in Appendix 4.1 to Chapter 4 of this book (see Figure 4A.1).

13. "We must also admit that there is a much wider interval in mental power between one of the lowest fishes, as a lamprey or lancelet, and one of the higher apes, than between an ape and man; yet this interval is filled up by numberless gradations" (Darwin, 1871/1952, p. 287).

14. " . . . man alone is capable of progressive improvement. That he is capable of incomparably greater and more rapid improvement than is any other animal, admits of no dispute; and this is mainly due to his power of speaking and handing down his acquired knowledge" (Darwin, 1871/1952, pp. 294–295).

15. Two oft-replicated categories of temperament are infants who are predisposed to be shy and withdrawn, and those who are more likely to be energetic and outgoing.

16. "Cause" has limited meaning in DLL theory. The presumed psychosocial causes of the problem patterns are components of a more complex total picture that includes heritable as well as experiential and existential factors.

17. The reader is asked to table questions about this brief sketch of DLL theory until it is discussed in more detail in Chapter 2.
18. A discussion of evidence suggesting that these instructions become hard-wired appears in Chapter 2.
19. The adult is responsible for responding appropriately to the child's developmental needs. Having sex with an adult is profoundly imbalanced and far too intense for a child to manage successfully. Hence sexual activity with a child automatically victimizes the child. The child is a victim even if he or she experiences pleasure (along with everything else) or sometimes initiates the sexual contact.
20. Marie did not include this on her list of presenting problems. When additional problems emerge while a case formulation is developed, they should, of course, be addressed by it.
21. The context specified that she had lost her identity, her self-concept as a rescuer. She needed to develop a new identity (i.e., to become a new person). Marie, like most patients, easily understood a simple metaphor for this difficult task.
22. In Appendix 4.1, more precise definitions are given for the A, B, C components of an event.
23. Definitions of the terms enmeshment and differentiation, and a description of the theory of affects and cognitions that parallel behavior, are presented in Chapter 4.
24. Defined in Chapter 4.

2

Case Formulation

WHY HAVE A CASE FORMULATION?

In practice, clinicians typically approach nonresponders by drawing upon a variety of established techniques (encouraging expression of affect, enhancing communication, teaching assertiveness, teaching better-modulated cognitive processes, etc.). When a given technique fails to achieve the desired result, clinicians may combine techniques at will, planning to stick with whatever works. Similarly, some experienced physicians develop "cocktails" of medications that can have good effects even after the recommended procedures for a single drug or therapy approach have failed. Advocates of these methods of treatment augmentation have argued that theory, or understanding the relation of the intervention to underlying causal factors, is far less important than the bottom line of results. The problem with using this "catch as catch can" approach with the nonresponder population is that results are often not forthcoming for them. Moreover, the history of science offers many examples to suggest that use of valid theory to organize facts can greatly enhance the ability to intervene in the domain under study.

THE NEED FOR THEORY THAT CAN
ORGANIZE INDIVIDUAL CASE DATA

Because I am respectful of the need to demonstrate effectiveness, and I am also a believer in theory, I regularly ask new graduate students to write an unsigned brief statement on the meaning of the words empirical and theoretical. Typically, over half of them write something to the effect that empirical means fact, while theoretical means fiction. Unfortunately, their impression is supported in today's intellectual climate. To illustrate, the online version of the *American Heritage Talking Dictionary* (1997) defines "theory" as follows: "Something taken to be true without proof: presupposition, assumption, postulate, postulation, premise, presumption, supposition, thesis, theory, hypothesis, speculation, conjecture. . . ."

It is true that theory begins as a guess, as a hypothesis. However, by stopping there, this popular understanding misses the point that valid theory can predict observable facts. In addition, any collection of relevant facts can be organized and interpreted by valid theory. Each informs the other to great advantage. This ability of theory to enhance fact and vice versa was clearly discussed by Poincaré (1905/1947). The connection has been the basis of most advances in science since the Dark Ages. Consider the stunning uses of theory to organize and predict facts that were offered by Newton and by Einstein. Who can count all of the ways that Newton's second law of motion ("Force equals mass times acceleration") affects everyday life? It has long been one of the core teachings of modern physics. Whereas Newton provided theory that enhanced the ability to predict and control objects visible to the senses, Einstein's theory provided many predictions that violated "common sense." For example, he suggested that space moves matter and matter bends space. One of the many implications of that theory is that gravity bends light. When astronomers subsequently observed a precisely predicted "change" in the position of a star during an eclipse of the sun, Einstein's theory was, with considerable drama at the time, proven to be correct. For another stunning example, consider that Mendeleev's theory, which organizes chemical elements in a two-way table according to atomic number and weight, predicted elements that were "discovered" decades later. These classical examples show that the complex, iterative dance between data and valid theory enriches the meaning of each to an enormous degree.

The clinical implication of this discussion of the merits of using theory to organize facts is clear: Effectiveness may well be enhanced if the presenting symptoms can be understood and organized by a coherent theoretical structure. Ideally, such a theory will account for most or all of the presenting symptoms in a case, not just one or two.

ESSENTIAL COMPONENTS OF CASE FORMULATION

The Developmental Learning and Loving (DLL) theory directs the Interpersonal Reconstructive Therapy (IRT) case formulation method, which seeks to organize the presenting symptoms in relation to common psychosocial causal factors. The definition of "causal factors" in DLL theory is wide-ranging; several other variables, such as heredity, traits, states, situations, and free will, are considered to be among contributing causal factors. Methods for constructing a case formulation are discussed in the next several sections. At the end of this chapter, a brief review of the theoretical and research bases of DLL theory is presented.

In the cases examples in Chapter 1, DLL theory was used to develop case formulations that helped makes sense of the presenting symptoms. The results demonstrated that connections between relationships with key figures and presenting problems can be made through one or more of three copy processes: (1) "Be like him or her," (2) "Act as if he or she is still there and in control," (3) "Treat yourself as he or she treated you." A key figure is defined tautologically: If a person can be directly associated with the presenting problems via one or more of the three copy processes, then that person is a key figure. The assumed motivation for maintaining the copied patterns is to achieve psychic proximity to key figures, called Important Persons and their Internalized Representations (IPIRs).

By continuing to exhibit behaviors, affects, and cognitions that are linked to the values and rules of an IPIR, the patient hopes to achieve more and better psychological closeness to that loved one. There is usually a wish or fantasy to rewrite history so that things will have been as they "should have been," rather than as they were. The strategy appears to be that if the patient remains loyal, and provides adequate testimony to the rules and values of the IPIR, the desired rapprochement and harmony will be obtained. The problem patterns inspired in this way belong to the Regressive Loyalist (Red) part of the patient (see Figure 1.1 in Chapter 1). The Red agenda to reconcile with loved ones, to achieve psychic proximity, is summarized by this phrase: "Every psychopathology is a gift of love" (Benjamin, 1993). Copy processes are the *mechanisms* by which early relationships are connected to presenting symptoms. The gift of love is the *motivation* that sustains the copy processes. The working hypothesis is that the gift of love, the wish for psychic proximity, is a psychosocial causal factor in presenting problems within the nonresponder population.

The treatment implication of a DLL analysis is that the Red wishes and fantasies about the results of adhering to old rules and values will have to be given up and grieved for. Many of the habits associated with those wishes must be changed. The Growth Collaborator (Green) part of the patient (again, see Figure 1.1) is in charge of processes that will lead to letting go. DLL theory helps the IRT clinician choose interventions from treatment as usual (TAU) that will minimize Red and maximize Green. The intended result is that the patient becomes freer to learn new, more adaptive ways of relating to current people and situations. Once the Red no longer dominates the psyche, patients also may become more responsive to medications appropriate to their condition,

For example, Marie's anxiety, her depression, her sudden dependency, and her Axis III medical condition all related reasonably to relationships within her family of origin. Technically, her presenting symptoms constituted three DSM-IV Axis I disorders (Major Depressive Disorders, Generalized Anxiety Disorders, Panic Disorder) and one Axis III disorder (her medical condition). The DLL case formulation attempted to answer this key question: "Why was all of this happening to Marie right now?" Instead of having four "disorders" that must be addressed in turn, Marie was understood as a total human being presently exposed to specific stresses, which she coped with according to her constitutionally given and developmentally shaped propensities. Her Red parts provided evidence of her loyalty to family rules and values as they were inferred from what she experienced. Her identity was centered on the need to try to help others in the same way she always had done. Her problem patterns stemmed from her view that she should and could protect and preserve other family members. Rather than representing a "breakdown," her symptom picture was a homeostatic attempt to maintain equilibrium according to her own internal mechanisms and needs. That same adaptive principle was demonstrated in all four cases described in Chapter 1.

DOES DLL THEORY APPLY TO EVERY CASE?

DLL theory seeks to interpret clinically significant problems in terms of a gift of love. Although normal development also includes copy processes and gifts of love, DLL theory does not apply to all clinical presentations. Clearly, if someone has lost his or her frontal lobes, the resulting deficit in cognitive functioning is not caused by a gift of love. If someone has a tumor that alters endocrine function, his or her resulting disturbances are not organized by a gift of love. If someone has suffered central nervous system damage from exposure to toxic chemicals, his or her dysfunction is not primarily due to a gift of love. The form that any of these disabilities might assume could be affected by gifts of love, but a gift of love would not be a primary causal factor in the dysfunction.

The limits of applicability of DLL theory and the IRT approach have not yet been established. Clinical evidence to date suggests that this applicability is broad, but there is no claim that it is universal. IRT is specifically designed for patients with treatment-refractory disorders, and hence eligibility is established residually. If the patient has a chronic, severe, and reliably established psychiatric diagnosis, but refuses or is not responding to several appropriate trials of the treatments (medication and/or psychotherapy) usually effective for that diagnosis, he or she is considered a nonresponder. If DLL theory applies to a nonresponder, IRT is likely to be helpful. The clinician working with such a patient should attempt to address a maximal number of presenting problems with a coherent, integrated DLL case formulation.

The effort to account for the total symptom picture must not exceed available supporting data. Evidence must be credibly organized by highly specific, testable, refutable hypotheses involving copy processes and psychic proximity. For a given case, it may be appropriate to acknowledge a list of symptoms that have not been encompassed by DLL theory. There should be no intent to use IRT to treat symptoms unrelated to DLL theory. Examples of such additional symptoms might be abdominal pain associated with appendicitis or psychosis accompanying cocaine or alcohol overdose. Typically, there are several such symptoms in the complex presentation of a nonresponder.

HOW TO DEVELOP A DLL CASE FORMULATION

The Basic Information

The information summarized in Table 2.1 and Table 2.2 is needed to create a case formulation. The DSM information (Table 2.1) can usually be completed for nonresponders by reading their medical records. These people have already had many prior treatments and assessments. With the basic

TABLE 2.1. Survey for DSM-Based Case Assessment

Name, age, gender, race, marital status, occupation, living arrangements, any needed financial information.

Chief complaints (include reason for coming to the hospital or seeking outpatient treatment).

Who brought/sent this person to the hospital or outpatient treatment?

Onset and course of present illness.

Current social stresses and supports.

Previous psychiatric diagnoses and family psychiatric history.

Previous treatments; include hospitalizations, medications, psychotherapies.

Diagnosed medical illnesses; include major medical procedures, events.

Current symptom status: Suicidality, homicidality, depression, mania, anxiety, panic, thought disorder, self-mutilation, dissociation, drug or alcohol abuse/dependence, legal problems, other.

Checklist for DSM-IV Axis I clinical syndromes, and diagnoses.

Checklist for DSM-IV Axis II personality disorders, and diagnoses.

Checklist for DSM-IV Axis III, IV, and V (related physical disorders, recent levels of stress, and recent levels of functioning).

TABLE 2.2. Survey of Important Relationships

In the present[a]

Spouse/partner, mother (or equivalent), father (or equivalent), major siblings, children, coworkers, therapist and health care system, introject, religious institutions, the illness itself, other.

In the past[a]

Spouse/partner, mother (or equivalent), father (or equivalent), major siblings, peers, therapist and health care system, self, religious institutions, the illness itself, other.

[a]Each important relationship should be assessed for input, response, and (if possible) impact on the self-concept. ABCs (affects, behaviors, and cognitions) are included to the extent possible.

DSM information in hand, the DLL interviewer can attend primarily to questions raised in Table 2.2. It recommends a survey of important relationships in the present and in the past that are likely to relate to the DSM information via copy processes and psychic proximity. Detail on how to get the information highlighted in Tables 2.1 and 2.2 is provided in the subsequent discussion of Figures 2.1 and 2.2.

Two Different Modes for Gathering Information

There are two modes for gathering the information needed to develop a DLL case formulation: (1) the inpatient consultative mode, illustrated by the four cases described in Chapter 1; and (2) the outpatient therapy mode, illustrated by many other treatment examples throughout this book.

Inpatient Mode

The inpatient consultative mode seeks to develop a complete case formulation in a 90-minute interview, whereas in the outpatient mode, quite a few sessions may be needed to complete the survey outlined in Tables 2.1 and 2.2. Completing the assessment in a one-time consultation is often stressful for patients. On the one hand, they typically are deeply appreciative of the depth of understanding and of new revelations. On the other hand, it is not unusual for them to be disoriented and disorganized by the interview. This effect may be gone by the next day, but it sometimes lasts for a day or two. The interview exposes core motivations that have heretofore been unconscious or preconscious. These patients may see how much sense the formulation makes, but also may find it difficult to accommodate. For example, it can be overwhelming for patients to realize that they have spent a lifetime providing testimony to the influence of people they thought they hated. Or, it can be disorganizing to see that they have been totally focused on goals that are now impossible and of dubious value. Because of the unexpected power of these truths, it usually is better to do a one-time-only case formulation on an inpatient basis. In the protected hospital setting, there can be adequate aftercare, monitoring, and follow-up.

The inpatient mode is more structured and the interviewer is more active, because all of the case formulation material needs to emerge in 90 minutes. The Inpatient consultation begins as follows: "My name is _____, and I am the consultant your doctor mentioned. If you are willing, I would like to talk to you for about 90 minutes and see if I can see the world as you do." Administrative details are negotiated, and then the interview begins with an open-ended question: "What do you need? What would help?" Patients often are startled by this question. They usually expect "What is wrong?" But that would focus on pathology. "What do you need?" taps implicitly into the underlying motivation in terms that are conscious but perhaps not understood in all their implications.

For example, Marie, the woman who was hospitalized with "ultimate fear" that later was linked to terrifying childhood experiences, said, "I want to feel safe, and peaceful, and protected." Kenneth, the man with the "Courtroom Agenda," responded to the opening question by behaving, as became clear later, like his mother: "My wife has been stepping out on me." Jessica's response was to ask whether her voices, which played out her lifelong conflict in relation to her siblings, were normal. This reflected her fundamental confusion over whether to sacrifice herself by pleasing others, or whether to defy others by sticking up for her own interests. Patsy, the woman who could not hold firm in her resolve to get rid of an alcohol-dependent and abusive husband, said, " I want to be loved, to have a good husband, a good father to the kids." She was looking for—and, unfortunately, had found—a "stand-in" for her father. Her struggle centered on intimacy with cruel males. All four answered the simple question "What do you need?" with statements that directly reflected their central underlying conflicts. Outpatients will respond in similar ways to that initial question.

Outpatient Mode

An outpatient assessment and development of a DLL case formulation can proceed more slowly. The therapist explores and clarifies no more than the patient can embrace at once. Each outpatient session should end with the patient comparatively intact, able to engage in his or her normal activities. Broad outlines of a complete case formulation need not emerge before the third session, and the formulation may not be complete until later. The inpatient 90-minute consultative interview can be compared to jumping directly into cold water. The slower outpatient procedure for developing a case formulation can be compared to entering the cold water slowly, taking time to accommodate to the temperature before going further in. But for both inpatients and outpatients, the case formulation is always a work in progress—subject to revision with the arrival of new data.

Although the approach to the case formulation is slower for outpatients than for inpatients, it should not be too slow. The IRT method is so specific and data-based that a patient usually can sense or clearly see the case formulation him- or herself rather early. If the interviewer fails to acknowledge the emerging picture and to make a statement about what is to be done about it, the patient may become frightened and leave therapy abruptly.[1] By contrast, outpatients can be stabilized and become comfortable with the treatment if an organized case formulation is developed "with deliberate speed."[2] It should be presented in the context of a specific treatment plan that will address the issues marked by the case formulation (discussed later in connection with Figure 2.3).

Methods of Gathering the Basic Information

The left-hand side of Figure 2.1 provides a list of tasks involved in gathering information for the case formulation. To the right of each listed task, specific interventions that may be helpful are mentioned. As the clinician seeks to gather the information listed in Tables 2.1, and 2.2, and arranged sequentially in Figure 2.1, the style is open-ended. The touchstone topics are covered with a natural associative flow. The interview may seem disorganized to an observer, but it will tend to follow the order shown in Figure 2.1. For example, if the patient starts with a symptom, the interviewer explores the patient's experience of it and what was going on in the most recent episode. If the interviewer asks for very specific examples, this will lead to detail about relevant current events. In this sequence, the session will have progressed from the first to the second box under Task in Figure 2.1.

Exploring Episodes in Terms of Input, Response, and Impact on Self

Each episode should be explored in terms of input, response, and, if possible, impact on the self-concept. Input becomes clear following careful inquiry about the patient's perspective on what was going on. As the interviewer pursues descriptions of relationships marked for exploration in Table 2.2, all kinds of "input" emerges. As the interviewer listens to these stories, he or she does not act as a judge (deciding this or that person was right or wrong, good or bad, etc.). Rather, the interviewer assumes Sullivan's (1953) position of "peripatetic empathy," and attempts to see and feel as if he or she had been there. The interviewer means it when he or she says, "I want to see the world as you do."

Patient responses to perceived input can be assessed from detail in the narrative. Sometimes it is helpful to ask for a "verbal replay." The inter-

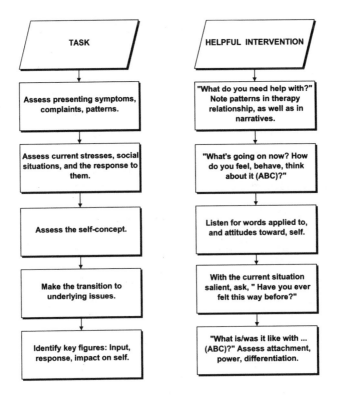

FIGURE 2.1. Making the case formulation: Information needed.

viewer might say, "Could you take me through that, so that I can follow right along? Please tell me what he said or did, then what you said or did, followed by what he said or did, and so on." "How did you feel?" and "What did you think?" likewise add important information about patient experience and learning. These questions explicitly probe for the affect, behavior, and cognition (the ABCs) associated with each episode.

Determining the impact of the various relationships on the self-concept is not so easy as assessing input and response associated with important relationships. People can usually tell an interviewer what was going on, and how they reacted to it, without a lot of difficulty. A good source of information about the self-concept is found in direct quotations spontaneously offered by the patient as he or she describes input and response to others. Examples of such informative remarks are "I am a loner," "I am gifted," and "God has it in for me."[3] Sometimes self-descriptions contradict one another (e.g., "I am worthless" vs. "I have a lot to offer"). Such evidence of ambivalence or conflict is important and should be included in the case formulation. Paying attention to exact words assures that the clinician will have good raw data. Specificity in language can define copy process easily. For example,

Patsy said, "When I lose my temper, I tear things." Later she reported, "When Mother lost her temper, she would tear things." Patsy showed no signs of connecting these remarks, but the use of the same language in each situation did provide direct evidence in support of the hypothesis that she was identified with (copied) her mother.

Identifying Links between Symptoms and IPIRs

Links between presenting symptoms and IPIRs must be identified. Depression is not just depression. Scarring one's arms with cigarettes is not just self-mutilation. Overeating and throwing up are not just phases in a binge–purge cycle. IRT treatment depends on understanding these markers in relation to fantasies and wishes associated with IPIRs. This understanding permits the treatment to be directed to the underlying relationship with the IPIRs, which needs to be transformed if the symptoms are to remit.

Connecting IPIRs to Axis I symptoms. The reader may find uses for the following list of likely connections between social perceptions (driven by IPIRs) and selected Axis I symptoms or group of symptoms. The list comes from clinical experience, DLL theory, and the literature. For illustrative purposes, key references are named.

- *Depression:* The individual is overwhelmed—trapped, blocked, helpless, and without recourse (Seligman, 1975; Breggin, 1994).
- *Depression:* The individual has experienced severe loss (e.g., van Doom, Kasl, Beery, Jacobs, & Prigerson, 1998; Harlow & Suomi, 1974; Blatt, 1998).
- *Depression:* The individual has incorporated a copy process that is manifest as relentless self-criticism, usually accompanied by perfectionism (Blatt, 1998).
- *Anxiety:* The individual is overwhelmed, but feels responsible for coping anyway (Zinbarg, Barlow, Brown, & Hertz, 1992).
- *Depression comorbid with anxiety:* The individual is overwhelmed. When depressed, he or she feels unable to cope. When anxious, he or she is still going to try.
- *Conceptual confusion:* The individual has received contradictory messages about something very important from a source that is powerful and perceived as credible. He or she has "learned" that his or her perspective is "wrong." In effect, "Noon is night."[4] Usually the confusion is about self-definition or love. (Some related papers have been reviewed in Humphrey & Benjamin, 1986.)
- *Mania:* The individual is persuaded on the basis of perceived history that he or she is (or has to be) very powerful and important (Fromm-Reichmann, 1959).

For a hospitalized patient, there is likely to be a current situation that reminds the patient of an IPIR's rules and values; hence the IPIR-related patterns have become reactivated.

Connecting IPIRs to Axis II symptoms. In an earlier book (Benjamin, 1996a), I have provided specific interpersonal descriptions of each of 11 Axis II disorders defined in the DSM-IV. The DSM criteria for each disorder are translated into interpersonal dimensions via the SASB model. The resulting interpersonal descriptions of the personality disorders are then related to prototypical IPIRs for each personality disorder.[5] The book shows how relationships with early caregivers can relate specifically to symptoms of specific personality disorders, and is recommended as a helpful adjunct to learning how to develop a DLL case formulation. Advantages of being able to draw connections from symptoms to IPIRs are illustrated here by comparing Passive–Aggressive Personality Disorder (PAG) and Borderline Personality Disorder (BPD).

In practice, PAG is often confused with BPD, perhaps because each disorder presents with entrenched comorbid depression as well as unremitting suicidality. Individuals with BPD and those with PAG also are often nonfunctional. Despite these similarities, the DLL analysis of their baseline patterns (Benjamin, 1996a, Chs. 5 and 11), and of the links to IPIRs,[6] suggests that the disorders have very different interpersonal origins and wishes. The treatment implications diverge because of their differences in perception and motivation that stem from differences in their histories. For example, patients with BPD can respond well to firm structure that is caring, specific, and constructive (Linehan, 1993). By contrast, for reasons explained earlier (Benjamin, 1996a), patients with PAG are likely to see structure focused on improvement as representing inordinate and intolerable control. If therapeutic structure is misread that way, a patient with PAG may feel compelled to self-destruct, in part, to "show" the clinician who is in control. Thus an intervention (e.g., warm structure) that is often helpful for BPD is anathema for PAG. The clinician who can use the recommended analyses to make the differential diagnosis between PAG and BPD is clearly in a better position to make optimal selections from TAU.

Connecting IPIRs to Axis III symptoms. Axis III conditions are treated primarily by an internist or other appropriate category of physician. IRT does not presume to treat Axis III medical disorders. However, as is recognized by the prevailing diathesis–stress model of disease, many medical conditions can be exacerbated by psychosocial or other stressful conditions. In addition, the rapidly growing discipline of health psychology is making additional important contributions to the understanding of connections between personality and disease. An example is the literature on hostility and cardiovascular disease (reviewed by Miller, Smith, Turner,

Guijarro, & Hallet, 1996). With some nonresponders who have Axis III conditions, therapists may find it helpful to try to connect these and other observations about stress and personality to IPIRs.

Another possible method for connecting Axis III conditions and IPIRs is offered by the Grace–Graham specificity hypotheses of psychosomatic disorder (Graham et al., 1962). In addition to addressing standard medical concerns, Graham's psychosocial explications involved careful inquiry about what was happening in a medical patient's life shortly before hospitalization. This was followed by clear and detailed exploration of what the patient wanted to do about it. Graham argued that the body would track these interpersonal perceptions and reactions with predictable specificity.[7] For a simple example, if a patient believed that he or she needed to maintain a state of hypervigilance[8] in order to fend off an attack that could materialize at any time, the likelihood of suffering from essential hypertension was increased. Graham's hypotheses were parsimonious, but provoked great controversy. Nonetheless, some readers may find them to be informative in selected nonresponder cases.

Using the Patient's Perception, Not Reality, to Drive the Case Formulation

Whether on Axis I, II, or III, the links between IPIRs and symptoms may be due to misperceptions rooted in the relationships with internalizations, to accurate perceptions of problematic situations, or both. In the development of the case formulation, the patient's perception makes the links, and it does not matter whether this perception is accurate. In other words, the individual reacts on the basis of his or her experience, which may not necessarily correspond to what actually happened. By contrast, when it comes to treatment, a realistic and accurate assessment—especially about current situations—is essential.

Obtaining Specific Details

As the interviewer seeks to understand the input and response from the perspective of the patient, specific details are vital.[9] Consider the way in which this interviewer followed up on a vague remark by a patient named Martin:

MARTIN: Work has been a stress lately. [This statement is too general either to SASB-code or to understand at a phenomenological level. Lack of detail requires the interviewer to project his or her own understanding of "stress."]

THERAPIST: What has been particularly difficult there? [A good follow-up question, designed to elicit specifics.]

MARTIN: My boss doesn't like me. [Again, the response is uncodable. Hostility is present, but little else is revealed]

THERAPIST: How can you tell that your boss does not like you? [This may move the conversation to better detail.]

MARTIN: He promoted me. [A surprise that is clearly informative, and never would have been guessed from the initial description of "stress."]

THERAPIST: Help me understand how that is a stress. [The interviewer continues to try to understand at a phenomenological level.]

MARTIN: Well, I am stupid and can't handle a desk job. He knows I do better in the warehouse. [Now, at last, there is some codable information. We at least know the patient puts himself down for alleged lack of competence.[10]]

THERAPIST: What convinces you that you are stupid? [No assumptions are made; further data are requested.]

MARTIN: I always have been. My mother and my father always called me stupid.

In this case, the link to the early figures was made spontaneously while the patient was talking about a present problem. The quest for specificity averted misunderstanding of the meaning of "stress," and also provided a segue to the past. The interviewer took that opportunity to move naturally to a key figure, even though the assessment of current situation was not yet complete. At that point, the probe "Tell me more about that, if you are willing," would probably plunge the interview into a discussion of relationships with early key figures. It is important to use the opportunity to discuss IPIRs as soon as they are mentioned. One can return to fill in any blanks about current situations later. In general, the interviewer seeks to obtain information about as many of the factors listed in Tables 2.1 and 2.2 as possible, but priority is given to spontaneously offered trails to potential key figures.

Asking Questions That Lead to Information about the Past

If the path to the past does not emerge spontaneously, or in response to the question "Have you ever felt like this before?", it can be opened by a general question about the past—for example, "Tell me what it was like growing up?" To encourage specificity, the interviewer frequently pursues answers with such questions as these: "Can you give me an example of that? What set your father off like that? Could we go through a time like that from beginning to end? Can you say exactly what he said and did, and then what you said and did?"

Consider a fairly common statement: "Oh, my childhood was fine. I had a good relationship with my mother." This comment tells very little.

Was she quite controlling, and does the patient think that was good? Or did she give a lot of freedom, and does the patient think that was good? Was she blaming, and does the patient see that as a good way to have taught him or her morals? Or was she warm and very supportive of the patient's independence? Such ambiguities can be resolved by asking, "Tell me more about what was good about it. Can you give me an example?" Usually a patient responds to such inquiries with specific stories that give a very clear, highly evocative, and SASB-codable picture of the relationship.

It is most helpful for the interviewer to obtain examples of interactions with parents that illuminate patterns related to the basic dimensions of attachment, attack/recoil, control/submission, and self-definition.[11] Information about the quality of attachment can come with a question as simple as this: "Tell me, what might your mother say to you when she saw you first thing in the morning?" The nature and quality of maternal control may become apparent in the answers to "What if you displeased her? How did she discipline you?" The degrees of aggression may become apparent in the responses to "What did she spank with? How many blows? How often? What happened afterwards?" Attitudes about self-definition may be manifested in the answers to "What happened if you disagreed with her?" Details of such typical daily interactions reveal the family rules and values that are likely to have been internalized. If examples have been provided of interactions involving the basic dimensions noted above, copy process links to problem patterns are highly likely to become apparent to the patient as well as to the interviewer.

If the client is unable to provide a concrete example in a critical area, sometimes it is helpful to say something like this: "Well, let's say you are in the fifth grade. Can you picture the house where you lived? Can you imagine yourself in that house? OK. Let's start at the beginning of the day. Do you wake yourself up, or does someone wake you?" The interviewer can then proceed through the day, being sure to cover each activity at a very specific level (e.g., who chooses what to wear, who prepares breakfast, what conversation is like at breakfast if people eat together, who packs lunch, how the patient gets to school). The specificity of answers to such questions provides rich information about the patient's developmental learning experiences. Again, fruitful questions typically touch on the basic dimensions defined by attachment, attack/recoil, control/submission, and self-definition; they may also touch on the related issues of nurturance, trust, neglect, blaming, and affirmation.[12]

Occasionally, even a verbal walk though a day at age 10 fails, because a client will be unable to remember anything specific. Sometimes it then helps to ask, "Could you guess what she might have said?" For some reason, the invitation to guess can break the block and open the interview to a world of important detail. Another approach to impasse is to explain the purpose of the interview again:

"It is possible that this 'X-ray' will be too cloudy, or it will be negative. These questions are only an attempt to see if there is anything in your early learning that is affecting how you see and do things now. Sometimes there is a connection, sometimes not. Would you be willing to keep exploring this question, or should we change the subject?"

Some people do prefer to change the subject. They usually go back to their presenting issue. If they never become willing to collaborate and take some initiative, including providing some detail, the DLL assessment cannot proceed. IRT cannot operate in the absence of valid raw phenomenological data from the patient him- or herself.

Including the ABCs as Often as Possible

After the behavioral details about input and response are very clear, understanding of the story should be expanded in terms of its associated affect (A) and cognition (C), as well as the behavior (B). As noted in Chapter 1, the ABCs can be elicited by such questions as "What did you feel? What did you do? What did you think about that?" For example, Marie told of a time when her father had provoked three men in a bar, and they chased him home. The other family members literally hid behind Marie's skirts as she faced the intruders on their behalf.

THERAPIST: How did you feel about that?

MARIE: Actually, I was glad they came. I hoped they would get him.

THERAPIST: What did you do?

MARIE: I just stood there in front of my mom. My dad was behind her.

THERAPIST: What did you think about it?

MARIE: This is the way it always is. I am protecting us from what Dad does.

THERAPIST: What happened then?

MARIE: They called him names for hiding behind his wife and daughter. They said they were sorry they frightened me, and turned around and went back downstairs out the door.

Here in this brief story, unpacked for the ABCs, was Marie's lifetime pattern. She faced serious danger to protect others, and succeeded. She was frightened at first, but managed to take control. This episode was more benign than others. Sometimes, for example, she deliberately challenged her father to save one of her younger siblings from her father's savagery. For that, she received severe beatings herself. Marie felt she could take the paternal assaults better than the little ones. Rescuing was her assignment, her core identity. All of her stories showed the same pattern to one degree or another. If the interviewer allows the patient's examples to provide the raw data for the interview, such patterns become clear, and they reliably recur in many stories.

Touching on Missing Points

Before the assessment is complete, the interviewer comes back to any remaining items in Tables 2.1 and 2.2 that have not yet been covered. Such backtracking is accomplished by asking transition questions such as these: "Let's see, we haven't talked much about your wife. How are things going there?" Or "I need to switch gears here and ask you some diagnostic questions." In the inpatient consultative interview, covering major bases (spouse/partner and parents, at a minimum) must be done. By contrast, in ongoing outpatient sessions, time can be taken for treatment interventions (see Chapter 3) even if the case formulation is not yet complete.

Explaining the Case Formulation to the Patient

The left-hand side of Figure 2.2 lists tasks that help link present symptoms to relationships with the IPIRs. The right-hand side of Figure 2.2 lists specific interventions that may help realize the tasks listed on the left. Briefly, the tasks are to identify copy process links from presenting problems to the people who were mentioned when the procedures of Figure 2.1 and Table 2.2 were followed. Individuals who are linked via copy processes to the presenting problems are IPIRs.[13] Once the key IPIRs are identified, the clinician is in a position to develop a treatment plan that targets the relationship with these IPIRs.

The Copy Process Speech

Figure 2.2 specifies that copy process theory and the gift of love hypothesis need to be checked directly with the patient. Table 2.3 presents the copy process speech, which summarizes the DLL theory about how current behavior patterns reflect relationships with early important persons. In a consultative interview, and sometimes early in an outpatient therapy, the clinician quite literally gives the copy process speech. However, it is important that the speech be delivered in a context wherein a summary or feedback is requested by the patient or called for by the consultative context.

Avoiding the "Telling" Error When Making Links

The clinician who repeatedly delivers the copy process speech may commit a "telling" error, which is to be avoided. As often as possible, the DLL formula-

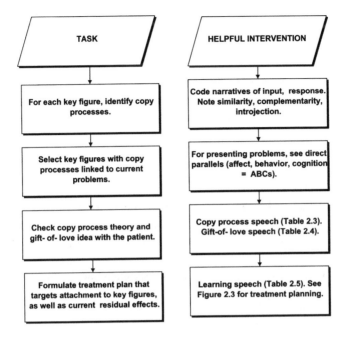

FIGURE 2.2. Linking the present to the past to construct the DLL case formulation.

tions should flow directly from patient material and should usually consist of no more than rephrasing and rearranging of the patient's words. Interpretation is done mostly with undistorted verbal mirrors[14] held directly in front of the patient. Except in the context of consultative feedback,[15] copy processes are better drawn from the patient than "told to" him or her with the copy process speech. Here is an example from a patient named Melanie of how to discuss copy processes without giving the speech.

TABLE 2.3. The Copy Process Speech

"I believe that everything makes sense. Usually problem patterns we have in adulthood reflect things we learned as children. The connections are often quite direct. What we do as adults often copies early patterns that we learned from our mothers or fathers or other important people in our lives. There are three ways to do it: 'Be like him or her,' 'Act as if he or she is still there,' and 'Treat yourself as he or she treated you.' For example, I notice that you say you are [a perfectionist], and you have been talking about how your [father] also [was a perfectionist]. . . . Do you see other connections? . . . Here are some that I see, although they will need further checking."

THERAPIST: So once again you are in a situation where you are carrying most of the burden and still coming up short.

MELANIE: Yes.

THERAPIST: Remind you of anything?

MELANIE: Yeah, sure. That's the way it was with my mother. I took care of everything and still was the bad guy.

THERAPIST: So her version of things is still in play?

MELANIE: I guess.

THERAPIST: How do you feel about that?

MELANIE: Disgusted. I can't believe how I keep doing this.

THERAPIST: Shall we talk about what you might do to start changing this pattern?

At this point, the outpatient interview switches to some techniques discussed in Chapter 3 under the heading of a flow chart for coming to terms. The present point is that copy processes can be woven into the narrative by the patient and consolidated by the therapist as illustrated here. "So her version of things is still in play?" marks a copy process even as it simply describes what the patient just said. Learning is more effective if recognition of copy processes comes directly from patient data, with cuing and consolidation from the therapist. This facilitates learning better than "telling," as the following dialogue illustrates:

THERAPIST: So once again you are in a situation where you are carrying most of the burden and still coming up short.

PATIENT: Yes.

THERAPIST: It sounds like you are copying your relationship with your mother as you relate to your husband.

There is a chance with this "telling" that the patient may feel cornered and become defensive. By contrast, a "mirroring" interpretation may lead directly to affect and cognitions that offer an entrée to new change.

The Gift-of-Love Speech

Table 2.4 presents (1) the DLL theory of copy processes; (2) Bowlby's (1977) description of internal working models, which suggests a mechanism for copy processes; (3) the patient's reasons for seeking psychic prox-

TABLE 2.4. The Gift-of-Love Hypothesis and Speech

Copy processes. Parallels between the problem presentation and early patterns with loved ones are best established by SASB codes of the patient's narrative. Links are via one or more of the three copy processes: "Be like him or her," "Act as if he or she is still there and in control," and "Treat yourself as he or she treated you." The SASB model offers predictive principles that can describe each of the copy processes.

Internal working models. Bowlby's hypothesis of internal working models and recent studies of internalized representations support the hypothesis that the child develops an IPIR of the parent and then relates to it. What once was an interpersonal interaction has become intrapsychic.

Psychic proximity. Copy processes are maintained by wishes for psychic proximity to IPIRs. By acting according to an IPIR's perceived rules and values, the patient attempts to receive the IPIR's approval. "If I do this well enough, long enough, faithfully enough, *then* maybe you will love me." The purpose of the gift is to be loved at last. Appeal to earlier "relationships" represented by IPIRs is more likely in less secure individuals, as well as in individuals under stress.

The speech. "So you see that in many ways, you are being faithful to the rules and values that you learned when you were little. The question remains: Why do we do that? Why do we keep on following those old ideas, especially when they don't work so well any more? Well, often it is because without realizing it, we are trying to 'get it right' with [Dad, Mom, brother, etc.]. It is like we do it the way they seemed to want it, in hopes that they will approve and be pleased. It is as if we hope that maybe things could be better after all. Does that make any sense?"

imity; and, finally, (4) the gift-of-love speech. This gift-of-love speech summarizes points 1 to 3 in terms that make sense to patients when presented at a time when their relationships with the driving IPIRs are salient. It is delivered at the end of the consultative interview to mark the therapy task ahead. Again, the preferred mode for delivering the gift-of-love speech in outpatient therapy is to minimize such "telling," and instead to draw it out of the ongoing narrative. A patient's own data make the point. For example, here is the story of Lacey, a woman who had lived a life rife with abuse and exploitation. She was famous for her rages:

LACEY: I can't believe this has happened again! Here I am out on the streets once more. And nobody cares a bit. I am so furious I want to kill him. And my mother too. This is just like with it was with her. I know I mix up my mother stuff with him.

THERAPIST: You feel the main issue here is your anger with your mother?

LACEY: Yes. I am just so frustrated. I just keep getting into this situation again and again.

THERAPIST: What would you like to tell your mother?

LACEY: That she is a lousy, rotten mother who didn't deserve to have children.

THERAPIST: Could you be more specific about what you are mad about?

LACEY: That I never could please her. That I took care of her, I took care of the house, I gave her all my money, and yet she never did a thing for me when I got in trouble.

THERAPIST: She expected and accepted a lot from you, but wasn't there when you really needed her.

LACEY: Yeah, and on top of that, she found something wrong with everything I did.

THERAPIST: What would you like from her now?

LACEY: A little concern. A little caring.

THERAPIST: So underneath all your hurt and anger is the wish that at last, she would be more loving.

LACEY: It is the least she could do. She should be a decent mother for once.

THERAPIST: So your wish to tell her off, your need to let her know how bad things are for you, is mostly about wanting her love?

LACEY: Yes. But telling her off has never has worked. She just turns things back on me. I guess it is not going to work this time either.

At this point, Lacey was getting ready to block a pathological pattern (raging at loved ones) and to begin coming to terms as described in Chapter 3. Notice that the gift-of-love interpretation of her rage flowed from the dialogue as the therapist kept asking questions focused on her experienced underlying wishes. The patient described the gift of love in her own words.

The IRT theory of underlying motivation must be supported by data for each IRT case. Patients are not "told" what their motivation is. Like any scientific hypotheses, the DLL descriptions of copy processes and psychic proximity are constantly subjected to checking and refinement by data from the clinical narrative. If a patient rejects the gift-of-love hypothesis, a therapist does not push it. The treatment can nonetheless proceed with the procedures discussed in Chapter 3. There is much work to be done on understanding the copy process links to problem patterns in affective and behavioral as well as cognitive ways. The reasons for copying can be addressed later in therapy, especially as enabling the will to change (step 4) becomes the main focus. When the patient seriously struggles to break old habits and stop copying, discussions of the gift of love are likely to become more relevant and clear.

The Learning Speech

Table 2.5 presents the "learning speech" that is given during the consultative interview, and also at the end of the first outpatient therapy session. It explains the IRT approach. The patient has every right to know what the therapy is about before agreeing to participate in it. Here is the speech: "Therapy starts with learning to recognize your patterns, where they came from, and what they are for. Once you see that clearly, you can make a decision about whether to change. Finally, work can begin on learning new and better patterns." The learning speech and the other speeches in Table 2.5 are prototypes. Naturally they vary, depending on the case formulation and the verbal level of the patient.

The process of recognizing and then developing new and better patterns is easier said than done, of course. But the DLL theory and the IRT interventions summarized in Chapter 3 are usually very helpful aids to this therapy learning.[16] Unlike the copy process and gift-of-love speeches, the learning speech is repeated literally and often. The reason is that most patients want more than self-development from therapy, and the learning speech provides a vital corrective that keeps things in perspective.[17] Sometimes I call the learning speech the "Is that all there is?" speech. The name comes from a song of that name delivered years ago in a depressed style by Peggy Lee. The idea is that life offers only so much, and one has to accept this and get on with it. "That's all there is." At many points in therapy when the patient is disappointed in his or her progress, in therapy, or in the therapist, the learning speech is helpful. It is vital to remember the wisdom of this speech when the patient is demanding that the therapist perform magic. The therapy contract is summarized by the learning speech. Just delivering the speech at the beginning of therapy is not enough; the therapist needs to help the patient understand the collaborative nature of the process, as in the following example.

A student therapist was totally flummoxed about what to do about an agreeable but passive patient who would take no initiative at all in therapy.

TABLE 2.5. The Learning Speech

"Interpersonal Reconstructive Therapy starts with learning to recognize your patterns, where they came from, and *what they are* for. Once you see these things clearly, you can make a decision about whether to change. Finally, work can begin on learning new and better patterns."

The patient was fixated on a childhood incident of alleged sexual abuse in peer play. Her main way of interacting in therapy was to ask the student therapist what he wanted to know. As the student therapist jumped through hoops trying to come up with questions, the patient typically would give very general, monosyllabic answers. The patient's theory was that the sexual abuse caused her to be afraid of men, and therefore she was sad and lonely. To protect herself from further abuse, she explained that she would engage men by "becoming" whatever they were interested in. When they eventually responded to her compliance and wanted to pursue a relationship with her, she would promptly reject them. Therapy had been stuck there when the student first tried the learning speech. It made no difference. The patient still did not agree to look at this pattern and see whether it had any meaning, other than that it was the residual effect of sexual abuse by a peer. She would not participate in the process of developing a DLL understanding of her pattern that might reach "closer to home."

In supervision, I noticed that the patient's pattern of focusing exclusively on what the other person wanted, and being completely passive, seemed to characterize the therapy relationship too. The student therapist agreed that the patient was indeed using her "seductive" habits, and we decided that to continue therapy in this vein would be to enable a problem pattern. Unless the patient could transcend her attempts to figure out and provide what the therapist wanted (and then later refuse it), she was inappropriate for IRT. If drawing the comparison between her dating pattern and the therapy process did not engage her interest in learning more about her patterns and possibilities for change, termination was the only reasonable choice. There would be no point in having a therapy that simply repeated a problem pattern. When the student therapist reviewed this perspective with the patient, she understood and became willing and able to participate more actively in IRT.

The story underscores the fact that responsibility for progress in the IRT learning model is shared by patient and therapist. The therapist works hard to bring to bear his or her knowledge and skills. He or she therefore charges a fee or is paid a salary for services rendered. The therapist is not like an auto mechanic. Under no circumstances can the therapist carry more than "half the variance." Learning is under direct control of the learner. He or she harbors the Green (the part of the patient that wants to change—see Figure 1.1); the genetic templates; and the motivations and energy to do the hard, sometimes terrifying, sometimes boring work. The therapist is, at best, a highly collaborative and supportive coach or teacher. Change will happen primarily at the initiative of the patient. It will be manifested slowly over time, accompanied by much hard work and some regressions. Therapy process can be greatly facilitated by the therapist, but is never determined by him or her. The learning speech keeps all this in perspective. There are many difficult times the patient will need to be reminded of its fundamental truth: "That's all there is."

METHODS OF DEVELOPING
A DLL-BASED TREATMENT PLAN

Figure 2.3 outlines stages in developing a treatment plan. First, a DLL case formulation links problem patterns to key figures, as described in Figures 2.1 and 2.2. Figure 2.3 suggests that the problem patterns can be addressed in any of three ways.

The first is TAU without regard to copy processes. Medications and/or empirically supported therapies (ESTs) that promise quick and effective relief are used. Since IRT is difficult and time consuming, it makes no sense to use it if the simpler, quicker ways work.[18] Ordinarily, IRT is for nonresponders, which means that candidates are defined after TAU has failed. However, when a therapist is developing a treatment plan, if the effective and efficient methods for addressing a problem pattern have not been tried, it is a good

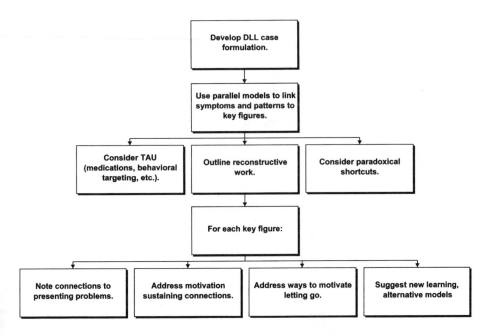

FIGURE 2.3. Formulating a treatment plan.

idea to consider the simpler route. An example would be a well-defined phobia that has recently appeared, requires immediate attention, and has not been treated by the usual behavioral methods. A trial of a standard behavioral treatment for phobia would be in order (e.g., Beck, 1997).

Another branch on the treatment-planning diagram is to choose a paradoxical shortcut that may achieve a quick result. These interventions attempt to turn the gift-of-love motivation that has been supporting the problem patterns around, so that they support good adjustment instead. This device is frequently used in crisis handling, discussed in Chapter 7.

An example of a paradoxical shortcut is offered by a woman who smoked to calm herself. She wanted to stop smoking for health reasons. When she participated in a DLL consultative interview, she discovered that she smoked in the same way that her mother did. She had long been aware that her mother was jealous, cruel, and negligent. Fortunately, the patient was not deeply attached to this mother, because she had been raised by a more loving aunt. The thought that smoking was testimony to her attachment to her mother was so alien that the patient never touched a cigarette again. Similarly, a man who had not been faithful to his beloved wife and children learned that he had been copying his "no-good profligate" father. With that realization, he moved summarily and comfortably to marital fidelity.

In sum, the paradoxical-shortcut technique seeks to make it clear that a problem behavior is an overt sign of love for and submission to a person believed to be hated. The resulting tension between the new perspective and the old habit can serve to ruin the "desirability" of the problem behavior. This sudden type of "cure" from insight is rare, but not impossible. If it can be achieved, IRT can be finished in one session. Unfortunately, the attachments to IPIRs are usually deeply ingrained—probably neurologically[19]— and it is not often easy to make such changes simply by recognition of copy processes.

The third and most central method of treatment planning shown in Figure 2.3 is systematically to address each key figure and the presenting symptoms associated with him or her. The main components of this process appear from left to right at the bottom of the figure. First, the copy process links are registered. Next, the specific motivations that sustain the copy processes are considered. Then ways to encourage letting go of the associated wishes[20] are assessed. Finally, methods of learning better alternatives are chosen. The treatment planner can draw from any technique from TAU in ways that meet these standards, and that realistically could be implemented in a given case.

For example, Marie's copy process analysis suggested that her terror, depression, dependency, and chronic diarrhea were related to living with her father IPIR. These symptoms were also related to the family's belief that she was the only one who could handle him and protect other family members. Marie's treatment needed to center on her attachment to her father and all that went into it. Additional considerations included the fact that her mother abandoned her, leaving her exposed and alone in the face of severe stress. Marie needed to come to terms with these abuses, and to have strong support and understanding for the position that she was in. She needed to progress through the five therapy steps, with the core issues being the tasks of grieving for (1) the loss of a decent childhood, and (2) the loss of the hope that her father and family could be or could have been more loving. She would need ultimately to let go of—to come to terms with—these aspects of her past. Then she could move on to learning new ways of relating that could enrich her remaining years.

It probably should be noted that this treatment plan did not include much focus on Marie's sexual abuse. The sexual abuse per se was not related to her anxiety as directly as were her father's episodes of throwing her and others through doors or walls and down flights of stairs. Rather than creating terror and pain, the sexual abuse offered moments of tenderness, intimacy, and pleasure with this otherwise frightening figure. Having him relate to her in a nonviolent, pseudo-caring way was as bizarre as her assignment of being the one, a child, who could influence, handle, and manage him. How could a young girl understand how this terribly violent, always displeased, and frequently out-of-control man could unpredictably became loving and a source of intense pleasure? The sexual abuse probably increased her loyalty to him, further trapping her in the role of self-neglect and sacrifice on behalf of others. In that sense, the sexual abuse was extremely destructive. However, to discuss it as if it were the core trauma would be to confuse her further.

ASSESSMENT IN IRT

A DLL Case Report Based on the Interview Method

The preceding sections have shown that the main IRT assessment method is an interview that follows the DLL principles and the methods discussed in connection with Tables 2.1 and 2.2 as well as in Figures 2.1, 2.2, and 2.3. This information can be presented in the following recommended outline for a DLL-based case report:

- Summary of presenting problems and the history of treatment.
- Current social circumstances.
- Developmental history.
- Treatment recommendations.

The treatment recommendations section includes DLL hypotheses about copy process links between the presenting problems, on the one hand, and the associated current problem patterns first learned in relation to early important figures, on the other. These, and their underlying motivations, are then addressed systematically, as suggested in Figure 2.3.

The Need for a Clear, Well-Documented, Nonjudgmental Report

A DLL case formulation summary requires no prior knowledge of DLL theory or IRT from the report reader. This is a taxing requirement, but it is important because it forces the report writer to provide compelling, self-explanatory data in support of the DLL hypotheses and the recommended treatment interventions. Jargon is avoided; for terms unique to IRT (e.g., "IPIR"), "translations" into everyday language are provided.

Explanatory detail is included, but no more than is necessary to explain the basis of the case formulation clearly. Any time specific descriptions of sensitive topics (sexual abuse, legal matters, highly confidential family material) are included in a report, they should relate clearly and compellingly to the case formulation. Otherwise, it may be better to omit them.[21]

The report writer does well to imagine that the patient, the patient's lawyer, and a hostile cross-examiner are reading the report. This mindset helps assure that the report will be clear, dignified, relevant, constructive, and (if required) easily defensible. These goals can be reached if the report writer focuses on the questions asked; supports positions with compelling detail that is noncompromising; distinguishes hypotheses from facts; and writes with a constructive, nonjudgmental tone.

Here is an example of a report that asks for too much faith from the reader. A person who had not heard the supporting detail and who did not understand copy process links could dismiss these conclusions as having no substantive basis whatsoever.

> Many of the patient's problems were shaped in childhood. The patient's suicide attempt, tendency toward harsh physical punishment, rigidity and inflexibility, and trouble in her marriage were exacerbated by her early social experience. Work toward recognizing patterns and where they came from may be beneficial in helping the patient overcome maladaptive ways of functioning.

It is better to say nothing than to say so much without explaining it. An informative report would detail clearly, for example, how this particular suicide attempt grew out of specific patterns in relation to specific important other people. Each of the patient's other symptoms should likewise be linked to well-established, easily described, clearly recognizable interpersonal learning experiences. Once the supporting detail explains the case formulation, the treatment section can detail how each of these problems might be addressed. When preparing such a report, the writer depends on having elicited extensive relevant detail and on having excellent notes available.[22]

Here is an example of an improved version of this report:

> The patient's mother was highly critical, frequently calling her worthless, and telling her nobody would ever want to live with her. Over the years, the mother enforced many rules and backed them with harsh punishments. The most common method was to administer several kicks in the shins. The patient learned that following her mother's rules helped avoid these outbursts of rage. Compliance therefore provided a measure of predictability and safety. Continuing in the same role, she has chosen a husband who is also critical and punitive. When he rages, she believes she has failed to follow some important expectation, and criticizes herself. Her recent suicide attempt was a response to her belief that she is unworthy and that nobody would want to be with her. During the consultation, she was able to see that this perspective exactly reflected her mother's stated opinion. In addition, the patient recognized that she treats her children with the same harshness she experienced in her own childhood. In fact, she administers the exact punishment that she experienced: several kicks in the shins.
>
> A long-term psychotherapy might help this patient better understand these links between her current difficulties and her earlier learning about herself and others. If she could develop a perspective that included more compassion for and understanding of herself as she faced those difficult situations, she might feel freer to chose to live her life differently. She could learn that she is using harsh control with her children, and accepting criticism and rejection from her husband without protest, because she believes that her mother was right about her. As she engages in these self-destructive behaviors, she demonstrates that she is willing to stick to her mother's values and rules.
>
> In a supportive psychotherapy that focused on such echos from the past as they appear in her current life, the patient might modify her perspective and learn, for example, that she has many worthy attributes. If she rejects automatic obedience to the views of these important other people, and tries to make her own judgments about herself, she might come to appreciate her many strengths. These include being an attentive and loving mother and an effective employee. She could realize that she has a right to be treated with dignity. During this process, she also might decide to change some of her own behaviors. For example, she might conclude that she does not want to subject her children to the same painful experiences she had. At that point, she might become willing to take advantage of available parent training, so that she can learn more adaptive parenting styles.

Use of Traditional Assessment Methods

Widely accepted measurements of symptoms, such as the Symptom Checklist 90—Revised (Derogatis, 1977), the Beck Depression Inventory (Beck, Rush, Shaw, & Emery, 1979), and the like, can provide excellent additions to the "symptoms" section of the DLL assessment. Perceived current social relationships and relations with IPIRs can be associated with the SASB Intrex (Benjamin, 2000b). This is a self-rating instrument that codifies perceived relations with others according to the SASB model. Computer-generated output characterizes each relationship and uses some of the predictive principles to link one relationship with another.[23]

SCIENTIFIC BASES OF THE DLL
CASE FORMULATION METHOD

What Needs to Be Proved?

According to the EST standards discussed in Chapter 1, all that needs to be proved is that IRT is more effective (efficacious or efficient) than a control condition. This compares to showing that a drug brings symptom relief in comparison to a control condition. However, those who believe effectiveness can be improved if it is known how and why a treatment works would add the demand that there be clear statements and tests of how the intervention affects causal factors. This introduction of theory compares to understanding exactly how a drug affects independently established causal factors of a symptom.

The Causal-Factors Assumption in DLL

In DLL, there are two components to the description of causal factors of problem patterns in nonresponder patients: (1) Presenting problems correspond directly to patterns developed in relation to IPIRs via the three copy processes. (2) These copy processes are motivated by the wish for psychic proximity to the IPIR (the gift of love).

Direct Tests of the Causal-Factors Assumption

The validity of these hypotheses can be tested by carefully assessing problem patterns and relating these to perceived relations with internalizations of current and past important figures.[24] As treatment continues, assessments of the present and wished-for relationships with identified key figures should show the changes said to be required for success. For example, at the end of treatment, the successful IRT patient should rate his or her relationship with a key IPIR in terms of friendly differentiation (discussed in detail in Chapters 4 and 9), rather than in terms of hostile enmeshment or angry alienation (either of which is likely at the beginning of treatment). Wishes in relation to key figures also should be changed in the direction of peaceful self-definition. Leslie Greenberg has successfully identified such changes by using SASB to assess change processes in emotion-focused psychotherapy (Greenberg & Foerster, 1996). Finally, any observed changes in internalizations should relate directly to predicted changes in symptoms.

Formal Definitions to Assure That the Case Formulation Links
Presenting Problems to Patterns with IPIRs

- Presenting problems: Problems noted by the patient or clinician that are related to the request for treatment. These are translated to symptoms characteristic of DSM disorders.
- Symptoms: DSM criteria (not disorders[25]) that are fulfilled by the presenting problems.
- Problem patterns: Interpersonal and intrapsychic patterns[26] associated with an IPIR that can be linked to symptoms.

The clinician connects *presenting problems* to diagnostic criteria listed in the DSM-IV. These diagnostic criteria describe *symptoms*[27] (e.g., American Psychiatric Association, 1994, pp. 2–3). Collections of symptoms mark *disorders*. Examples of symptoms that mark disorders on different axes include anxiety on Axis I; the need to have others comply with one's idea of how things should be done on Axis II; headaches, diarrhea on Axis III. Despite the fact that the diagnostic criteria in the DSM-IV are descriptive and without attributions of cause (American Psychiatric Association, 1994, p. xxiii), symptoms are generally considered to be markers of underlying psychopathology (e.g., Janicak, Davis, Preskorn, & Ayd, 1997, p. 6). The DLL case formulation centers on DSM-relevant symptoms, and it does make causal attributions.

These distinctions narrow the focus of the DLL case formulation sharply to the presenting problems (not disorders),[28] and expresses them in conventional symptom descriptions from the DSM. The DLL case formulation uses clear descriptions of interpersonal and intrapsychic patterns (problem patterns) and copy process theory to relate presenting problems to IPIRs.

The Performance Model: The View That IPIRs Interfere with Mechanisms Invoked by TAU

The requirement that each symptom be specifically linked to an IPIR suggests that relationships with IPIRs function as causal factors. This section bypasses that requirement and instead provides an alternative model, called the performance model. Under this model, relationships with IPIRs are seen as motivational factors that interfere with the ability of TAU to address symptoms. This alternative may be more acceptable to readers who prefer to make sharp distinctions between psychosocial and biological disorders.[29] They may argue that the psychosocial variables defined as IPIRs are unlikely to relate in a causal sense to physiological or neurochemical events that generate symptoms characteristic of such clinical syndromes as depression.

Retaining the firm distinction between biological and psychological factors, these readers may nonetheless find the performance interpretation of IRT to be useful. They need only invoke this reasoning: IRT can help nonresponders react favorably to medications and other forms of TAU by changing the psychosocial and intrapsychic motivation that has been overshadowing the power of TAU. Such patients' wish for reunion with their key figures has been far more important to them than maximizing their current function and well-being. Once their devotion to outdated wishes and habits softens through treatment with IRT, TAU can prevail. There need be no necessary connection between IPIRs and symptoms.

The performance model is illustrated by a self-sabotaging figure skater, who understands and resolves his fear of success after treatment. The skater goes on in subsequent years to win gold medals. According to this model, the intrapsychic factors that interfered with his successful performance would have had no necessary connection to skating per se. The same improvements would have been observed if the individual's specialty were skiing, playing a musical instrument, or performing any other complex skill. The "symptom" of poor skating or skiing or violin playing was not directly, and especially not physiologically, connected to an IPIR. The will to execute these skills in optimal ways was impaired by the relationship with the IPIR, not the skills themselves.

Consider how this performance model would apply to a nonresponder depressed person. The DLL analysis could argue that the wish to claim the approval of a highly critical IPIR may outweigh anything an antidepressant can do for such a person. No matter what his or her chemistry, the patient will choose to be relentlessly self-critical as he or she follows the perceived rules and values of the IPIR. Similarly, the patient may also be unable to benefit from assertiveness training, placing a higher priority on complying with the IPIR's rules that he or she shall not "back-talk." The quest to be loved and accepted on the IPIR's terms will carry each day. The depressed person's daily performance is impaired by his or her outdated motivation in relation to the IPIR. However, after resolving the relationship with the IPIR (using IRT processes summarized in Chapter 3), the patient may be able to make good use of assertiveness training and mood-elevating drugs.

Under the performance model, there is no need to argue that a relationship with an IPIR shows any specific connection to any particular symptoms. The perspective argues only that relationships with IPIRs *interfere with* the ability of TAU to be effective with nonresponders.

The Causal-Factors Model: The View That Relationships with IPIRs Are Specifically Related to Symptoms

Advantages of Thinking of Relations with IPIR as Causal Factors

Why make a distinction between a performance and a causal-factors interpretation of the DLL model? Both implicate motivation, and both imply that treatment should give priority to these motivational factors. The short-term answer to that question may be that it probably makes little functional difference. However, the two models have different long-term implications for theory, research, and practice. Whereas IRT can be applied effectively now under the performance model, it could potentially become even more effective and efficient as connections between symptoms and IPIRs become better understood at physiological and neurological as well as psychological levels. In addition, the causal-factors interpretation of DLL theory has more logical coherence, and this usually turns out to be helpful in science.[30]

Here, then, are some reasons to entertain the causal-factors interpretation of DLL theory.

• *The causal-factors perspective is based on a testable, refutable rationale concerning observed connections between IPIRs and presenting problems.* The causal-factors perspective is offered as a hypothesis, not as ultimate truth. That hypothesis can be tested and refuted. There is no requirement to accept it on faith, or out of loyalty to any ideology. To date, clinical data are highly supportive of the claim that symptoms can usually be linked specifically and reasonably to IPIRs. For more formal tests, independent observers could rate a tape of an IRT-adherent DLL interview, and agree on the identity of key figures. They also would be likely to see that the symptoms do relate via copy processes to the relationship with the IPIRs. Data come directly from the patient, and connections are usually affirmed by the patient. Understanding the DLL case formulation does not require special language, special training, or acceptance of unclear assumptions. An intelligent reader without special training could reasonably assess the content validity of the case formulations for the four cases described in Chapter 1.[31]

• *The causal-factors perspective provides a clear method to define IPIRs. Again, an IPIR is directly associated with problem patterns that directly relate to presenting problems.*[32] Without direct links between key figures and symptoms, the psychosocial clinician has no specific reason to discuss one historical figure or another. By contrast, tightly linking IPIRs and symptoms by a specific rationale increases precision and accuracy of therapeutic focus. For example, Jessica's siblings, who heretofore had been completely ignored in her treatment, were defined as key figures because of their direct link to her devotion to suicide and other self-sacrificing behaviors. The siblings might not have been recognized as central if the assignment to link symptoms and IPIRs had not been accepted by the DLL interviewer.

• *The causal-factors claim allows the clinician to see the patient as a whole person who is trying to adapt to dilemmas that arise in relation to the IPIRs, rather than as a collection of signs of breakdown.* When a patient like Jessica has symptoms of more than one clinical syndrome, conventional practice suggests that she has two or three DSM-defined Axis I disorders, such as Major Depressive Disorder With Psychotic Features, Generalized Anxiety Disorder, and Panic Disorder. Under the DLL case formulation, it all fits together. Jessica's depression, anxiety, and arguing voices all corresponded sensibly to patterns associated with her IPIRs of her siblings. The causal-factors model provides an integrated view of her entire presentation.

• *The causal-factors claim attempts to focus the treatment sharply on presumed underlying causes. If these presumptions are correct, treatment effectiveness should be improved over that of approaches focusing only on symptoms, or simply on general motivational factors.* Under the conventional model, symptoms are targeted independently by procedures that have demonstrated efficacy or effectiveness in treating them. For a given patient, there can be several procedures for the several symptoms or classes of symptoms (e.g., anxiety, depression, thought disorder). Under DLL case formulation, the internalizations rather than the symptoms are the focus of treatment. Symptom change is expected naturally to follow changes in relationships with the internalizations. For example, Marie would understandably become less anxious after she no longer believed that her identity in life was to protect her family from violence.

Relationships with IPIRs Shape Symptoms

The reader is reminded that the causal-factors model is offered in a broader context that also considers temperament, history, situation, state, and more. Links to the perceived relationships with IPIRs encourage expression of the symptoms and contribute to their shape. Relationships with IPIRs do not account for 100% of the variance, even in cases for whom DLL theory applies well. The relevant model from biology is found in studies of the effect of experience on gene expression. There is rapidly accumulating evidence, for example, that brain development is affected importantly by experience (Kolb & Whishaw, 1998).

To illustrate, the fact that Jessica suffered from voices in the first place may have depended on an inherited propensity to fantasize. That tendency is probably encouraged by perceived rejection and isolation, as was the case for Jessica. The quality of the voices is also likely to have been affected by experience (Benjamin, 1989). For example, familial habits of ignoring context and communicating in rapidly shifting, absolutistic terms—"good or bad," "right or wrong," "win or lose"—probably help give voices the unyielding, contradictory quality they typically have.[33]

Clearly, much work needs to be done to further articulate and test these causal-factors hypotheses about the impact of relationships with IPIRs on symptoms. Again, readers who object to the causal-factors inter-

pretation may nonetheless find IRT useful by using the performance interpretation of DLL, described earlier.

Compatibility of Copy Process Theory with Genetic, Cellular, and Behavioral Data

DLL theory increases the specificity of Bowlby's idea of internal working
models by describing them more precisely in terms of the SASB model, and
by linking them directly to presenting problems. To review, copy process
theory details three ways to connect IPIRs and problem patterns. A problem pattern (1) imitates an IPIR (e.g., a micromanaging patient had a
micromanaging mother); (2) was an understandable reaction[34] to IPIR
qualities (e.g., an oppositional character had a micromanaging mother);
and/or (3) treats the self as the IPIR treated the patient (e.g., a person with
a micromanaging mother micromanages him- or herself). As will be shown
in Chapter 4, there can be minor variations on these copy process themes.
Suppose a man seeking treatment was not micromanaged by anybody, but
nonetheless micromanages himself. A copy process is present if he saw his
mother micromanage and criticize herself as she tried to deal with his violent father. Although he is not treating himself as she treated him, he imitates her manner of treating herself.

Copying is a widely studied phenomenon at many levels. For example,
at the genetic level, DNA carries the basic instructions, and RNA facilitates
the copy process needed to build new cells like the originals. Copying at
the behavioral level is easy to see among young children.[35]

In sum, there is substantial evidence that copying is a centrally important process at the genetic, cellular, and behavioral levels. DLL theory
merely applies this understanding by claiming that the particular quality
of an IPIR is likely to show up in the behavior, affect, and cognitions of
the perceiver. Copy process theory is a parsimonious explanation for a
significant amount of the variance in description of psychopathology. It
was discovered[36] through extensive clinical interviewing that involved
coding[37] of the interpersonal and intrapsychic dimensions of the problem
patterns, and discussions of spontaneously mentioned persons in patients' worlds.

ADDITIONAL DETAIL ON DLL THEORY AND ITS EMPIRICAL BASES

The balance of this chapter is about empirically informed attachment theory, which has so greatly affected the development of DLL theory and related IRT interventions. Readers who are presently not concerned about

the theoretical and empirical background can go directly to Chapter 3 from here.

Psychic Proximity and Bowlby's Theory of Attachment

The law of parsimony might suggest that centering on the concept of psychic proximity when one is trying to help patients give up patterns is needlessly complex. Why not think that problem patterns, though they may have been learned in relation to early attachment persons, are permanently encoded habits? Perhaps, like learning to ride a bicycle, patterns of social interaction are preserved for many years without practice or functionality. Hard-wired habit formation is probably part of the reason why copy processes are sustained, and why they are so difficult to change. Moreover, earlier-learned responses become more salient at times of stress, whether the stress is due to sickness, inordinate challenge, or something else. Just as a skier who recently learned parallel turns goes back to snowplow when encountering terrain beyond his or her abilities, so an adult may fall back on early patterns of interaction when the social world becomes especially challenging. One could leave DLL theory at that, and conclude that therapy is a matter of breaking old habits and learning new ones.

Sensible and parsimonious though that interpretation may be, it does not apply well to nonresponders. Almost all of them have had medications to help manage affect, as well as behavioral coaching to change their habits. Still, their problem habits do not change. There is every reason to believe that most such patients have had good treatments according to the state of the art. Waiting for someone who is even more expert at augmenting medications or even more skilled at designing behavioral programs, is not a likely solution for them. When a patient is unable to change interpersonal and intrapsychic habits despite good coaching and appropriate chemical support, it is more reasonable to conclude the old patterns must be serving an adaptive purpose that overwhelms their costs.

As has been said before, the DLL functional analysis proposes that attachment supports the desire for psychic proximity to an IPIR. Patterns of interaction with such internalizations are directly related to patterns in the original actual interactions. Internalizations serve some of the same purposes served by original or current attachment persons. For example, proximity to current loved ones or to internalizations of current and past loved ones can provide reassurance when needed, and also can be a desired goal in itself. Hugging a loved one is good if a person is frightened, but also can be appreciated as an end in itself. Mental processes replay family scenarios (Sullivan, 1953).

A nonresponder's version of love does not look like the normative version.[38] Nor is his or her attachment is not likely to be what Bowlby calls secure attachment. But it is all this patient has. He or she reaches for it and hopes for the best. The minimal result of providing testimony to the rules and values of the IPIR is that the nonresponder derives whatever security he or she can from proximity to it. The optimal fantasied result would be that the actions will be acknowledged by the IPIR and a loving union will take place.

Chapters 5–9 provide details on various ways to try to help the nonresponder let go of such problem wishes and develop new and more adaptive internalizations. The therapy relationship, discussed in Chapter 5, is a major contributor to this change process. One of its functions is to recapitulate the developmental process in a circumscribed way. Hence it is important to provide further details here about normal developmental processes as they have been described in the attachment literature. Understanding how attachment functions, and appreciating the meaning of Bowlby's "dance" between dependence and independence, can be very helpful to both the clinician and the patient.

Bowlby's Theory of Attachment

After carefully observing mother–child interactions, and studying children who had lost their mothers, John Bowlby proposed that attachment to the mother is a reflexive phenomenon that is not dependent on receiving food. Bowlby (1969) detailed the building of the bond between the mother and infant, and effectively described the many long-term developmental problems that result if the bond is impaired or disrupted. Massive numbers of research and clinical studies have confirmed and extended his thesis that the quality of the early bond reverberates throughout life. A creative theoretical integration of some of these findings was prepared by Hazen and Shaver (1994).

Bowlby's description of attachment has been confirmed in infrahuman as well as in human primates. Suomi (1999, p. 181) makes this clear: "Indeed, virtually all of the basic features of human infant behavior that Bowlby's attachment theory specifically ascribed to our evolutionary history could be observed in the normative mother-directed behaviors of rhesus monkey infants described by Hinde and other primate researchers." Suomi goes on to provide details:

> Virtually all infants in these species spend their initial days, weeks, and (for infant apes) months of life in near-continuous physical contact with their biological mothers, typically clinging to the mothers' ventral surface for most of their waking (and all of their sleeping) hours. Rhesus monkey neonates clearly and consistently display four of the five "component instinctual responses" that Bowlby . . . listed as universal human attachment behaviors. . . . All of these response patterns reflect efforts on the part of the infant to obtain and maintain physical contact with or proximity to its mother.

Rhesus monkey mothers, in turn, provide their newborns with essential nourishment; physical and psychological warmth . . . ; and protection from the elements, potential predators, and even other members of the social group, including pesky older siblings. During this time a strong and enduring social bond inevitably develops between mother and infant—a bond that is unique in terms of its exclusivity constituent behavioral features, and ultimate duration. (1999, p. 182)

The monkeys' behavior after early infancy is likewise consistent with that of human children, according to Suomi:

As they grow older, most monkey infants voluntarily spend increasing amounts of time at increasing distances from their mothers, apparently confident that they can return to the mothers' protective care without interruption or delay, should circumstances warrant it. Their mothers' presence as a secure base clearly promotes exploration of their ever-expanding physical and social world . . . On the other hand, when rhesus monkey infants develop less than optimal attachment relationships with their mothers, their exploratory behavior is inevitably compromised . . . ; this is consistent with Bowlby's observations regarding human attachment relationships . . . (1999, p. 183)

Suomi also discusses neurochemical correlates of the attachment bonding process: "Several studies have documented that initiation of ventral contact with the mother promotes rapid decreases in hypothalamic–pituitary–adrenal (HPA) activity (as indexed by lowered plasma cortisol concentrations) and in sympathetic nervous system arousal (as indexed by reductions in heart rate), along with other physiological changes commonly associated with soothing" (1999, pp. 182–183).[39]

Bowlby's Description of the Dance between Dependence and Independence

Suomi's (1999) review includes the primordial features of Bowlby's theory of attachment. Developing an attachment bond is a crucial first developmental step. It provides the basic security needed to leave the parenting figure and explore the environment during the second developmental step. Bowlby described a paradoxical "dance" between dependence and independence at this stage. If there is a good attachment, the child has the courage to separate from the mother, explore the world, and build his or her own separate strength. The resulting functional independence that follows stable dependency is also vital to survival.

When the attachment bond is not reliable and effective in providing security, the infant becomes pathologically independent or dependent. Detailing all that is known about the results of poor attachment in monkeys and humans is far beyond the present scope. However, Harlow's research on infant monkeys on the extremes of attachment failure is worthy of special note by those who work with severely disordered individuals. Monkeys deprived of social contact from birth were hyperaggressive and sexually inappropriate (Harlow & Harlow, 1967). If impregnated artificially, they tended to be abusive and inattentive to their own infants, sometimes even killing them (Harlow, Harlow, Dodsworth, & Arling, 1966). Despite the severity of the social impairment observed simply in the absence of opportunity to develop a mother–child bond and to play with peers, Griffin and Harlow (1966) found that these monkeys were not impaired in terms of their learning capacity. Hence there can be severe social damage if attachment fails, but this is not necessarily associated with a breakdown in the ability of the brain to process information.

These studies of extreme isolation demonstrate that social experience is needed for proper expression of the preprogrammed social reflexes described by Harlow and by Bowlby. In other research by Harlow, more lengthy and complete social deprivations yielded more intractably withdrawn and inaccessible monkeys. The four monkeys that had total social isolation for the first year of life were terrorized, seemingly overwhelmed, by simple removal from their opaque cages.[40] Their priority appeared to be to withdraw from whatever was going in whatever ways were possible. Lacking social models to copy and direct their unfolding social reflexes, they developed "no interaction" as their norm. They copied what they knew, which were inert cage walls and their own bodies. This barren, autistic[41] world comprised the "rules and values" that directed their extraordinary avoidant behaviors.

The Normality of Copy Processes and Psychic Proximity

A focus on the relevance of attachment and imitation to social development was suggested long ago by Darwin (1871/1952, pp. 289, 291). Copy processes are normal developmental processes. Seeking psychic proximity is a normal developmental process. Pathology is determined by what is copied, and by the amount of security associated with the IPIRs. A normal person can copy good models that teach modulated social behavior, and that provide the security needed to develop a functional and sociable independence.[42]

The Relation between Attachment Theory and DLL Theory

Ideally, the reader can now see that DLL theory is a specifically detailed version of attachment theory. DLL theory centers on Bowlby's concept of internal working models and calls them IPIRs. DLL theory increases the specificity of Bowlby's concept by describing internal working models more precisely in terms of the SASB model, and by specifying connections between IPIRs and problem patterns via copy processes and the predictive principles of the SASB model.

Various biological reasons and mechanisms assure that internalization will occur. The "rules" are that the attachment person is vital to security, and that security is vital to willingness to learn to become skilled and independent in a well-socialized way. Normal persons copy patterns that encourage both security and independence. Persons with pathology have copied patterns that do not; hence their internalizations need change in therapy. As old internalizations diminish in importance, new ones develop. The therapist and benign others are internalized during therapy. The therapist should attempt to provide the basic security needed for new learning, while also facilitating independence with increasing consistency. To do this, the therapist needs to have a firm understanding of the "dance" between dependence and independence. Such an understanding will help the therapist choose more effectively when to lean in the direction of control, and when to emphasize autonomy.

NOTES

1. For example, a highly perceptive student therapist had a clear case formulation by the end of the first session. The therapist said nothing about the formulation for the next three sessions, however, because she was following the warning not to move "too rapidly." The patient terminated abruptly after the fourth session, declaring that "there was no connection" between her and the therapist. A review of tapes of the sessions suggested the contrary: There was an intense but painful connection. Although deeply empathic about the woman's distress, the therapist offered no concepts to help the patient understand how she might begin to deal with what she was seeing—namely, that she had married a frighteningly exact copy of her mother.

2. Three sessions constitute an approximation of a good balance between "too much too soon" and "not enough to calm and stabilize the patient."

3. The Structural Analysis of Social Behavior (SASB) codes, explained in Chapter 4, can help the interviewer link such statements to the patient's interpersonal world. For example, "I am a loner" is coded WALL-OFF. It implies either NEGLECT in the history, or a position antithetical to excessive CONTROL. "I am gifted" may reflect reality, SELF-LOVE, or possibly arrogance (BLAME). "God has it in for me" may be coded as resentful compliance (SULK) in relation to overwhelming hostile power, which probably can be found in relation to important others. The context will affect the codes, but typically they are reliable when all coders have access to all the data.

4. W. Shakespeare, *The Taming of the Shrew*, Act IV, Scene V.

5. This is done by using SASB predictive principles plus clinical experience.

6. In that book, the terms DLL and IPIRs are not used. Nonetheless, the concepts are invoked throughout.

7. The IRT procedure of systematically assessing input and response is an ex-

plicit extension of the teachings of David Graham, who was chair of the Department of Medicine for over a decade at the University of Wisconsin–Madison. Although David's hypotheses about psychosocial attitudes and psychosomatic disorder were unconfirmed by formal clinical trials, I have found them to be extremely useful, both personally and in my practice.

8. DLL analysis would add "because of an explosive internalization."

9. It is best if the narrative provides enough detail that the content can be SASB-coded (see Chapter 4). Use of the SASB model directs the interviewer's attention to critical features in each story: identity of the interactants; focus of the interaction; love and hate; and enmeshment (control/submit) versus differentiation (emancipate/separate). The reader does not have to learn to SASB-code, presuming that he or she is able intuitively to attend to specific critical interpersonal features of the narratives.

10. The predictive principles of the SASB model, presented in Chapter 4, immediately suggested some antecedents to the poor self-concept that apparently interfered with this patient's ability to accept a promotion.

11. These are opposing poles that define dimensions of the SASB model.

12. These are examples of points on the SASB model that consist of varying combinations of the underlying dimensions.

13. It is essential to establish that no such links are forced by the interviewing method. It is completely possible that the interview will yield no evidence of copy processes. Alternatively, there may be copy processes, but they may show no discernible links to the presenting problems. The method is so simple and straightforward that one might wonder why copy processes have not been noted previously. The answer probably is that what is copied is interpersonal dimensionality, not "external" attributes (gender, profession, cultural preferences, etc.). Without SASB coding and its demand for relentless focus on specific interpersonal dimensionality, I might never have noticed the generality of copy processes.

14. I hesitate to say "mirrors," because to some it means playing on illusions. That definitely is not what is done in IRT, wherein "mirroring" means reflecting the patient's own signal directly back to him or her. Here is the relevant part of the *American Heritage Talking Dictionary* (1997) definition of "mirror": "Something that faithfully reflects or gives a true picture. . . . "

15. And sometimes in emergency situations, as discussed in Chapters 3 and 7.

16. Therapy learning takes place in the three modes: affective, behavioral, and cognitive.

17. The IRT therapist is always open to any patient's desire to decline IRT. Patients' disappointments and preferences are discussed readily, and other options are freely offered. Of course, the therapist takes care to assure that this is not done in an abandoning or punitive way.

18. An exception to this assertion would be a case in which the patient has the needed resources, and makes a fully informed choice to work in more depth on his or her personality structure in IRT.

19. At the end of this chapter, there is a brief discussion of possible neurological consequences of problem attachments.

20. It is not possible to briefly summarize recommendations on this unfamiliar but vital topic. Please see Chapter 8 for more details.

21. An exception to this is that information required by legal or ethical standards must be included. An example would be newly uncovered, current sexual abuse, which would require reporting according to local norms.

22. I find it convenient to make a transcript on a laptop during a session. With this method, I can maintain eye contact with the patient, and concentrate on the interview itself. Tape recordings or scribes can serve the same function. The requirement for substantial verifiable detail adds considerably to the burden of a consultation. Without it, the data-based authenticity of the DLL formulation is weakened.

23. An introduction to this technology is provided in Chapter 4 and its Appendix 4.6. The Intrex manuals (Benjamin, 2000) and Pincus and Benjamin (in preparation) give enriching detail.

24. Such hypothesis testing is made possible by use of Intrex ratings of perceived relations in various states (current, past, wished-for, feared, etc.).

25. Again, note that the DLL requirement is to use diagnostic criteria, not categories. Even the presenting problems of people who qualify for the nonspecific label Personality Disorder Not Otherwise Specified can be described by items from the nearly 100 descriptors listed for the various personality disorder categories.

26. It is recommended that the patterns and the links be made in terms of SASB codes and predictive principles.

27. Contemporary research and clinical presentations frequently use the terms "symptoms" and "signs" without making any explicit distinction between them. The *American Heritage Talking Dictionary* (1997) defines these two words identically. Each "signals the existence of something else: indication, earmark, evidence, notice, sign, symptom, token, trace, warning, clue, foretoken, hint, signal, mark, suggestion." Sometimes the following distinction is made: A symptom has been identified by patient report, and a sign has been identified by objective observation. Sometimes a symptom is a definite marker of a disorder, while a sign is a suggestive indication.

28. I am indebted and grateful to Paul Pilkonis for making it clear that IRT needs to do this.

29. A widely recognized advocacy for a biological–psychosocial dichotomy appears on the Web site of the National Alliance for the Mentally Ill (http://www.nami.org).

30. Science abounds with theories that are helpful, but that fail in logic and/or to accommodate all agreed-upon facts. That condition is unavoidable, because a valid theory takes time to construct, to test, and to be adjusted to newly emerging facts. A valid theory is always "a work in progress." That progress is maximized if serious attention is given to logical consistency with constant reference to confirmed observations. Einstein's struggle with his "universal constant" is a good example of such a process. He initially added it post hoc to his equations to describe a constant universe, which seemed logical and consistent with experience. Then he retracted it. Recently, some have argued that he was right in the first place. The process of refining the theory continues.

31. Readers may assume that an author has integrity in providing such case descriptions. Interestingly, the psychologist ethics code provides much detail on

how to change cases to protect confidentiality, but says nothing about authenticity. If readers had been present at those consultations (or were to view the videotapes), they would know that the descriptions are accurate in clinical substance. If present (with ethical clearance, of course) at any randomly selected consultation, readers would probably see that the copy process and psychic proximity logic applies well, except for cases excluded in ways described in the earlier section "Does DLL Theory Apply to Every Case?"

32. These links are usually made via SASB codes and predictive principles, and by connections suggested earlier in the subsection "Connecting IPIRs to Axis I Symptoms."

33. If careful, systematic assessment of such psychosocial conditions could be made, along with ongoing studies of genetics, neurochemistry, and structure in the brains of psychotic individuals, understanding of voices would probably be enriched.

34. That is, it reflected complementary, opposite, or antithetical SASB predictive principles.

35. Imitation, or observational learning, has been studied carefully (for an arbitrarily selected recent example, see Forman & Kochanska, 2001). A contemporary review of efforts to link imitation or observational learning to internalized representations in monkeys and humans is offered by Suddendorf and Whiten (2001). The neurology of this process has also been of considerable interest (Iacoboni et al., 1999).

36. I decided to use the term copy process after a discussion with my youngest daughter, who is a veterinarian. As she explained, "Cancer is basically from copying errors," I suddenly understood how prevalent and important copying is in life processes. My descriptions of interpersonal copy process do not involve "errors." Instead, recognition of copy process in psychopathology highlights the dominant role that copying normally plays in human development.

37. Using the SASB model.

38. It is important that clinicians understand this point, or else they will have great trouble thinking of destructive patterns as acts of "love." Optimal patterns of love are defined in Chapter 4, and in the associated discussions of therapy goals in Chapter 9.

39. The passage from Suomi (1999) are reprinted by permission of The Guilford Press.

40. Personal observation, University of Wisconsin Primate Laboratory, 1955–1959.

41. Use of this word does not imply that social isolation is the usual cause of autism in humans.

42. A formal definition of normal behavior is suggested in Chapter 4. Use of the definition of "normal" in setting and assessing therapy goals appears in Chapters 4, 5, and 9.

3

Choosing Interventions

A BRIEF SUMMARY OF THERAPY
RULES, STEPS, AND PROCESSES

Every intervention in Interpersonal Reconstructive Therapy (IRT) attempts to invoke a maximal number of elements of the core algorithm, first described in Chapter 1. To review, the core algorithm specifies that each intervention offers and facilitates (1) accurate empathy; (2) maximal support for the Growth Collaborator (Green), and minimal support for the Regressive Loyalist (Red); (3) a focus on key aspects of the case formulation; (4) articulation of detail about input, response, and impact on the self for any given interpersonal episode; (5) exploration of any episode in terms of affect, behavior, and cognition (the ABCs); and (6) implementation of one or more of the five steps from the therapy learning hierarchy.

Whereas the first five facets of the core algorithm describe the basic IRT therapeutic style, the sixth involves the five steps of therapy change (see Figure 3.1 on p. 88). These steps are so central to the approach that an entire later chapter of this book is devoted to each. The therapy tasks most appropriate to each of the five therapy steps are sketched in this chapter.

The linchpin of IRT—the target of each facet of the core algorithm—is the process of coming to terms with Important Persons and their Internalized Representations (IPIRs), which organize the problem patterns. Coming to terms compares to working through in traditional psychodynamic therapy. Once the patient has experientially recognized and appreciated the meaning and consequences of his or her relationship with key IPIRs, he or she is free to learn new and more adaptive patterns. This chapter provides a flow chart for coming to terms (see Figure 3.2 on p. 90), which details how to focus on this central therapy task.

For the times when therapy seems stuck, there is a flow chart for exploring blockers to change (see Figure 3.3 on p. 98). This diagram helps a clinician choose interventions that guide the process back to coming to terms. Finally, if stalemates—especially those involving crisis—cannot be broken by the recommended procedures, IRT switches from the focus on problem internalizations to traditional symptom management. This procedure is summarized in a flow chart for switching to symptom management (see Figure 3.4 on p. 104). Figures 3.1 to 3.4 are discussed in more detail later in this chapter.

The chapter closes with an overview of who is suitable for IRT, a definition of adherence while practicing IRT, and a discussion of various administrative issues.

THE CORE ALGORITHM

Trainees often say that it is overwhelming to be asked to attend to all six facets of the core algorithm. Nonetheless, such expertise is required if IRT is to be effective with nonresponders. Without the ability to read what is going on in light of the case formulation, therapists can become frustrated with lack of progress. Even worse, they can become mincemeat as they try to deal with a subset of nonresponders who are skilled in the art of biting the hand that feeds them. Acquiring proficiency in IRT methods of dealing with such dilemmas compares to mastering any complex skill. It takes time and effort. Although a person can play the piano after relatively brief training, nobody would suggest that this person is an expert piano player after just a few lessons and a little bit of practice. On the other hand, just as a good piano player might quickly learn to play the organ, there can be good transfer of learning for therapists who have practical experience with interpersonal and intrapsychic concepts. But no matter what the initial level of skill, it still takes some time and practice for the core algorithm and the flow charts to be implemented reliably.

A therapist new to IRT might begin by practicing one skill at a time. If necessary, strengthening the habit of working from a baseline of accurate empathy should be the first step. Next, it is vital to learn to develop a case formulation. Once empathy and a case formulation are well established, a therapist learning IRT might concentrate on identifying Red and Green events (see Figure 1.1) in the narrative and therapy process. Then he or she might begin to practice shaping the empathic responses so that they support Green and minimize Red. When this skill is starting to become "second nature," the therapist might turn to another facet of the core algorithm, such as attending to the balance among ABCs. With repetitive focus and practice first on the separate facets, and then on simple combinations of facets, the six core skills eventually come together. The therapist has expertise in IRT. If the reader's experience parallels that of many IRT supervisees, cases that have long been "stuck" will clearly begin to move in Green ways.

RULE 1: WORK FROM A BASELINE OF ACCURATE EMPATHY

Empathy in IRT

In general, empathy can be defined as warm and compassionate paraphrasing that any reasonable observer would agree corresponds to what has been said. For approaches like IRT that include a case formulation, accurate empathy must also be consistent with the case formulation.

Empathy is the cornerstone of almost any psychotherapy. Particularly helpful discussions of empathy and the correlated attitude of deep respect for the patient appear in Teyber (1997) and in Greenberg, Rice, and Elliott (1993). Therapists who have not been trained to attend carefully to empathy will be richly rewarded by reading Teyber's and Greenberg et al.'s references on this basic skill. There is little question that empathy enhances the therapy alliance and therapy effectiveness (Horvath & Symonds, 1991; Horvath, 1994a; Hellerstein et al., 1997).

Empathy in IRT is defined by Structural Analysis of Social Behavior (SASB), and by the parallel models for affect and cognition (see Chapter 4, Appendix 4.1). According to the SASB model, empathy involves friendly focus on the patient that clearly respects his or her personal autonomy.[1] It is saturated with understanding, caring, and interest in the person who is being listened to. As the patient discloses and the therapist listens empathically, the therapy relationship becomes stronger. The patient develops an attachment to the therapist that flows naturally from being well understood.[2] The therapist is also likely to develop an attachment.[3]

Beyond Listening: How to Phrase an Empathic Reflection

The fundamental principle of operant conditioning[4] objectively describes an effect of empathy: Interested listening increases the likelihood that whatever is being listened to will remain the focus of conversation. This phenomenon is linked to behaviorism by the following folk tale: B. F. Skinner was subjected by his students to operant conditioning during a lecture. The originator of modern behavior theory was programmed to move to a specific corner of the lecture hall as he spoke. Unbeknownst to him, his students had conspired to listen with rapt attention whenever he approached that particular corner, and to put down their pencils and become restless when he moved away from the designated spot.[5] Years later, this phenomenon was described in terms of social influence theory (Johnson &

Matross, 1977). The Skinner fable and social influence theory imply that it makes a difference when and how empathy is expressed. Empathy is generically helpful, but, like any powerful factor, it also has the potential to make things worse (e.g., Pugh, 1999).[6]

Empathy that conforms to the core algorithm in IRT is called Green empathy. Selective empathy that enhances Green, some might say, does not "accept" the patient as he or she is. In that case, Green empathy would not represent empathy as described by Rogers (1951). That is correct. Although the IRT therapist has the deepest respect and liking for the patient, he or she does not presume to accept that patient entirely "as is." There is no attempt in IRT to provide what Rogers (1951) called "unconditional positive regard." What is totally embraced and warmly encouraged by the IRT therapist is the patient's Green. What is actively minimized whenever possible is the patient's Red. Of course, the patient collaborates in defining Red and Green. He or she understands and agrees to try to contain or become freer of Red and to build Green. The therapist's carefully focused empathy, then, amounts to working on what the patient has asked for and agreed to. By mindfully expressing Green empathy, the IRT therapist makes sure that the power of understanding is neither wasted nor misdirected.

Using Empathy to Highlight Many Therapy Steps at Once

A maximally effective form of empathy implements many elements of IRT at once. Here is an example of an empathic therapist response that enhances collaboration (step 1), describes patterns (step 2), blocks a maladaptive pattern (step 3), and addresses the will to change (step 4).

Jason saw himself as destined for permanent placement in a mental hospital because he was chronically and inconsolably depressed. He felt severely neglected and unloved as a child. He was convinced it was too late for him to receive the loving energy he needed to get his psychological engines running. He believed he was a ghost, a figure from the land of the dead, condemned to walk the earth without ever touching or being touched by anyone. The DLL case formulation suggested that this perspective was encouraged by past lessons to the effect that if he was competent and vital, Jason made his disabled and depressed brother feel worse. Whenever he sparked with life, Jason was told by his parents that he was inconsiderate of his brother, and that he should be quiet or go away. Jason's adult life had faithfully followed that instruction. One day he remarked, in the midst of his report of ongoing emptiness and loneliness, "There is still a pesky part of me that is alive." Jason said he did not know how to access this part of himself, but he was quite sure that "deep down," it existed. After a number of exchanges that explored this conflict, the empathic IRT therapist summarized:

"You want to be alive.
To be alive, you must be loved.
To be alive is to be pesky.
To be pesky is to be not loved.
Therefore, you cannot be alive. "

Jason's response to this level of understanding of the dilemma was to become more hopeful. By clearly viewing his own impossible injunction against himself, he began to become more willing to let go of his problematic internal rules. He took an early step in his long journey back to the land of the living. Ultimately he had to come to terms with the fact that he was loyally adhering to the injunction not to have spark, but rather to be quiet, alone, and out of sight. He was seeking approval and love by giving up his will to be lively. The syllogism nailed the Red and invited the Green to come out. It was an interpretive reflection based directly on the patient's own words and phenomenology.

RULE 2: SUPPORT THE GROWTH COLLABORATOR (GREEN) MORE THAN THE REGRESSIVE LOYALIST (RED)

The terms "Red" and "Green," shown in Figure 1.1, are allegorical devices that refer to interpersonal and intrapsychic habits learned in relation to loved ones. Problem patterns are Red, and normal patterns are Green.

The Regressive Loyalist (Red)

The Red name applies if interpersonal and intrapsychic habits are connected to problem patterns. The Regressive Loyalist is identified by following the trail from problem behaviors though copy processes back to early important caregivers (the IPIRs). The perceived rules and values of these key figures support the problem behaviors via the gift of love. Recall that the gift of love refers to the wish for reconciliation and rapprochement, which the patient hopes will be the results of loyal adherence to the rules and values of the IPIR.

Red behaviors almost always reflect a baseline of hostility, and/or excessive enmeshment or differentiation.[7] Patients usually ask to change[8] behaviors, affects, or cognitions associated with hostile behaviors, or behaviors that are imbalanced on the intimacy–distance dimension. Behaviors from the SASB cluster model that typically describe the Red include IGNORE, ATTACK, and BLAME when focusing on another person; WALL OFF, RECOIL, and SULK when focusing on self in relation to another person. According to the affect model that parallels the SASB model of social behavior (see Appendix 4.1), affective responses predicted for these Red interpersonal positions respectively include **Disregard, Hate,** and **Scorn;** Alienated, Terrified, and Agitated. The expected cognitive styles typical of the Regressive Loyalist, according to the parallel cognitive model (again, see Appendix 4.1), include **Distract, Destroy,** and **Condemn;** Scattered, Shut Down, and Secretive. The SASB model also describes the expected introject when Red focus on other is directed inward upon the self: *SELF-NEGLECT, SELF-ATTACK,* and *SELF-BLAME.* The affect and cognitive models do not presently spell out the parallels. They follow this model: A person engaged in *SELF-BLAME* would have an affect of *Self-Scorn,* and a cognitive style described as *Self-Condemn.* Red imbalances on the vertical pole of the SASB model could include too much control (e.g., omnipotent aspirations or delusions), submission (e.g., abject defeat, spineless compliance), or emancipation or separation (e.g., chronic disconnection from others).

The Red can be compared, in part, to the id in classical psychoanalysis. Both the id and the Red are powerful, often work at the level of the unconscious, pursue goals that are not currently appropriate, and ignore reality. Unlike the id, Red is interpersonally based and is not the direct result of sexual or aggressive impulses. It can also be formally assessed via ratings of key figures, problem patterns, and objective coding of the therapy narrative (see Chapters 2 and 4).

The Growth Collaborator (Green)

The Green name is appropriate if the interpersonal and intrapsychic habits connect to normative therapy goal behaviors. These have been defined as friendly, moderately enmeshed, and moderately differentiated.[9] The SASB-based descriptions of these normative behaviors include AFFIRM, ACTIVE LOVE, and PROTECT when focusing on another person; DISCLOSE, REACTIVE LOVE, and TRUST when focusing on self in relation to another person. According to the affect model that parallels the SASB model of social behavior (see Appendix 4.1), affective responses predicted for these Green interpersonal positions respectively include **Accept, Love,** and **Nurture;** Centered, Delighted, and Hopeful. The expected cognitive styles typical of the Growth Collaborator, according to the parallel cognitive model (again, see Appendix 4.1), include **Understand, Enhance,** and **Concentrate;** Expressive, Optimistic, and Well-Directed. The SASB model also describes the expected introject when Green focus on other is directed inward upon the self: *SELF-AFFIRM, SELF-LOVE,* and *SELF-PROTECT.* The affect and cognitive models do not presently spell out the parallels. They follow this model: A person engaged in behaviors describe by the model point *SELF-PROTECT* would have an affect described as *Self-Nurture,* and a cognitive style described as *Concentrate on Self.*

Like the Regressive Loyalist, the Growth Collaborator can also be traced back through copy processes to important early caregivers. The perceived rules and values of key figures that support normal behaviors are Green; hence normal as well as pathological behaviors are gifts of love. In such cases, reality is so supportive of normative patterns that they take on their own momentum in adulthood. Unlike Red patterns, Green patterns yield their own rewards, and are not so dependent on fantasized hopes in relation to internalizations from the past.

The Green resembles the ego of psychoanalysis, but does not share the assignment of negotiating between the primitive desires of the id and the demands of society as interpreted by the superego. Rather, the Green has the job of implementing therapy learning about patterns, where they came from, and what they are for. The Green also must decide to change and to learn new patterns. Like the ego, the Green does have the job of engaging in realistic and healthy interactions. It also must integrate affect, behavior, and cognition. Like the ego, the Green is a helpful observer, a "good parent," an effective "executive." Important aspects of Green (as well as Red) relationships can be rated on the SASB Intrex questionnaires, and tracked by observer coding of the therapy narrative.

Recognizing That Key Figures Facilitate Both Red and Green

It is important to remember that Red and Green are not necessarily associated with a specific person or role. Red and Green patterns can come from the same IPIRs. Consider the following mixed picture.

Nancy had long been on disability leave for neck pain, which she said was the result of botched surgery for a neck injury. She had been tried for years on nearly every known psychoactive medication, and recently had exhausted her psychiatrist with frequent phone calls to the psychiatrist's home. These were accompanied by dramatic, suicidal actions. Nancy's current list of prescriptions included a dosage of pain medications that suggested the equivalent of severe alcoholism. Until the injury to her neck 2 years ago, Nancy had functioned extremely well as a production supervisor. At the same time, she had received a major promotion to the international office. Since then, she had been nonfunctional because of her problems with her neck, many surgeries, and an oppressive assortment of other medical and psychological disorders.

In the DLL interview, it became clear that Nancy believed she could not function well because this would affirm her father, who had been abusive and neglectful in the extreme. She believed that her dysfunction was an indictment of his actions. She also thought that her suffering would adversely affect her father's position in the afterlife. Nancy identified with her mother, who had suffered greatly at the hands of her father. In addition to bearing heavy psychological burdens, Nancy and her mother were very intelligent and had advanced rapidly in their jobs. Each had had misfortunes that resulted in disability just as they were about to be promoted to the highest level of their respective professions. Nancy's mother had used alcohol to cope; Nancy's neck pain required ever-escalating amounts of benzodiazepines. Identification with her mother was capped by the fact that her suicidality emerged when she reached the same age at which her mother had died.

Nancy's identification with her mother was both Red and Green. Her former life, which had been filled with accomplishments and good friends, was Green. The copy processes that led her to suffering and severe disability were, of course, Red. Recognition that a key figure is often a source of strength as well of problem behaviors makes the case formulation more accurate and appropriately complex. In addition to avoiding the temptation to dichotomize key figures into "good" and "bad," therapists also need to be aware of their own case formulations, so that their nonverbal as well as verbal messages can consistently work on behalf of their patients' Green.[10]

Examples of Red and Green Empathy

It would be very easy inadvertently to provide Red empathy for Kenneth (Chapter 1), who dwelled endlessly on his wife's unfaithful duplicity. His therapy behaviors were almost 100% in the blaming category. Kenneth was given empathic support for his pain over his wife's perceived infidelity, and his outrage at those he thought were involved in it. Expression of this empathy was important, so that Kenneth could know the therapist was paying attention and really did want to help. However, no matter how justified his anger might have been, such empathy would support Red if Kenneth saw it as support for his position of making demands of and condemning others. In such a case, an IRT therapist tries to minimize that effect as he or she seeks to find every opportunity to support Green. Consider these examples of how a therapist might have done this with Kenneth.

Red Empathy

When Kenneth described his wife's alleged infidelity, the interviewer might have said, "She was a sneak," or "Her lying made you furious," or "Your marital rights [to have sex with her] were denied," or "Your marital contract was violated." Any of these comments would have accurately reflected what Kenneth said, and would have met the generic definition of accurate empathy. They would have been received most enthusiastically by Kenneth. However, they also would have inflamed his Red pattern of blaming, and therefore would not have been consistent with rule 2 (maximal support for Green and minimal support for Red).

Green Empathy

Examples of empathic responses that would conform to rule 2 might have included: "Despite all your checking, it was impossible to control her," or "You felt that your marital rights were being defiled, and you wanted to make her obey," or "The fact that she refused to obey either you or the pastor was more than you could bear." All of these would have met the generic standard of accurate empathy, and yet they would not have unduly inflamed Kenneth's Red. They would have been close enough to what he was saying to make collaboration possible, and they would also have begun to teach him about his problem patterns. In this way, they would have begun to build Green.

Red Empathy at First, Then Green

If an IRT therapist cannot frame reflections in Green, then he or she goes ahead with pure Red, but tries to enlist collaboration and other Green behaviors as soon as possible. Again, here is an example of how this might have been done with Kenneth:

THERAPIST: It seems morally right to have everybody know how very wrong she is. [Red]

KENNETH: Absolutely. What she did is completely out of line. [Red]

THERAPIST: It is easy to see why you are so angry. [Red] Still, I wonder if we could spend a little time exploring what else might be behind the intensity of your feeling about this? [Green]

KENNETH: What do you mean? What else is there to say? [Red]

THERAPIST: Well, you have been quite angry for several weeks now, and it seems like nothing is changing. [Green]

KENNETH: Right. She won't even talk to me any more. [Red]

THERAPIST: So if we talked about you—your expectations of marriage and where they came from—we might figure out another way to approach this problem. [Green] Would you be willing to try that? [Green]

KENNETH: I guess so. What do we do? [Green]

From here, the therapist could have elicited Kenneth's views of marriage and his early learning about it. The answers would have led to the case formulation for Kenneth described in Chapters 1 and 2.

RULE 3: RELATE EVERY INTERVENTION
TO THE CASE FORMULATION

Rather than using a technique to address a particular symptom, IRT requires that chosen techniques be determined by the case formulation. For example, consider a depressed patient who despairs over his or her long-lasting dysphoria and lack of hope. According to some practitioners of CBT, it would be good to use evidence from the patient's own narrative to point out that things are not so bad after all. This would challenge the depressive cognitions with evidence from the patient's own life, and help him or her develop a more realistic and positive attitude.

If, however, this patient is organized by patterns and wishes typical of Passive–Aggressive Personality Disorder (PAG), this version of CBT would probably be iatrogenic. An individual with PAG (Benjamin, 1996a, Ch. 11) is likely to have burned out from trying to meet the impossible expectations of someone who failed in the caregiver role. The person with PAG is primed to see caregivers as cruel and neglectful, and is unlikely to submit to or agree with them in any way. If this is the case, then pointing out evidence that the patient is doing better (e.g., "You were able to go shopping this weekend; you did go out with friends on Friday night") is likely to deteriorate into an argument. The citation of evidence may be seen as the therapist's trying to "toot his or her own horn." If so, the patient with PAG will have to "one-up" the therapist by further defeating the therapy and regressing into more depression and anger. Believing that his or her symptoms prove the therapist to be incompetent and neglectful, the patient with PAG "wins" by deteriorating.

The case formulation for a patient with PAG suggests that a high priority should be placed on not saying anything that could be seen as coercive, and on making it clear that any progress belongs to the patient and not to the therapist.[11] Hence the IRT therapist will be more likely than usual to empathize with the depressed Red. At the same time, he or she is hyperalert to flickers of Green in the narrative. For example, suppose the patient says, "I had a terrible weekend," and proceeds to provide details. The IRT therapist reflects the pain, supporting the Red. Then the IRT therapist might say, "Was it like that all weekend, or were there moments when you were able to take control of yourself?" The question nods to the Red and then asks for Green. The language chosen marks a known antidote to helplessness[12] and depression. Here is an example of how to catch and affirm signs of Green without stomping on the patient's ownership of it:

PATIENT: Well, I discovered that even though I could not get out of the depression, I could at least keep it from getting worse when I decided to clean my apartment.

THERAPIST: You found moments when you could affect how you felt.

This therapist remark clearly gives credit to the patient and experientially affirms the idea that he or she has control of what happens.

A large number of clinicians and trait theorists consider the planned impact on others to be an important descriptor for personality. For example, a person may take care to wear the right clothes and say the right thing as a way of making others react more favorably to him or her. The substantial academic literatures on faking good, faking bad, social desirability, blame avoidance, and so on, are consistent with this idea that such an individual is a public relations (PR) manager for him- or herself. According to DLL theory, people who have a PR orientation probably learned from important caregivers that approval and affirmation are available via impression management and manipulation. The formulation could apply to individuals with Histrionic Personality Disorder. They often have a template that requires them actively to entertain and elicit admiring responses from others (Benjamin, 1996a, Ch. 7). Similarly, people who qualify as having Narcissistic Personality Disorder (Benjamin, 1996a, Ch. 6) can become quite coercive of others' responses to them. Clearly, the pattern of being a PR manager can be found in some nonresponders.

But not all nonresponders exhibit such a concern with PR. Some have learned relatively little about making a difference or influencing others. One can hardly see oneself as a PR manager if one does not have a sense of a self that is effective in at least some ways. Individuals with Dependent Personality Disorder (Benjamin, 1996a, Ch. 9) belong to the subgroup of patients who do not specialize in impression management.

According to DLL, the pattern of impression management, like any other problem pattern, can be included in the case formulation. Without evidence that manipulation is a feature of the case presentation, therapist efforts "not to be manipulated" may be inappropriate. A suicidal person may, for example, be responding to powerful internal distortions, and may not be concerned about the impact of suicidality on the therapist. In that case, to react as if the patient is manipulating rather than struggling with ancient impulses (or both) could be an error. Every intervention should relate to the specific case formulation.

RULE 4: PROVIDE DETAILS ON INPUT, RESPONSE, AND IMPACT ON SELF

Using Specificity to Channel the Therapy Process

Better data support better case formulations, which should improve outcomes.[13] Requests for specific verbal "replays" of an episode should include detailed interpersonal descriptions of input, response, and impact on the self. Three scenarios are offered here to show how supporting detail can send the therapy process in different directions.

In the first scenario, suppose a mother says something like this: "I was upset and yelled at the kids today." In order to process such a statement in terms of the DLL case formulation and the treatment plan, it is important for the therapist to ask, "What was going on that led to that?" In response to this request for input, the patient, Dolores, might say that the kids were late for school and were watching television instead of getting ready.

The clinician might then inquire, "What did you yell?" The details in her answer to this question about her response would probably draw a line between normative parental irritation and pathological behaviors that would be likely to injure the children. Dolores might report that she yelled, "You kids are going to be late for school if you don't get dressed right now." This descriptive statement is not problematic, the IRT clinician would conclude.

Then, for impact on the self, the therapist might ask:

THERAPIST: How did that make you feel?

DOLORES: Like I am getting to be just like my mother.

THERAPIST: Tell me more about what she did at times like this.

Dolores might then report that she never would have been late in the first place, because the slightest deviation from expectation would have been met with several blows with a belt. The discussion might turn to her memories of disciplinary experiences and her decision never to do that to her children. Before the end of the session, the therapist should return to Dolores's initial self-criticism of her own parenting. In this first scenario, the differences between what she yelled and what her mother would have done could be affirmed, even celebrated. Not only would the emphasis on her task-oriented method of discipline improve her self-concept on a realistic basis, but marking the differences should help her separate from the internalization of her harsh mother. In providing this benevolent support, the therapist would help Dolores's self-esteem as she maintained her more benign parenting behaviors.

The importance of specificity is underscored by realizing what a different turn the therapy would take if the conversation had been the same up to the point of Dolores's response. In a second scenario, suppose she were to answer, "I told them they were lazy dogs and would never amount to anything. I said I would whip them if they were not completely ready in 10 minutes." Now, when asked how she felt, Dolores might report, "Well, not so good. But I was relieved that they did hop to."

In this case, the therapist might ask whether this situation seemed at all familiar. Dolores might associate it with a parent who placed ultimate value on his or her control of children, including Dolores. In that case, it would be important to help Dolores recall how she felt when subjected to the harsh parenting. She would need empathic support as she remembered her own beatings and recalled how badly those damning words damaged her sense of herself. If possible, her discomfort at being the victim of these aggressive child-rearing practices could be used to contain her own repetition of them. In this second scenario, the memory of childhood beatings, viewed with support from the therapist, would provide a new and more realistic perspective. This, in turn, might help Dolores decide to stop repeating the pattern with her children, and eventually to distance herself from her reassessed IPIR.

Details might have taken this conversation in still another direction. Suppose for a third scenario that Dolores remained so attached to her abusive parents that she could not use the associations to her past to contain her own parenting. She might observe, "I deserved it, and so do my children." Individuals still deeply attached to an abusive IPIR will often find it difficult to take a perspective sympathetic to themselves. For them, more time is needed to experience the therapist's support before they can envision rejecting the abusive ways of their parents. Several sessions of reviewing and reexperiencing the beatings might be needed before Dolores could experience how inappropriate they were. As that became apparent, Dolores (or any patient with a similar history) could make the decision to stop repeating the pattern with her children. Later, she could even let up on the residual effects of self-attack. It is important again to note that as therapy progresses, child-abusing patients are more likely to become empathic on behalf of their children before they become supportive of themselves.[14]

Knowing When to Ask for Specific Details

In general, the more specific the narrative, the better the therapy. But, as usual, good procedures can be used in destructive ways. Specificity is no exception. Asking for more and more specific details must be clearly relevant to the case formulation. There are times when asking for specific details is contraindicated because it is not relevant to the case formulation, and also will needlessly diminish the patient's self-esteem. For example, once I interviewed a man who struggled with strong wishes to rape young girls. He had been arrested for doing this once, and presently was on probation and in a treatment program. My interview centered on his current life circumstances and his tragic personal history. I asked essentially nothing about the details of what he had done or what he wished to repeat. It was perfectly clear to me that the rape fantasies had to do with having the power to terrorize females, and that this reflected a copy process from his own history. It really was not relevant exactly how he would frighten them or exactly what he wished to do with them. Those details would have added nothing to the DLL case formulation and the treatment plan. The patient was greatly moved by the interview, especially because he had previously had no idea how much his violent and imbalanced sexuality was related to his relationship with his mother. His regular therapist, who was present, felt that the session was extremely helpful and remarked, "I could not believe how nice you were to him. I expected that you would humiliate him by making him go through all the details."

RULE 5: ELICIT ABCs ASSOCIATED WITH THE NARRATIVE

In Chapter 4, there is a discussion of predicted parallels among the SASB model (which, as its full name indicates, is a model of social behavior), a model of affect, and a model of cognitive style. These models invoke the idea that behaviors that have proven successful in evolutionary history (e.g., attachment, control, separate territory) are accompanied by affects and cognitions that support them. If these three systems have evolved in parallel and if they support one another, clearly they all should be explored in the discussion of any given episode. As previously noted, the ABCs rule reflects that reasoning. It specifies that any narrative about input, response, and impact on the self should include all three aspects: affect, behavior, and cognition.

In the chapters on the five steps of therapy, many examples are given of the ABCs rule. It is easy to operationalize. As a given scenario is being developed in terms of input, response, and impact on the self, the clinician elicits a description of what happened and then makes sure that the following three questions have been asked and pursued (in one form or another and in any order): "What did you do, what did you feel, and what did you think?" Questioning in all domains will deepen the experience for the patient and lead more expeditiously to relevant associations for the therapeutic process.

RULE 6: RELATE EACH INTERVENTION TO ONE OR MORE OF THE FIVE STEPS

The Learning Speech and the Five Steps

The learning speech (Table 2.5) describes the quintessence of the IRT therapy model. One of any number of variations on this speech might be: "Therapy involves learning about your patterns, where they are from, and what they are for. Understanding your patterns might lead you to decide to change, and then you can begin work on learning new patterns that may work better for you." According to IRT, "that's all there is." This simple summary of the therapy process provides a way to deal with a large number of difficult dilemmas in therapy. Again, the five steps of the therapy learning process are described in depth in Chapters 5–9. Discussion here is limited to consideration of their hierarchical arrangement, a reiteration of the need to match interventions with the case formulation for each patient, and the main therapy tasks for each step.

Approximate Hierarchical Order of the Five Steps

The approximate hierarchical order of the five steps emerges naturally: (1) There must be collaboration to begin the work. (2) Learning about patterns defines the work. (3) Blocking problem patterns has to happen before new ones can be established. (4) Profound change cannot happen until the person is less ambivalent about giving up old ways. (5) As new patterns are learned, the therapy goals are achieved.

Any of the later stages can invoke earlier steps. A patient is unlikely to learn about patterns (step 2) if he or she does not collaborate in the process of exploring them. Problem patterns are unlikely to be blocked (step 3) if they cannot be recognized (step 2). For example, people with Anorexia Nervosa who do not see anything wrong with their eating habits are unlikely to block them. Similarly, patients who misuse substances but who deny they have a problem are unable to begin work on restricting their substance use.

Violations of Hierarchical Order

The hierarchical order of the five steps is not absolute. Sometimes new patterns are learned before the will to change is in place. Sometimes collaboration is not complete until the will to change has been initially engaged. Sometimes problem patterns are not fully blocked until new alternatives have become well practiced. A common example is seen when a person learns to assert rather than attack and enjoys the more benevolent reactions that follow the new behaviors. After a few positive experiences, the patient will want to behave in the new rather than the old ways. Unfortunately, this widely known behavioral technique does not often work with nonresponders, who are likely to be more emotionally invested in behaving like beloved but hostile IPIRs. For them, the hierarchy holds. They must come to terms with the sustaining IPIRs before they will be free to enjoy the reward of new, more constructive behaviors.

Interventions That Are Constructive for One Person but Iatrogenic for Another

At IRT workshops, I am sometimes asked questions like these: "What do you do when a patient with Borderline Personality Disorder becomes angry at you?" Or "What can I do with a patient who has Bulimia Nervosa and an out-of-control spending habit?" These persisting and distressing behaviors are the hallmarks of nonresponders, and it is easy to see why clinicians ask these questions. However, such questions miss the central thesis of IRT—namely, that every intervention is based on the case formulation. It is not possible to hear about a symptom and directly suggest an intervention based on IRT. Rather, the symptom first has to be understood in terms of the case formulation. Then an intervention can be chosen.

This means, among other things, that for a given symptom (e.g., chronic anger at the therapist), an intervention that may be effective with one patient may only make things worse with another. For example, if anger is a temper tantrum learned in an enmeshed relationship with an inappropriately indulgent mother, then ignoring it[15] and just sticking to the task of working on the related IPIRs should be effective. The therapist may say, "Having a tantrum usually worked with your mother, but our work here is entirely different. Let's get to it. What are you wanting from me now, and how can we address this in a way that is going to work better for you?"

On the other hand, suppose the anger is triggered by perceived abandonment (e.g., when the therapist obviously has other patients, can't schedule an appointment at the desired time, goes on a trip, etc.). In this case, the underlying panic needs to be identified and addressed. Discussion of relevant IPIRs, using procedures for coming to terms, should be ideal. Palpable reassurances about the constancy of the therapy relationship will also be needed. Collaborative development of alternative responses to panic about abandonment may help the patient engage in better self-management. Collaborative agreements that yield more access to the therapist when things go well, and less access when things do not go well, may help. Various other interventions appropriate to either of these scenarios are discussed in the five chapters on the five therapy steps.

A Summary of Therapy Tasks at Each of the Five Steps

In Figure 3.1, the five steps are linked to recognized therapy techniques from various schools of therapy. These techniques are grouped into two categories: self-discovery and self-management. For example, in the self-discovery group (shown in the center of the figure), there are examples of activities that encourage deep levels of experiencing. These include telling stories, reexperiencing, grieving, and accepting. In the self-management group (shown on the right-hand side of the figure), there are some suggested activities that engage willfulness and encourage active decision making. Examples provided include being honest, changing self-talk, choosing new internal models, resisting urges to retreat, and practicing new patterns.

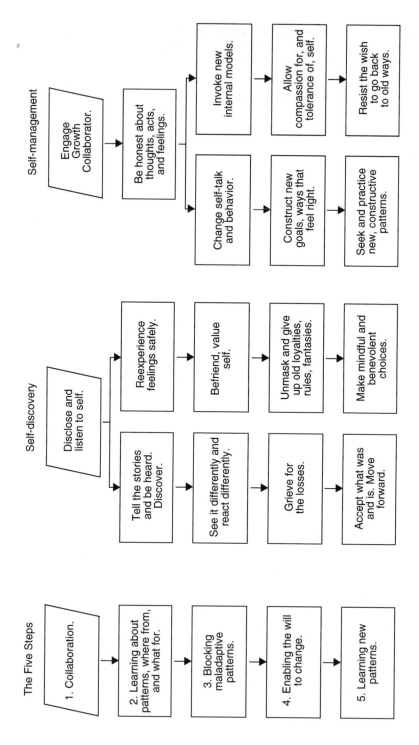

FIGURE 3.1. Therapy steps and tasks.

Self-management

Engage Growth Collaborator.

Be honest about thoughts, acts, and feelings.

Invoke new internal models.

Allow compassion for, and tolerance of, self.

Resist the wish to go back to old ways.

Change self-talk and behavior.

Construct new goals, ways that feel right.

Seek and practice new, constructive patterns.

Self-discovery

Disclose and listen to self.

Reexperience feelings safely.

Befriend, value self.

Unmask and give up old loyalties, rules, fantasies.

Make mindful and benevolent choices.

Tell the stories and be heard. Discover.

See it differently and react differently.

Grieve for the losses.

Accept what was and is. Move forward.

The Five Steps

1. Collaboration.

2. Learning about patterns, where from, and what for.

3. Blocking maladaptive patterns.

4. Enabling the will to change.

5. Learning new patterns.

88

Therapy activities in the first group are more likely to be drawn from the so-called psychodynamic schools of longer-term therapy, whereas activities in the second are more likely to come from briefer approaches—CBT (Beck, 1999), interpersonal psychotherapy (IPT; Weissman, Markowitz, & Klerman, 2000), and other empirically supported therapies. Individuals preferring the first set of activities typically expect therapy to be "a happening," a place where there are intense experiences in therapy followed by feeling better afterward. Individuals preferring the self-management approaches typically expect therapy to be a place where one gets sensible instruction on how to "pull up your socks and get on with it." These distinctions are trends, not absolute dichotomies. Psychodynamic therapists do sometimes invoke plans for self-management. Behavioral, CBT, and IPT therapists do sometimes discuss early events and encourage expression of affect, even if those particular interventions are not emphasized in the manuals for these types of therapy.

Critics of the first approach note that people often enjoy the therapy experience, but not much happens to improve life outside of therapy. Critics of the second approach note that some people get rapid symptom relief, but may relapse quickly. Others do not respond at all. In IRT, both classes of interventions are required; self-discovery/experiencing and self-management are equally important. Talking about the past is primarily focused on targeting the will to change (Red), while discussions of self-management activities are primarily devoted to building Green. Again, the distinction is not absolute. IRT presumes that understanding the Red can facilitate better self-management. For example, a patient may say, "I don't want to be like him any more. I am never going to do that again." But better self-management can also lead to better understanding of the relationship with an IPIR. For example, a patient might say, " As I do it this new way, I see that she could have done it this way, too. How much easier that would have been on all of us."

FLOW CHART FOR COMING TO TERMS

Figure 3.2, a flow chart for coming to terms (i.e., helping the Growth Collaborator come to terms with the Regressive Loyalist), describes the heart of the reconstructive work in IRT. The IRT therapist tries to facilitate reconstructive work as often as possible. If not engaged in reconstruction as shown in Figure 3.2, the IRT therapist follows procedures designed to return the therapy to the activities shown in Figure 3.2. Flow charts in Figures 3.2, 3.3, 3.4, and 7.1 (as well as other tables and figures in this book) provide general guidelines. The recommendations should not be taken as rigid instructions. Clinician judgment is the arbiter of optimal combination of procedures described in figures and tables, and by the core algorithm.

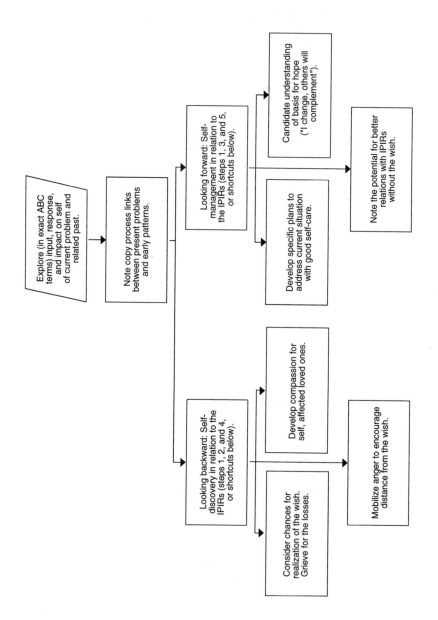

FIGURE 3.2. Coming to terms.

90

Reviewing a Current Problem Episode, Using as Many Facets of the Core Algorithm as Possible

Figure 3.2 shows that the core therapy work begins by examining a current problem episode in terms of interpersonal input, response, and impact on the self. There is elaboration in terms of all systems: affect, behavior, and cognition. Connections between this episode and the past are reviewed, usually in terms of copy processes. Once the past connections are identified, the work can turn directly to the underlying motivation for the problem patterns—namely, attachment to the related IPIRs.

Reviewing the Current Problem and Its Copy Process Links

Suppose Marie, introduced in Chapter 1, were to start a session with a report that after she talked with her daughter on the phone yesterday, she had a panic attack. Figure 3.2 suggests that it would be good to explore what was said in that conversation, how Marie responded to it (in terms of the ABCs), and how it affected her self-concept. Suppose it is established that in the phone call, Marie learned that her daughter is very happy in her new marriage, but that her son-in-law's job will force the young family to move to a distant city. Marie is scared about their leaving and expects that she will feel quite useless and alone without her daughter and grandchildren.

This is a serious problem for any grandmother, but it does not normally create a full-blown panic attack. The case formulation for Marie has established that she needs to take care of people in trouble as a way of dealing with her own anxiety. This pattern emerged from a time when she was terrified to be alone with her father and discovered that she could feel better if she focused on the task of protecting her younger siblings. From the perspective of her case formulation, it makes sense that Marie still becomes anxious when she loses contact with people she takes care of.

Branching into Self-Discovery Activities

Once the problem issue is fully developed and linked to the past via copy processes, the therapy can go in one of two directions. The first group of therapy techniques (shown in the center of Figure 3.1, and on the left-hand side of Figure 3.2) have to do with self-discovery. They address underlying motivation directly. In Figure 3.2, the process of self-discovery begins with the box, Looking backward: Self-discovery in relation to the IPIRs. The looking backward branch draws most heavily on the self-discovery techniques listed in Figure 3.1 for steps 1, 2, and 4 from the therapy learning hierarchy.[16] Disclosure and listening are basic collaborative activities (step 1). Learning about patterns (step 2) is best achieved by telling stories, being heard, and discovering. Difficult feelings can be reexperienced in a safe setting. Enabling the will to change (step 4) focuses on unmasking and letting go of loyalty to old rules and values. Once the patient decides to let go, he or she must grieve for the losses. Finally, the patient can move on to form new loyalties and new patterns. It is vital to note that the internalized representations are what the patient gives up, not the here-and-now relationships with the people who have been internalized.

Consider how this model could be applied to Marie's panic attack after her daughter's phone call. If Marie were to use this session to deepen self-discovery, the conversation would turn to related incidents with her terrifying father and her passive mother. In general, Marie needs an opportunity in a safe setting to extinguish her anxiety over thoughts and memories of his assaults on her and other family members. Going through many episodes with the accurate, empathic support of the therapist could help Marie begin to realize affectively that her father is no longer a threat to her or her siblings. Her mother no longer needs Marie's protection and guidance. After a lifetime of saving others against all odds, she has a right to be peaceful and to be safe from threat of bodily harm. It makes sense that she has no idea of who to be if she is not a rescuer. In IRT, steps 1, 2, and 4 are practiced again and again until the patient not only understands at all levels (ABCs) what shapes his or her problem patterns, but also gets ready to give up the hope of rewriting history—of living childhood again on better terms.

In addition to emphasizing steps 1, 2, and 4 in self-discovery, the left-hand side of Figure 3.2 mentions some possible "shortcuts" to reconstruction. The shortcuts do not usually bring sudden reconstruction, as the term might imply. However, they can be especially powerful and therefore can shorten the process of coming to terms.

The first suggested shortcut is to conduct a "thought experiment" with the patient and help him or her construct a fantasy scene wherein the wish is realized. Often patients are unable to do this because they simply cannot imagine the impossible. Then the therapist can have some creative fun making up such a scene. For example, Marie's therapist might have Marie imagine meeting her father in heaven, and hearing her father say:

> "Oh, Marie, I am so glad to see you. Please accept my apologies for all of those horribly violent beatings and for my inappropriate and confusing sexual approaches. I realize it has made life very difficult for you. I am so very sorry, and wish I had it to do over again. You can bet things would be altogether different. I would not be threatening at all, and I would instead be a devoted and loving father. Is there any way I can make it up to you? I love and respect you so much I would do anything at all to set it right."

Patients' reactions to such a scenario can vary. Some will chortle. Some will sob. Some will "freeze." Most will then become very contemplative. If urged to elaborate on the therapist's first draft of the fantasy, they may or may not join in. If asked how they feel about the scene, they will usually begin to realize that they have truly been reaching and hoping for the impossible. Once they see the absurdity of their hopes, it may be easier to give them up. The slow work of grieving for the fact that what never was, never will be, can then begin. In addition to grieving for what the IPIR never can do or be, there is grief over the losses that have affected the self, such as losses of time, energy, and opportunities. Grieving is the final step of coming to terms. When that grief work is finished, the internalization no longer has any power. Normal grief after loss of a loved one takes about 1 year. There is no reason to expect that grief over loss of an IPIR should happen any faster.

Figure 3.2 suggests another shortcut: developing compassion for oneself and for presently affected loved ones, such as lovers or children. For example, Marie needs help in developing compassion for herself as a small girl who was given an assignment that apparently was impossible for the only other adult in the household, her mother. It must have been terrifying, for example, to fend off the strange men who invaded the family home in pursuit of her father. On the other hand, it must have been reassuring to learn that she could manage such a situation, and that the men were kind to her as they mocked her father's inappropriateness. The outrageous assignment of coping with her out-of-control father was given pseudo-credibility by her "successes." Her success in the role should not be overlooked, because it had a lot to do with why she adapted it for a lifetime. Although Marie believed she could "cope," the threat posed by her internalized representation of her father was ever-present, chronic, and severe. The physical and mental pain he inflected was very real. Unrelenting anxiety would be a most natural and expectable consequence.

In therapy in the present, Marie needs a lot of help and support to develop the courage to recall scenes in which she or her siblings were thrown through walls or down stairs. As she details the input, response, and impact on herself, she should be helped to feel appropriate (i.e., vulnerable) feelings about those scenes and to think about them clearly. Realistic cognitive processing of the story necessarily will lead Marie to the realization that she was in an extremely abusive setting, and that it was wholly unreasonable for her to have to cope with it. Sympathy and a wish to protect herself from those internalizations can be facilitated by the therapist's strong demonstration of compassion for her.

Simultaneously with this work on developing a supportive and rehabilitative view of the abuse experience, Marie can be encouraged to change her loyalties to the past by reflecting on what this has done to her adult relationships. She already knows that she married and separated from a husband who was like her father. After IRT, she may be freer to choose a more benevolent new partner. As she becomes more able to let go of the protector role, it may be easier for Marie to relate to her children and grandchildren in more playful and less "overdetermined" ways.[17]

A third shortcut for coming to terms is to mobilize any anger at the IPIR on behalf of distance or differentiation from it. According to SASB theory, aggression is employed for modulation of space and supplies (actual and psychological). If the anger involves focus on another, it is for the purpose of control. If anger is fundamentally reactive, it is for the purpose of achieving distance. An IRT therapist does not think of anger as a fixed amount of energy that has to be unloaded somewhere or somehow. Rather, anger has evolved to implement control or distance. The fountain of anger is unlimited whenever interpersonal context and internal loyalties call for it.

This interpretation of anger suggests that anger can help a patient come to terms if it facilitates differentiation from a problem internalization. Anger can be harmful if it facilitates enmeshment with a problem internalization. Marie's anger was largely inspired by a wish for distance from her threatening father. For this reason, it was possible to free up her interest in sexuality by noting that by being uncomfortable sexually, she had been allowing him to continue to have control over her. Mobilizing her anger at her father seemed to help her distance herself from this aspect of his internalization.

Unfortunately, when anger is Red, therapist facilitation of anger becomes iatrogenic. Suppose, for example, that Marie's pleasant sexual encounters of adolescence with her father had been ongoing from a very early age until age 16. In this case, she might have become severely addicted to the relationship with him and be unable to do much other than be a needy victim. Then her anger might have the intrapsychic goal of bringing him closer to her and ultimately restoring their sexual connection. In this case, therapist facilitation of anger would be a mistake. It would excite the Red and condemn Marie to a life of fantasy devoted to the past and frustrated with the present.

Branching into Self-Management Activities

The second group of therapy activities that can facilitate coming to terms is shown on the right-hand side of Figures 3.1 and 3.2. These have to do with self-management. They seek to enhance the strength of the Growth Collaborator. Figure 3.2 indicates that looking forward is most often facilitated by therapy activities classified at steps 1, 3, and 5 in the learning hierarchy. Step 1 (collaboration) is required no matter which branch is chosen. According to Figure 3.1, step 1 includes any intervention that facilitates the Green, or Growth Collaborator.

Figure 3.1 also mentions that step 3 (blocking maladaptive patterns) is facilitated by therapy techniques that encourage changes in self-talk and consciously chosen changes in behavior. Step 3 suggests another self-management device that helps block maladaptive behavior: choosing a new and better internal model. In Figure 3.1, it can be seen that step 5 (learning new patterns) necessarily involves the selection and practicing of new patterns. It also draws upon techniques that help the patient resist the wish to regress and go back to old ways.

Here is how these self-management techniques might be applied in Marie's case. Consider the therapy session that began with Marie's report of a panic attack after her daughter's phone call. The work should begin with collaboration on the goal of trying to understand the panic reaction. One possibility is to help Marie manage panic attacks by changing her self-talk. She might learn to say to herself:

"Now wait a minute. I realize I won't be able to see them every day and help them with whatever has come up. I'll miss that, but I don't *have* to have them to be OK myself. The feeling that I do is from a long time ago, when things were very different. Dad is no longer alive. Dad is not going to beat anybody up. The kids don't need me for protection from that, and I don't need to have them need me, just because at one time I could keep it together only if I had to keep it together for others. Dad, take a hike. Butt out of this. I am dealing with my daughter and my grandchildren on my own terms now."

According to Figure 3.1 (step 3), maladaptive patterns can also be blocked by deliberately invoking new models. Here group therapy can be particularly helpful, because members can model a variety of problems and solutions. Somebody in the group might model control of panic in ways that Marie admires. Sometimes patients in individual therapy can use models from literature or the other arts. Occasionally the therapist might suggest a movie or a play that provides a relevant model. Self-help books (see Norcross, 2000) can be particularly useful in this context, too.

According to Figure 3.1 (step 5), seeking and practicing new and better patterns are great ways to use self-management to cope with a problem behavior. Marie and the therapist could work together to develop alternative behaviors in response to panic about the departure of her daughter and her family. Marie might develop a list of things to do when she panics. Since taking care of others and being taken care of are the organizing issues for Marie, her list should concentrate on self-care. Marie might have some favorite "indulgences," and they should be high on the list. Nurturant and caring friends should be noted and called to make "dates" at such times. If Marie has no helpful friends, then cultivating some should become a priority. The therapist may need to become a very active coach in this.

Next, Figure 3.1 (step 5) suggests that Marie could benefit by learning that she does not have to take care of others in order to feel safe herself. If she does not understand what drives her, she might, for example, be tempted to become embroiled in friends' family troubles and rebuild her rescuer identity. This probably would not help Marie's Growth Collaborator, since there is a high likelihood that the troubles of friends will be unending and sometimes totally out of control. In those relationships, Marie would be functioning mostly with her Regressive Loyalist.

However, if Marie were to take her considerable skills in caregiving and turn them to structured, socially sanctioned helping, that might be Green. Marie might, for example, make a fantastic employee or volunteer in such organizations as Scouts, Big Sisters, Eldercare, or the like. There is nothing pathological about taking advantage of one's acquired expertise, as long as the motivation is not overdetermined, and therefore at risk of getting oneself or others into further trouble because there are no boundaries on the assignment.

After tagging steps 1, 3, and 5 as particularly relevant to self-management, Figure 3.2 lists three shortcuts that may accelerate self-management in coming to terms. The first, to develop specific plans to address the current situation with good self-care, has been discussed above. The second suggested shortcut is to receive instruction in complementary theory. Even if the clinician and the patient do not appeal to the SASB model explicitly, the folk wisdom behind it nonetheless can be incorporated here into the therapy process. For example, anyone can understand that a person who freely offers help and advice is going to be likely to find people who seek it.[18] Hence, if Marie presents as a problem solver, she soon will be surrounded by people with problems. Now if Marie decides that she would rather build new friendships based on play and not on trouble, then she needs to understand that a playful orientation is more likely to be matched by return play. Instead of choosing work/volunteer/social organizations that involve helping, Marie should, if this is appropriate to her stage of therapy, choose organizations that offer activities for people who have similar interests. All kinds of clubs offer such opportunities (e.g., sewing circles, hiking clubs, photography groups). The therapist would actively encourage this social homework, but the choice would be up to Marie.

The third shortcut to better self-management is to recognize that improved relations with IPIRs are very likely to improve actual current relations with the very people who were internalized. Once the expectations based on old rules and values are gone, the patient is free to relate to family members in more cordial ways. Marie's father, as noted in Chapter 1, was deceased by the time she was hospitalized. However, if he were still living, and if Marie were able to truly distance herself from the terror that was appropriate in childhood, she might be able to visit her father with relative equanimity. She might now see him as a frail old man who had his own injuries and who made some very bad choices over a long period of time. Nonetheless, he would still be her father. She could deliver a minimum of filial propriety, and she could do it without becoming upset.

Strange as it might seem to people not familiar with psychopathology, patients are relieved to know that they can (if they so choose) learn to be "nice" to the people who abused them, without also being vulnerable. The last thing an IRT therapist wants to do is increase a patient's alienation from family members. The reason, as has been explained in so many contexts, is that attachment to family members gives them tremendous influence. It is foolhardy not to try to use that power for the benefit of everyone. On the other hand, if a patient elects not to reconcile with his or her family, the IRT therapist supports that decision too—as long as the patient is free from the dictates of the internalizations. Forgiving is a very personal decision that clearly belongs to the patient.[19]

FLOW CHART FOR EXPLORING BLOCKERS TO PROGRESS

The most common version of a stuck therapy can be paraphrased as "I understand all this, but my feelings just won't change." Figure 3.3 presents a flow chart outlining steps that can be taken to try to come unstuck and return to the core task. This multistep intervention begins with a summary and acknowledgment that the process is stalemated. Red and Green are deadlocked—or, worse yet, Red still predominates.

Resolving the Impasse Directly

According to Figure 3.3, the first step in coming unstuck is to summarize the impasse and context. Here is an example: A paranoid patient named Judy functioned adequately in a technical job that required little social interaction. She had been very anxious and without friends for several years before starting IRT. Neither psychotherapy nor antipsychotic medications brought relief from her intense and unhappy alienation. She believed that people hated her because they thought she was homosexual. After several months in IRT, she had made some progress in daring to transform acquaintanceships at work into friendships. But she still was quite vulnerable to feeling rejected and shunned. During one session, she reported she had felt that everyone at her church group the previous night hated her. She said:

JUDY: It has been this way forever, and it never will change. People will always think badly of me.

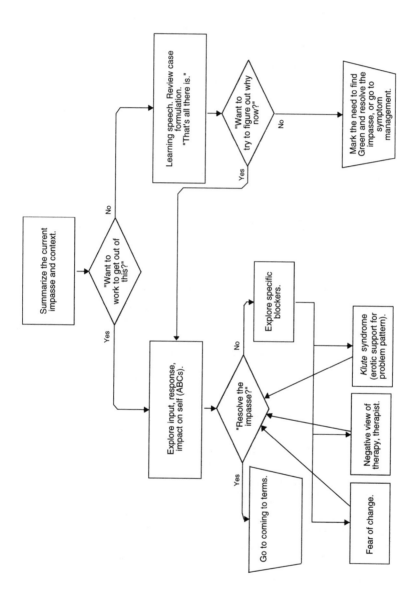

FIGURE 3.3. Exploring blockers to change.

THERAPIST: You're feeling shunned again. It seems like it's always been that way and always will be that way.

JUDY: Yes. I know this has something to do with my mother, but honestly, I just cannot help feeling this way about myself.

THERAPIST: So it does not help to recognize that your mother rejected you, and so that is what you expect from others.

JUDY: Not really.

Next, the therapist went to the first question presented in a diamond-shaped box in Figure 3.3 ("Want to work to get out of this?").

THERAPIST: Are you willing to take a closer look at this and see what might be going on?

JUDY: I suppose so.

THERAPIST: OK, good. Please recall how you felt last night when you decided that everybody hated you.

After Judy described the situation, the therapist asked for more detail about her reaction in terms of the ABCs. The therapist saw no connections to the IPIR and then asked about context:

THERAPIST: Tell me about yesterday. What was going on?

JUDY: Not much. It was a regular day. I went to work and then went home, had dinner with my mother, and then went to church group.

THERAPIST: You had dinner with your mother?

JUDY: Yes, I always do.

THERAPIST: How did that go?

JUDY: Same as always. Except she did not want me to go to church group.

THERAPIST: She did not want you to go out?

JUDY: No. She said she wanted me to watch TV with her. She seemed upset that I was going, but I went anyway.

It appeared that nurturing new friendships at the church group was upsetting both the mother and the patient's Regressive Loyalist.

THERAPIST: How did it feel to take care of your own needs when she did not want you to go?

JUDY: Not good. I was afraid she would be mad at me.

THERAPIST: (*Silence*)

JUDY: Well, maybe that is why I felt so uneasy.

THERAPIST: Could be.

JUDY: I suppose that I was thinking I was bad to go, because Mother thought so, and then I just assumed the others thought so too.

THERAPIST: That could be. You imagined your friends saw you as your mother did.

JUDY: Oh, darn, I keep doing that. I know I need to watch for it.

THERAPIST: That's a good idea. And you can look for data, too. For example, did your friends say anything to indicate how they felt about you being in the group?

JUDY: Not really. One said she was glad I came.

THERAPIST: (Silence)

JUDY: So there it is again. I think I also felt I was being "unfaithful" to Mother, and so I punished myself.

This sequence illustrated progression to the top box on the left-hand side of Figure 3.3. Input, response, and impact on the self were explored carefully. There was excellent collaboration in developing connections that explained the return of Judy's paranoia. Once the relevant background had been highlighted, the patient needed very little help to see the impact of her IPIR. Having resolved the impasse, she went directly from there to coming to terms. She was becoming increasingly comfortable with doing things separately from her mother. This kind of self-generated insight is common after the patient understands the case formulation well.

When probing such an episode for connections to an IPIR, an IRT therapist is careful to word questions in ways that support Green without offending Red more than necessary (core algorithm rule 2). For example, this patient's therapist did not say, "How did it feel to realize she did not want you to take care of your own needs?" That might have sounded as if the therapist were attacking the mother, and thus could have irritated the Regressive Loyalist. Irritated Red could make the patient feel guilty and stay blocked. By contrast, the reflection "take care of your own needs when she did not want you to go" would merely have stated the facts. The clean objectivity would have helped the patient's Green see that her mother did not support her normal efforts to develop friendships with peers.

Exploring Specific Blockers

Negative View of Therapy or of the Therapist

If exploration of input, response, and impact on self does not take the process back to coming to terms, Figure 3.3 suggests that a negative view of therapy or of the therapist may be a problem. It stands to reason that if the patient does not like or feel safe with the therapist, there will be little progress. This potential blocker is easily explored by a question such as this: "How do you feel about our work together?" The therapist should listen carefully to the answer. If the patient expresses negative views, the therapist looks first at him- or herself to see whether the criticism is accurate. He or she should paraphrase all complaints, no matter how embarrassing they might be. If the negative evaluation is valid, this should be acknowledged. If there has been a misunderstanding, the therapist should clarify it. Perhaps the therapy model needs explanation. Maybe the therapist meant something different, but did not say it clearly enough.

There will be times when the patient seriously distorts a therapy event in which the therapist's contribution to the problem was negligible. Negative feelings about the therapist in this case probably reflect negative feelings about an earlier important figure. This is otherwise known as "transference" and is frequently observed.

Finally, if the patient's family frequently expresses hostility to the idea of therapy or the therapist, IRT may be seriously compromised. The reason is that family members almost always constitute the most powerful IPIRs. If they mobilize against the treatment, the Regressive Loyalist or Red often becomes so large that the patient panics and has to terminate.

Figure 3.3 makes it explicit that in IRT, negative feelings about the therapist or therapy—whether valid or not—are a problem to be resolved before therapy can continue.

Fear of Change

Figure 3.3 suggests that another common blocker is fear of change. When people realize how their problem patterns have been driven by loyalty to old IPIRs and they decide to give up their outdated solutions, they typically feel lost. In fact, this loss of identity can induce genuine panic. The problem and suggested solutions are discussed at length in Chapter 8.

Fear of feeling the feelings associated with change is a very common specific blocker. For example, Marie might be very reluctant to stop rescuing others, simply because she knows that will make her anxious. The last thing she wants is to feel anxiety again like that she felt in relation to her father. She has spent many years believing that she is a protector, not a vulnerable and helpless person needing protection. If she stops protecting others, then her original feelings are likely to come flooding back. Yet she must do this in order to reconsider (in regard to the ABCs) the old beliefs in ways that allow her to come to terms with the internalization of her father.

The Klute Syndrome

Sometimes nonresponders have unwittingly but regularly associated sexual satisfaction with their problem patterns. For example, an abusive spouse or partner may be aroused by the act of abusing. A lonely person may feel sexual only if alone. Someone who fears being humiliated may have sexual fantasies that involve humiliation. If present, this connection can severely compromise the potential for constructive change. The *Klute* syndrome is discussed at length in Chapter 8.

When the Patient Does Not Want to Work on Breaking the Impasse

The right-hand side of Figure 3.3 details what happens if the patient does not want to explore the current impasse collaboratively. If that happens, the therapist can only deliver the learning speech (see Table 2.5), along with this message: "This is what is offered. There is nothing more. If you want to pursue it, I'll help." The attitude can be compared to that of a restaurant owner who has to tell a demanding customer the limits of the menu: "If the menu is not OK, there is nothing more we can do. We can't offer what we don't have." Some patients have fantasies that without much effort on their part, therapy will "fix" them and the world around them. It is most constructive to be very honest about the inability of IRT to realize those fantasies, even while the therapist knows that these patients may not like the task-oriented attitude of the IRT approach

If a patient is reengaged in IRT by the learning speech, then Figure 3.3 shows that the process goes back to the "Yes" loop on the left-hand side. On the other hand, if the patient continues to refuse to look into possible reasons for the impasse, Figure 3.3 suggests that the therapist needs to explain that there has to be some Green, or IRT cannot continue. If collaboration cannot be elicited, therapy goes to symptom management, described below.

When the Patient Is Willing, but Stays Stuck

If the session ends before the patient agrees to go back to the core work of coming to terms (Figure 3.2), the process can be resumed at the next session. So long as life-threatening, legal, or ethical problems are not the subjects, some specific impasses can be left unresolved. The patient and therapist may agree to return to the them later when it may be more convenient or appropriate. IRT does not demand that every issue be pursued to the last detail at any given point in time. It is usually best to follow the flow of the patient's preferences. If a problem is important, it surely will show up again, even if it was discussed once and not resolved. The procedures in Figure 3.3 can be repeated at a later session when the problem comes up again. Altered perspectives on the self that may have developed in the interim may make a difference. This time, the patient may be better able to work on coming to terms with the attachment to an internalization that organizes the repeating problem.

Sometimes the impasse is not worked out because the case formulation is incomplete. Perhaps the therapist and patient have missed the power of an additional IPIR, even though the case formulation is accurate and prior work has been relevant. If so, connecting a problem pattern to a newly named IPIR can unblock the process.

Another possible explanation for failure to resolve the impasse by following procedures in Figure 3.3 is that the therapy has not been IRT-adherent. Consultation or supervision by a certified IRT therapist is one way to be sure that the approach has been properly implemented.

FLOW CHART FOR SWITCHING TO SYMPTOM MANAGEMENT

Figure 3.4 describes a multistep intervention called "switching to symptom management." It is particularly appropriate if life-threatening situations cannot be managed immediately by appeal to the procedures in Figures 3.2 (coming to terms) and 3.3 (exploring blockers to change). A flow chart focused on how to approach blockage involving life-threatening situations appears in Chapter 7. More details about handling emergencies are provided in that chapter. Switching to symptom management can also be appropriate if the therapist and patient find themselves in a long-term stalemate, even if there are no emergencies.

Marking the Need for Green

According to Figure 3.4, when it is necessary to switch to symptom management, there is an acknowledgment that the Growth Collaborator (abbreviated as GC in Figure 3.4) is nowhere in evidence. The therapist must make it very clear that the therapy cannot proceed without a collaborative connection with the part of the patient that wants to function well. The case formulation is reviewed, and the therapist explains that if the patient cannot connect with the Green, a different approach is required. Continuing therapy without better results would be like continuing to take a medicine that is not working. While discussing this proposed change in the approach, the therapist gives the patient every opportunity to go back to the work of coming to terms. Consider this sample explanation:

> "So it looks like what we have been doing has not been helping. We may have to deal with your suicidal wishes by hospitalization and possible changes in medication. Maybe we need a consultant or a cotherapist. But first, let's talk about our alternatives within this learn-

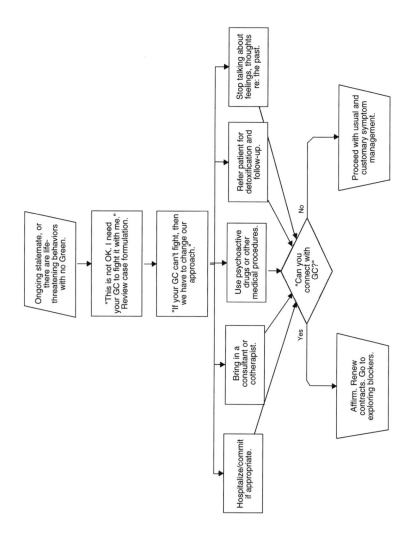

FIGURE 3.4. Switching to symptom management.

104

ing model. We have agreed that you become suicidal whenever you do well, because when you were a child, every success was viciously attacked by your stepfather. If we pursue that hypothesis, we might find out, for example, that right now you are reliving that scene because you just got a promotion. If your stepfather is involved in your suicidality now, your wish to attack yourself amounts to agreeing with him. If you don't like that thought, you might want to reconsider the plan to attack yourself. This is an example of how we could look at this if we stay with the learning model. Ultimately, the goal would be to understand this so completely that you can let go of these destructive ties and feel free of the control he has of your psyche."

Sometimes such a clarification suffices to help the patient return to the work of coming to terms. Readers may wonder whether this is a "telling" error, described in Chapter 2. Exceptions to the "no telling" recommendation can be appropriate in emergency situations. The reason is that quick results are mandatory, and directly invoking the case formulation can be effective at temporarily blocking dangerous behaviors. In subsequent sessions, the slower process of coming to terms can take place. If framing the crisis in terms of the case formulation is not successful, Figure 3.4 details important (not all) features to consider in proceeding to switch to symptom management.

Changing Medications, Hospitalization/Commitment, or Bringing in a Consultant or Cotherapist

When warranted, hospitalization/commitment, changing medications, or bringing in a consultant or cotherapist are presented to the patient as possibilities. The IRT therapist gives clear instructions that explain how these services can be received. Further discussion of these standard interventions appears in Chapter 7.

Once the switch to symptom management has been implemented, all talking about the past stops. The therapist explains that reviewing stories and trying to understand connections between the past and the present is not helping. It may even be making things worse. Patients who have been indulging their Red parts in therapy will not like this decision at all. If talk about the past is forbidden, it becomes harder to nurture the fantasy of reliving it better. On the other hand, patients who find that discussing the past reactivates painful memories may be relieved.

The switch to symptom management necessarily means that the case formulation no longer dominates intervention decisions, and IRT ceases for the short term. If the switch to symptom management effectively blocks the intolerable symptoms and adequately mobilizes the patient's Green, IRT can resume. If no Green reappears, the switch to symptom management becomes permanent. If the treatment is no longer based on the case formulation, it is not IRT. Long-term return to symptom management by any accepted practices terminates IRT.

Focusing on Symptoms That Interfere with Learning

Figure 3.4 includes as an alternative "Refer patient for detoxification and follow-up." This is a special case of switching to symptom management that can be invoked before IRT even begins. Since IRT is fundamentally a learning approach, factors that interfere with normal learning preclude IRT. Patients who are overmedicated with alcohol, prescription drugs, or street drugs are poor candidates for learning in IRT unless and until these conditions can be better moderated. Alcohol and drugs also may interfere with the will to learn new patterns. Acute psychosis unquestionably rules out effective new learning. However, if psychotic symptoms subside, IRT can be useful (as the case of Jessica has illustrated).

If the decision is to refer patients with chronic and intensive alcohol and/or drug use for management of their substance dependence problems, there are a number of treatment possibilities. Approaches might include (1) 12-step groups, such as Alcoholics Anonymous (AA) or Narcotics Anonymous (NA); or (2) CBT or other treatments that have documented effectiveness. For example, Ouimette, Finney, and Moos (1997, p. 230) showed that "12-step [i.e., AA or NA] patients were somewhat more likely to be abstinent at the 1-year follow-up; 12-step, [CBT], and combined 12-step–[CBT] treatment programs were equally effective in reducing substance use and improving most other areas of functioning." Miller, Meyers, and Tonnigan (1999, p. 688) focused sharply on motivation for change by working with family members. They showed that in a randomized clinical trial of three approaches, "a community reinforcement and family training . . . approach . . . [that involved] teaching behavior change skills to use at home . . . was more effective in engaging initially unmotivated problem drinkers in treatment (64%) as compared with the more commonly practiced Al-Anon (13%) and [another family-based] intervention (30%)."

Once a patient has agreed that drug or alcohol use is a problem and begins to control it by participation in an effective program, he or she can begin concurrent IRT. If the ability and will to learn are not compromised by chemical dependencies, the IRT approach can enhance response in the symptom-oriented treatments. For example, suppose that a man with a drinking problem is willing to join AA and to work the program. Furthermore, suppose the DLL analysis shows that in his use of alcohol and in his behaviors when drunk, he is copying his hated stepfather. Work on the relationship with the internalization of his stepfather can help him choose to take better advantage of the techniques he learns in his alcohol treatment program.

The judgment of what constitutes reasonable control of alcohol or drug use is difficult. It is suggested that patients participating in IRT keep their blood alcohol level below the legal level for driving. Other limits might be negotiated on a case-by-case basis. Naturally, it is difficult to monitor compliance without collaboration. If evidence emerges that IRT learning is impeded by drug- or alcohol-related patterns, IRT switches to a policy of zero tolerance, described in a special paragraph of the consent-to-treatment form presented in Appendix 3.1. If a zero tolerance policy is in place, a decision to use is a decision to terminate IRT for a significant period of time. Six months of randomly tested, monitored sobriety would be an example of a condition required to resume IRT with any hope that the needed learning could take place. Another possible condition suggesting readiness to use IRT well would be graduation from a symptom-focused treatment program.

WHO IS ELIGIBLE FOR IRT?

Because of its complexity and length, IRT is recommended for nonresponders. However, not all such patients can use IRT well. The capacity for IRT can be compromised by several factors, which are discussed here.

Compromise Associated with Motivation

One of the more serious problems for IRT is the patient who is dangerous to self or others and is completely out of touch with any Green. An example of such a patient was Nancy,[20] the chronically suicidal, erstwhile successful production supervisor. Nancy's self-sabotage was supported by her belief that her suffering assured her father's place in hell. This provided her with enormous reassurance. Furthermore, her addiction to pain medications seemed an entirely appropriate response to abuse from yet another male caregiver (the surgeon who, she maintained, had botched her neck surgery). She had no perceived incentive to change her views or behaviors. In the complete absence of any evidence of a wish to change, Nancy was not an acceptable candidate for IRT.

Another factor related to lack of motivation that can rule out IRT is, as indicated earlier, a patient's being deeply affected by familial hostility to the idea of therapy and/or the therapist.

Compromise Due to Interference with Learning Capacity

Some symptoms preclude IRT because they interfere too much with learning. If such symptoms are successfully addressed by other procedures, IRT may proceed. Acute psychosis (with Axis II comorbidity) or heavy use of certain drugs or alcohol are examples that have been discussed above.

Some symptoms that interfere with learning lack the potential for remission, and these permanently rule out IRT. Examples include insults to cognitive function, such as disabling head injury or major central nervous system damage from exposure to toxic chemicals. Even if there are no identified problems with chemical states or defective central nervous system functioning, IRT defaults to symptom management when presenting problems do not remit after a reasonable trial.[21]

There is a minimum level of intelligence required for using IRT, but exactly what this is remains unknown. Readers who work with mentally disordered persons of limited verbal skills might try IRT, using the simplest possible language[22] and planning corrective learning experiences within an institutional milieu. For example, if a mentally retarded patient has been neglected by key attachment figures, nurturant attention from staff and other patients might help build new, better-socialized internalizations. If such a patient is defiant in reaction to overcontrol by attachment figures, minimizing arbitrary demands and maximizing the possibility for rewarding choices might prove helpful.

DEFINING ADHERENCE WHILE PRACTICING IRT

An intervention is considered IRT-adherent if it implements one or more rules from the core algorithm and does not violate any of them. Adherence to rules should be assessed in context. For example, early in therapy it is sometimes necessary to "cozy up" to the Red because there is so much of it (as discussed in the section on rule 1). Red empathy can be IRT-adherent if it is required by context and if it is accompanied by a message that supports Green. An example of how to do this has been provided in the discussion of Red and Green empathy for Kenneth (again, see the section on rule 1).

In supervision, the most commonly observed failure to adhere to IRT is that a therapist does not attend to the case formulation. This error is usually easy to recognize as a well-intended effort to use a standard procedure to address a symptom. As has been said repeatedly, symptom-focused interventions may or may not be consistent with the case formulation. For example, if a therapist "points out" a problem pattern, the observation may be used well by some patients. A secure person who simply needs some feedback for corrective learning could benefit from this. On the other hand, pointing out may be seen as an unbearable criticism by other patients. A highly self-critical person may use "pointing out" as another reason to condemn him- or herself, and settle more firmly into a transference that views the therapist as a critical IPIR. Appeal to the case formulation should help the therapist know when pointing out may be helpful and when it may be iatrogenic.

In eventual research study, checklists and rating scales that tally degrees of adherence to or violation of the core algorithm may be developed. For clinical training purposes, however, it is relatively easy to determine whether an intervention conforms to the core algorithm. A supervisor can review a printout of the six rules and get a sense of how well each was implemented in a given session.

ADMINISTRATIVE ISSUES

Administrative issues such as missed appointments, ending sessions on time, requests for reduced rates, or deferred payment frequently come up in therapy. These and other issues are reviewed in detail below. In general, the IRT therapist negotiates such matters in a collaborative manner. Of course, many patients invite a power struggle over these issues. It is one of the ways they have of testing who the therapist is, and whether or not they "matter." Their tests often are Red and so it is especially important the therapist respond in Green ways. If it is not possible to negotiate a solution to key administrative problems, the IRT therapist simply describes his or her boundaries, and the patient can then choose whether to participate in IRT.

Consent to Treatment

Appendix 3.1 presents the consent-to-treatment form that I currently use for outpatient work. It includes and goes a bit beyond current local ethical and legal requirements concerning the need to inform patients about terms and conditions of psychotherapy. Each practitioner will need to modify such a form according to his or her own system needs and preferences. Among the more unusual features of this consent form are the warning about the potential impact of disclosure to insurance companies or employers, and the description of the highly informed degree of control the patient has in such a release. Whether the patient signs the contract or not, I believe it is important that he or she has this information, and that I keep my part of the agreement.

Timeliness and Missed Appointments

To illustrate the collaborative attitude in resolving administrative problems, consider the possible issue of patients' being late to appointments or missing appointments. For me, this is not a problem unless the case formulation suggests that it is a significant event. The truth is that there usually are plenty of other things to do if I am not in a session. The time is there and available to the patient if he or she wants to use it. However, I become concerned if missing or canceling becomes a pattern. Then the problem is discussed in relation to the case formulation.

If a therapist is working for an organization that requires a large number of billing hours, being lenient about canceled appointments may be difficult or impossible. In that case, the conventional procedure of charging for missed sessions if there has not been adequate prior notice is recommended. There are probably still other settings where the usual requirement of 24 hours' advance notice for cancellation is appropriate.

Telephone or E-Mail Contact between Sessions

Availability by telephone or e-mail between sessions can be important to the stability of the therapy relationship, but it is not to be used as a substitute for therapy. Such contact is only for a brief "check-in," with the option to schedule an emergency or extra appointment if needed. If I am called or e-mailed for an inappropriate purpose, I shorten the contact and discuss it at the next appointment. If someone does not "get the message," I treat this as a problem pattern and approach it with the procedures outlined in Figures 3.2 to 3.4.

Failure to Keep the Contract to Pay for Therapy

The rules about money are not lenient. Although it is easy to use the time from a canceled appointment in constructive ways, going unpaid for completed work offers no such satisfactory alternative. The IRT therapist provides intense and thoughtful focus on the patient's concerns. The purpose is to help the patient learn to escape from his or her cage by gaining awareness and choice that could lead to greater satisfaction in his or her love relationships and at work. Therapy is not about love for sale or free love, either. The therapist is neither an ersatz parent, nor a banker who provides interest-free loans. Rather, the therapist expects to be paid the agreed-upon fee for his or her work to help the patient learn to love and work with more satisfaction.

Collecting fees keeps the nature of the therapy relationship in proper perspective. For that reason, it is best to hand billing statements directly to patients, rather than to engage in "discreet" mailing (which allows the pretense that money is not part of the relationship). Trainees need to have supervised experience in learning to handle the psychological problems of billing and collecting.

Most therapists accept a percentage of cases at a reduced fee or no fee. But far more patients than one could possibly work with want to have therapy on such terms. In fact, many seem far more comfortable asking the therapist—a relatively new person in their lives—to finance their therapy than to ask their own family members. When therapists or agencies volunteer to provide for indigent cases, that is appropriate. However, the rules are defined by agencies or therapists according to their own internal policies, resources, and needs. Those rules have been agreed upon independently of any particular therapy, and before therapy begins. The choice of who gets low-fee or no-fee therapy should not be determined by defaulters, whether they be patients or insurance companies. If brief attempts fail to support a nonpaying patient in his or her decision to give therapy a higher priority,[23] the therapist needs to provide suggestions for available alternative places to seek treatment at low or no fees.

Frequency of Sessions and Time to Termination

It is fair for people to ask how long IRT will last. For a long time, I have explained that a year is a minimum and 2 years are average, but that 3 years are not unusual. As I have been sharpening the concepts of IRT and focusing relentlessly on underlying motivations, I believe that people are responding more rapidly. A few reconstructions have recently taken place in less than a year.

Once a week is a reasonable rate of treatment. There are times, especially early in therapy with persons who exhibit life-threatening behaviors, that two or three times a week may be more appropriate. Toward the end of therapy, there is often tapering of the therapy dose to once every 3 or 4 weeks by mutual agreement.

Assessment Methods and Record Keeping

As indicated in Chapter 2, it makes sense to begin and end psychotherapy with assessment of symptoms according to the medical model. There are many available brief rating scales of depression, anxiety, thought patterns, and so on. For example, the Symptom Checklist 90—Revised (Derogatis, 1977) and the Beck Depression Inventory (Beck, Rush, Shaw, & Emery, 1979) work well. A measure of personality disorders is usually appropriate, too. For this, there are also many options. I prefer the Wisconsin Personality Inventory (Klein et al., 1993) or the Structured Clinical Interview for DSM-IV Axis II (First, Spitzer, Gibbon, Williams, & Benjamin, 1997). At therapy termination, I find the Retrospective Assessment of the Therapy Experience (Strupp, Fox, & Lessler, 1968) very useful, because it asks for ratings of attributes presumed to be important (e.g., "On the whole I experienced very little feeling in the course of therapy") and asks sensible questions that seem very relevant to the therapy process (e.g., "How much do you feel you have changed as a result of psychotherapy?"), as well as straightforward important open-ended questions (e.g., "Describe the most important changes you have experienced").

For measures of relationships with important others in the present and the past, "before" and "after" assessments with the Intrex[24] (Benjamin, 1996b, 2000b) are highly appropriate. Further information about that approach is available in Pincus and Benjamin (in preparation).

Record keeping should be consistent with the DLL and IRT model. To facilitate adherence, I recommend a one-page outline, shown in Figure 3.5. The document asks the therapist to assess what is going on in the patient's life; what was discussed in relation to major IPIRs; what was done that could be classified at each of the five steps of therapy learning (recorded separately for therapist [T] and patient [P]); whether there was an emergency, and if so, how it was addressed; and a brief summary.

The summary should be written according to the time-tested medical algorithm, SOAP (S, subjective report of the patient; O, objective relevant data; A, analysis [from the DLL perspective]; and P, plans that were and will be implemented). For example, the summary for the paranoid patient who thought the people in her church group hated her might be as follows:

S: Feels hated by people in the church group.
O: Nobody said anything hateful. One person said she was glad the patient came. Paranoia was evident, but abated during the therapy session.
A: Her mother asked her to stay home that night, and so, given her difficulty with boundaries, she was probably imagining the group, like her mother, was angry. She also tends to feel that she betrays her mother if she is independent.
P: Connect expectation of hatred from church group to mother's expected anger about autonomy. Support right to be Green (friendly to mother, but separate).

The single page of Figure 3.5 encourages supervisees to stay close to the case formulation. It is a bit brief, but if completed electronically, it can be expanded to any desired degree. For even greater flexibility, I prefer to use the same items in a data base in Microsoft Access. It takes about 10 minutes after each session to enter the highlights of a session. The data base form is especially useful when one is trying to retrieve information. One can, for example, easily search for all sessions in which a particular IPIR was discussed, and thus trace the evolution of the view of the relationship over the course of therapy. Reports can be easily tailored to the situation. The summary section is long enough that it can serve as a succinct basis for responding to requests for case notes. The SOAP algorithm assures that the summary will conform to professional norms.

Session number and date	
Symptoms	
Participants	
Current events	
Responses	
Impact on self	
Spouse or partner	
Mother	
Father	
Siblings	
Children	
Work	
Collaboration—T	
Collaboration—P	
Pattern recognition—T	
Pattern recognition—P	
Blocking maladaptive patterns—T	
Blocking maladaptive patterns—P	
Enabling will to change—T	
Enabling will to change—P	
Learning new patterns—T	
Learning new patterns—P	
Transference	
Countertransference	
Old homework	
New homework	
Emergency?	
Address emergency	
Summary—line 1 (SO)	
Summary—line 2 (AP)	

FIGURE 3.5. IRT form for session summary.

Ethical Codes

Conformity to the ethical code of the therapist's profession is required. An example of a particularly well-developed code is that of the American Psychological Association (APA), available to all on the Web (APA, 2002). The APA code addresses the administrative issues discussed above, plus other important matters (e.g., conflict of interest, dual-role relationships, impaired providers, and conflicts between ethics and organizational demands).

WHERE TO GO FROM HERE?

Chapter 1 has reviewed the context in which psychotherapy is currently practiced, and provided case examples of nonresponders and an overview of IRT. Chapter 2 has provided detailed instructions for how to develop a case formulation. It includes the theory of psychopathology upon which formulations are based. This third chapter has given specific descriptions of IRT interventions. Chapter 4 describes the SASB model and its parallel models for affective and cognitive behavior. Readers who are not presently interested in SASB may go directly to Chapter 5, skipping Chapter 4. Some may choose to return to Chapter 4 later. Most of the remaining chapters (Chapters 5–9) are devoted to detailed explanation of each of the five therapy steps.

NOTES

1. SASB code AFFIRM, accompanied by an affect of warm acceptance and by a balanced, reciprocal cognitive style. Technical definitions of SASB codes in terms of three underlying interpersonal dimensions are presented in Chapter 4. Readers who elect not to learn SASB coding may either ignore footnotes with SASB codes, or interpret them according to ordinary rules of language.
2. That is, it is complementary, according to the SASB model.
3. Professional ethics and common sense put unequivocal limits on therapist attachment. I find that I often have an ever-deepening respect and genuine liking for patients as unique individuals. However, this has to be channeled strictly and without exception into the business at hand: a patient's therapy.
4. That is, what works is likely to be repeated.
5. I heard this story as an undergraduate student of G. A. Heise, who was an enthusiastic Skinner PhD student. Heise was a marvelous teacher, and is one of my favorite IPIRs.
6. Pugh found that in cognitive behavioral therapy (CBT), empathy that followed expressions of maladaptive statements was associated with worse outcome.
7. According to the SASB model, baseline positions in the Detached Group

(DAG) of behaviors include the following: **BLAME**–<u>SULK</u>–*SELF-BLAME*; **ATTACK**–<u>RECOIL</u>–*SELF-ATTACK*; and **IGNORE**–<u>WALL OFF</u>–*SELF-NEGLECT*. Or they may represent contextually inappropriate responding at the extreme of autonomy (**EMANCIPATE**–<u>SEPARATE</u>–*SELF-EMANCIPATE*) or at the extreme of enmeshment (**CONTROL**–<u>SUBMIT</u>–*SELF-CONTROL*).

8. Support for the SASB-based definitions of pathology and normality is found in the fact that people do not present with complaints about normal behaviors. Their symptoms almost always can be classified in the DAG, as described in note 7.

9. Baseline positions in the Attachment Group (AG) of behaviors are as follows: **AFFIRM**–<u>DISCLOSE</u>– *SELF-AFFIRM*; **ACTIVE LOVE**–<u>REACTIVE LOVE</u>–*ACTIVE SELF-LOVE*; and **PROTECT**–<u>TRUST</u>–*SELF-PROTECT*.

10. I have worked with utterly honest therapists who confessed they were aroused by patients who were in pain and needy. This is an orientation that should be changed, because the associated nonverbal messages are likely to encourage the patient's Regressive Loyalist (Red).

11. The IRT therapist is responsible for process, not outcome. Thus he or she works hard to deliver optimally effective interventions, but knows that outcome belongs to the patient. My students like the characterization of IRT as "cat therapy," meaning that the therapist puts out the "tuna fish" and the patient may or may not sample it. This attitude is absolutely essential when one is treating PAG.

12. Helplessness is associated with depression, both in the literature and according to the parallel affect and cognition models discussed in Chapter 4. Taking control of oneself is the introjection of the complement of helplessness. The IRT therapist's understanding of the SASB predictive principles helps shape the intervention in ways that pull for Green.

13. DLL case formulations are defined so specifically that this hypothesis can be tested. Until it is tested in a formal protocol, there is robust theory that helps guide the treatment in a consistent direction.

14. If the specific details of a narrative suggest child abuse, the therapist needs to attend to the abuse-reporting requirements in his or her area of practice. In some instances, it may be necessary to mark the behavior as abusive and invoke any reporting requirements. My strong preference is to make this observation and offer to work very hard with the patient to contain the abusive behaviors, in a manner that is very like the handling of suicidal tendencies. At some point, depending on clinician judgment and on local legislation and norms, one has to report problem behavioral tendencies, whether they involve suicidality, homicidality, or child abuse—to appropriate authorities. Every effort is made to do this in a way that minimizes damage to the most important tool of therapy, the therapy relationship.

15. I recall being astonished when Carl Whitaker would read his mail or fall asleep in family sessions that were replaying this scenario. As a young postdoctoral fellow, I had no idea what was happening; in retrospect, I better understand the effectiveness of the "intervention."

16. Any other step in Figure 3.1, on either branch (self-discovery or self-management), could also be relevant.

17. "Overdetermined" is a psychoanalytic word suggesting that behaviors in a

given situation are determined by more than meets the eye. From the psycho-dynamic point of view, the proverbial "black box" of behaviorism is chock-full of old expectations and rules. These suggest that the behavior will be affected by far more than the "stimulus" of the moment. When the "black box" is filled in this way, behavior is "overdetermined."

18. TRUST is the complement of **PROTECT**.

19. According to the *American Heritage Talking Dictionary* (1997), "forgive" means "1. To excuse for a fault or an offense; pardon. 2. To renounce anger or resentment against. 3. To absolve from payment of (a debt, for example)." Meaning 2 applies directly to IRT. Meanings 1 and 3 may also be required by the personal values of same patients.

20. Nancy has been discussed in the section on rule 2 of the core algorithm.

21. Defining what is "reasonable" has not yet been operationalized. If crisis behaviors are involved, a reasonable trial is quite short. In reality, IRT often does manage to contain crisis behaviors quite rapidly. The more challenging question of how long is too long arises when a patient (somewhat like Nancy) seems devoted to disability. This matter is discussed at greater length in Chapter 8.

22. I was surprised to see that on an occasion in continental Europe, when I was asked to speak through a translator and provide a DLL consultation for an institutionalized patient with marginal intelligence, it was possible to develop a sensible case formulation. The patient and staff agreed that the analysis was highly relevant to his problem patterns.

23. I let patients know that I do not send accounts for collection. The matter of paying or not is part of the therapy relationship. If we do not reach resolution, past-due accounts are my problem, and that is OK. However, I do not agree to provide future service for no fee unless unusual circumstances suggest that this is warranted.

24. Available from the University of Utah. Go to the university's Web site (http://www.utah.edu), and then search for SASB within the site. Or e-mail Intrex@Psych.utah.edu.

Appendix 3.1

Sample Consent-to-Treatment Form

Lorna Smith Benjamin, PhD, FDHC
Licensed psychologist, Utah and Wisconsin

1. Informed consent

By the end of the third session if not before, I usually will discuss with you my evaluation and treatment recommendations, along with some options for other approaches. You are entitled to receive information about the methods and techniques of therapy to be used, and to participate fully in specifying goals.

It is important to recognize that there can be periods of time during psychotherapy when you may become upset as a possible result of the discussions in therapy. This is a natural consequence of learning to recognize certain painful feelings. However, every effort will be made to help you cope constructively with these feelings and thoughts, and use them to facilitate your healing process.

Although the exact length of treatment is hard to predict, I will give you an idea of average duration for conditions similar to yours. At any time, you have a right to discuss your progress in treatment and your other treatment options. You may end treatment at any time. However, if your decision to terminate is unilateral, you are asked to return for one session to discuss that decision. The purpose of that session would be to clarify and perhaps rectify any misunderstandings. You also may seek a second opinion regarding any aspect of your therapy at any time if you wish to do so.

2. Confidentiality

The information provided by you during therapy and psychological evaluations is legally confidential except as required by law (Utah Statutes 62a [3–4, 78 [14a]). These exceptions include "threat of serious harm to self or others," as, for example, in the case of threats of behavior that might lead to child abuse, homicide, suicide, or grave disability. If such exceptions were to arise, I would notify you at the time.

In addition to these exceptions, you should know that I may consult with other practitioners, but will do so without revealing any identifying information. I also may occasionally make very carefully disguised reference to an aspect of your case when teaching mental health professionals or supervising professionals in training. I also might wish to write about an aspect of your treatment in a professional paper or book. If that description, always well disguised, were longer than just a few sentences, I would submit it to you and would not publish it until you gave written permission. You would be under no obligation to give that permission, and your refusal to do so would not compromise your treatment in any way.

Disclosure to insurance companies: Your insurance company will require some information about you. The billing statement that you receive from me will include the dates and length of your sessions, the procedure code (usually 90806 = individual psychotherapy, or 90847 = family medical psychotherapy), and your diagnosis. The latter will be from the American Psychiatric Association's *Diagnostic and Statistical Manual of Mental Disorders*, fourth edition (DSM-IV). I will discuss your diagnosis with you and show you the description of it in the DSM-IV. When you submit the statement to your insurance company, that action will constitute permission to me to release that information to your insurance company. If your insurance company requires more than dates, procedure, and diagnosis, I will forward my response to their request to you rather than to the company. You may then release that information to your insurance company, if you choose to do so.

You should be aware that in the future, when you apply for income disability, life insurance, other insurances, or some types of employment, you may be asked to disclose your participation in this psychotherapy and to release information about it to relevant persons or entities. In that event, I will prepare a response that I will forward directly to you, rather than to the person or entity who has your permission to request such a report from me. You will then be able to choose whether to include the information with your application or not.

3. Fees

Before your first appointment, you will be informed about my current fee for a 50-minute session. The fee will include an adminstrative charge, which can be waived if you choose to pay cash at each session.

There may be other charges for reports, letters, and lengthy phone contacts. You will be informed about those charges at the time they are incurred.

4. Missed appointments

I usually do not charge for canceled or missed appointments. I do appreciate the courtesy of being informed ahead of time if possible. If missed appointments or last-minute cancellations become a pattern, I reserve the right to implement a policy of charging for the missed time unless notified 24 hours in advance. You will be informed of this change before any such policy is put into effect.

5. Emergency situations

In an emergency, call me using the telephone numbers I give you at the first appointment. These include office, cell phone, and home, to be used in that order.

In the rare event that you cannot reach me rapidly enough through these channels, please call [name of hospital] at [phone] and ask to speak with a crisis worker. I assume that if you cannot wait for me to return a call in response to your messages left at one of my three voice mails, you will need hospitalization. If the crisis worker makes that judgment, please ask to be seen by one of the following psychiatrists on staff at [the hospital]: [Names]. Any others would be acceptable too, but these are the ones whose work I know most directly.

6. Addendum for: _____, whose signature here acknowledges a problem with street or prescription drugs and/or alcohol.

This therapy is a strength-building, learning approach, and such growth is greatly compromised by use of drugs or alcohol. If you wish to participate in this Interpersonal Reconstructive Therapy, you agree to a policy of zero tolerance. Any use of drugs or alcohol during this therapy for a person with an acknowledged problem is a decision to terminate the therapy process until you have again maintained sobriety for 6 (or, depending on circumstances, 3) months. In the event that there is a relapse, you agree to one additional session for the purpose of consolidating gains and considering (a) whether this therapy can resume after 3 or 6 months and (b) of plans for referral (e.g., long-term inpatient treatment for alcohol or drug abuse or dependence). You understand and agree that further treatment is your responsibility, once you have started this therapy, signed this contract, and then made the decision to terminate it by using drugs or alcohol.

7. Consent to treatment

I have read and understand the descriptions of informed consent, confidentiality, fees, missed appointments and emergencies. I consent to treatment under conditions in sections 1, 2, 3, 4, and 5. If I sign my name in the blank provided in section 6, that means I also agree to the terms described therein.

Print name: _____

Signature: _____

Date: _____

Countersignature by L. S. Benjamin: _____

Date: _____

Shortly after you add your signature to this form, it will be countersigned, and you will be given a copy for your records.

4

Structural Analysis
of Social Behavior
The Clarifying Lens

Structural Analysis of Social Behavior (SASB) is a technology that objectively measures perceived interpersonal and intrapsychic relations. The methods therefore make Developmental Learning and Loving (DLL) and Interpersonal Reconstructive Therapy (IRT) concepts amenable to research confirmation or refutation. The SASB model can also function as a lens through which the clinician sees patterns more clearly and connects them more precisely. These skills enhance case formulation, therapy process, and outcome.

SASB-BASED DATA

There are several ways of generating SASB assessments of Important Persons' Internalized Representations (IPIRs) and perceived interpersonal relations.

Intrex Questionnaires

The SASB Intrex questionnaires ask the rater to describe perceived self and others. Examples of Intrex items are "To become perfect, I force myself to do things correctly," and "He puts me down, blames me, punishes me." The rater chooses a number from 0 to 100 to show how well a given item applies or not.

120

When a rater assesses several key relationships in terms of the SASB Intrex items, the series provides a straightforward method to identify copy processes. As will become clear in the comparison of SASB predictive principles to copy processes, the questionnaires can quantify the degrees to which a rater is (1) being like an IPIR; (2) acting as if the IPIR is still there and in control; and (3) treating him- or herself as he or she was treated. Another of many possible uses is to assess transference by comparing the patient's ratings of the therapist to the patient's views of important others (Connolly et al., 1996). Results can be shown directly to the patient to facilitate therapy learning, kept as a record that informs the case formulation, and (with proper permission) entered into a research data base.

SASB Codes

Formal SASB codes are generated according to procedures detailed in a manual. They provide objective observer data suitable for research uses. Comparison of a family member's (or patient's) perceptions assessed by questionnaires to objective observer coding of videotapes of family (or patient–therapist) interactions can identify distortions in perspective among family members (Humes & Humphrey, 1994) or between patient and therapist.

SASB Software

Software is available[1] for processing data from the SASB Intrex questionnaires or from the formal SASB coding system. Approximately 200 publications[2] illustrate potential research uses of this interpersonal technology (see overviews by Benjamin, 1996c; Henry, 1996; Constantino, 2000).

Real-Time SASB Coding

During sessions, clinicians can create SASB codes according to a less microscopic and formal process, called "real-time coding." The present chapter concentrates on this less formal but clinically useful version of SASB technology. Discussions of the questionnaires, the formal research coding, and the software appear elsewhere (e.g., Benjamin, 1996b, 2000b; Benjamin & Cushing, 2000; Pincus & Benjamin, in preparation).

It is possible to be very good at IRT without understanding the SASB model or doing real-time coding. For that reason, readers need not continue with this chapter unless they choose to develop their skills in IRT at the more rigorous level facilitated by SASB. Another possibility is to skip this chapter on a first reading of this book, and return to it later.

REASONS TO MAKE THE EFFORT TO LEARN SASB

Imagine that a person has a good musical ear and is interested in learning to play the guitar. He or she reads some books and takes a few lessons. Within a relatively short time, the gifted person may be ready for home entertainment. However, if he or she wants to become an expert, then substantial amounts of practice (along with continued input from good books and/or teachers) will be required. Routine drill on basic skills is likely to be suggested. In addition, most conservatories of music require that future performers, teachers, and composers study music theory as well as music history. In music theory, students learn a lot about underlying structure. For example, they study principles of combining notes (chords), sequencing (rhythm), and more.

In their lessons and performances, musicians apply theory in many ways. One simple example is that they learn to transpose—that is, to play in keys other than the one written on the sheet of music. Another is that they can fill in missing chords if given only a melodic line. Common patterns and sequences are quickly recognized and understood. The proficient musician is able both to grasp the meaning of a very complex set of symbols, and also to add well-informed complexity to a very simple line. With a firm base of theoretical understanding and well-practiced skills in applying theory, greater artistry is possible.

The same is true for IRT. Learning the SASB perspective on the structure of interpersonal and intrapsychic patterns helps the clinician function at a higher level of expertise. When he or she recognizes and connects SASB codes of problem patterns, the accuracy of case formulations is improved. By referring accurately recognized patterns to his or her internal catalogue,[3] the clinician can choose better interventions. For example, even before there is a clear case formulation, knowledge of a suspected prototype can help the clinician provide an antidote that keeps the therapy process collaborative.[4] Of course, some experienced clinicians can do the same thing on the basis of intuition. Still, it is likely that any intuition can be enhanced with better articulation of underlying cues. Hence, learning and practicing skills in SASB online coding can be useful to experts as well as to novices.

ELEMENTARY SASB CODING: THE QUADRANT MODEL

The Three Dimensions Underlying All Versions of the SASB Model

The basic three dimensions of the SASB model are shown in Figure 4.1.

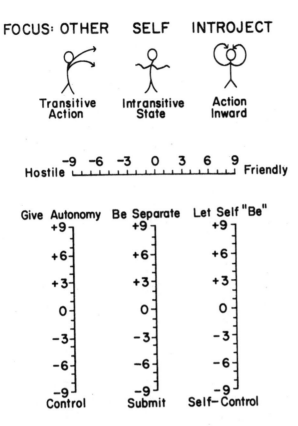

FIGURE 4.1. Three dimensions in interpersonal space. Focus is represented by the stick figures. Affiliation ranges from hostile to friendly on the horizontal scale. Interdependence, shown by the three vertical scales, has different names, depending on focus. If the focus is on other, interdependence ranges from **Control** to **Give autonomy**. If the focus is on self, it ranges from Submit to Be separate. If transitive focus is directed inward, interdependence ranges from *Self-control* to *Let self be*. From Benjamin (1986). Copyright 1986 by The Guilford Press. Reprinted by permission.

Focus

The first dimension is "focus," shown by the three stick figures at the top of Figure 4.1. At the left-hand side, transitive[5] focus on other is illustrated by the pointing figure. Focus on another is the primary job of a parent in relation to an infant, and hence behaviors coded as having a focus on other are called "parentlike." Developmental data (e.g., Benjamin, 1974) support this choice of name. It is important to note that the parentlike domain according to SASB includes a wide variety of behaviors, not just "control," as some assume. For example, friendly listening (a basic therapist behavior) involves transitive, friendly, autonomy-giving focus on other. Friendly listening is parentlike,[6] but not controlling.

Focus on self, shown by the middle stick figure, involves an intransitive[7] state of being. Focus on self in this way is characteristic of infants, and hence this group of behaviors is called "childlike." This term does not have the negative connotations sometimes attributed to the word. According to SASB, a mature adult in a healthy, balanced relationship shows about 50% parentlike behaviors, and 50% childlike behaviors.

Introjected focus, shown by the right-hand stick figure, involves turning transitive focus inward. The self is the focus of the person's own transitive action. The introjective process[8] was named by Sullivan (1953) as important to the development of a self-system.

Affiliation

The second dimension of SASB analysis is "affiliation," shown on the horizontal axis of Figure 4.1. Hostile interactions appear on the left-hand side, and friendly ones on the right. The names for hostility (and friendliness) vary, depending on focus. For example, in the cluster version of the SASB model that is presented below and used in footnotes throughout this book, maximal transitive hostility is called ATTACK. Maximal intransitive hostility is called RECOIL. Transitive hostility that is introjected is called SELF-ATTACK. The respective friendly opposites of these three points are ACTIVE LOVE, REACTIVE LOVE, and SELF-LOVE.

Interdependence

The third dimension of SASB analysis is "interdependence," shown by the three vertical axes at the bottom of Figure 4.1. The vertical dimension has different names, depending on the type of focus being described. Figure 4.1 shows that if the focus is on other, interdependence ranges from **Control** to **Give autonomy**. If the focus is on self, interdependence ranges from Submit to Be separate. If transitive focus is introjected, interdependence ranges from *Self-control* to *Let self be*. In the cluster version of the SASB model, enmeshment is described at the CONTROL/SUBMIT end of the interdependence scales, and differentiation is depicted at the EMANCIPATE/SEPARATE end.

The online SASB coder learns to "hear" therapy narrative and process in terms of these three basic dimensions. As will be explained below, the dimensions can be combined in various ways to create categories with more familiar names, such as BLAME or **136. Put down, act superior.** Another option is to listen for SASB dimensions without translating to categories. That nonverbal but still precise method compares to the technique of asking listeners to turn a dial to the right if they like what a speaker is saying, and to the left if not. The continuous measure provides immediate, fine-grained feedback that is fully comprehensible but does not require finding exactly the right words to express it. The skilled SASB coder has two mental dials that assess the affiliation and the interdependence dimensions, respectively. When focus is added to the intersection of those judgments, the event has been understood in ways that can invoke the predictive principles.[9] Intuition has been clarified in a way that can sharpen the accuracy and relevance of the clinician's next intervention.

Example of Online Coding with the Quadrant Model

SASB coding begins by selecting or constructing a brief phrase that summarizes a person in a relationship that needs to be assessed. To illustrate basic SASB coding, consider Kenneth, the blaming patient described in Chapter 1. Almost all of Kenneth's messages were angry attempts to change his wife's errant ways—for example, "My wife has been stepping out on me." Most of his stories simply provided details to support this allegation. His focus was exclusively on her. It did not take the DLL interviewer long to see that Kenneth's process during his marital crisis had the same underlying dimensionality as did his mother's when she was abandoned by his father. Kenneth and his mother did not have much else in common, so his identification with her was not obvious. If the connection had not been noticed, the interviewer might not have elicited so much detail about what it was like when Kenneth's father left his mother. Yet it was that this part of the interview that Kenneth mentioned when he later left a tearful message asking to discuss his similarity to his mother. Recognition that they both used blaming to deal with abandonment not only provided the core of the case formulation, but also had a deep emotional impact on him.

The three dimensions of Figure 4.1[10] generate the quadrant version of the SASB model, shown in Figure 4.2. The next four subsections show how to code Kenneth's blaming of his wife on this quadrant model.

Dimension 1: Focus

It is easy to agree that as he engaged in blaming his wife for infidelity, Kenneth was focused on other, represented by the pointing stick figure at the top left-hand side of Figure 4.1 and by the top third of Figure 4.2.

Dimension 2: Affiliation

Clearly, Kenneth was hostile toward his wife. His position would be on the hostile (left-hand) side of the horizontal axis.

FOCUS ON OTHER

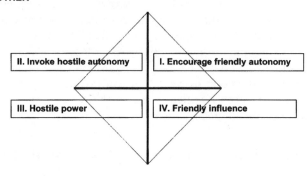

FOCUS ON SELF

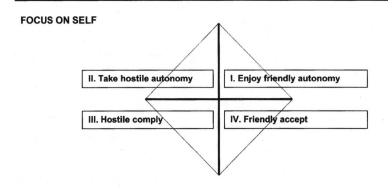

INTROJECTED FOCUS

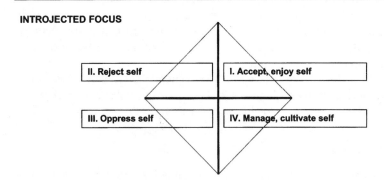

FIGURE 4.2. SASB quadrant model. For each type of focus shown in Figure 4.1, this figure defines the intersections of the affiliation and interdependence axes. For example, Kenneth's blaming involved focus on other that was hostile and controlling. Hence, in this figure, it is represented by **III. Hostile power.** From Benjamin (1979). Copyright 1979 by the William Alanson White Psychiatric Foundation. Reprinted by permission.

Dimension 3: Interdependence

Since Kenneth was focused on other, his interdependence would be classified on the vertical dimension ranging from **Control** (at the lower end of
the vertical dimension in Figure 4.1) to **Give autonomy** (at the upper end).
Kenneth's efforts to control his wife would place him at the control (lower)
end of the vertical scale.

The Three Dimensions to Yield Classification on the SASB Model

These three decisions have shown that Kenneth was (1) focused on other,
(2) hostile, and (3) controlling. Together, they would place him on Figure
4.2 in the lower left-hand quadrant of the "focus on other" group, labeled
III. Hostile power.[11]

How SASB Classification Differs from Inspection of Categories

Note that the category **hostile power** was not chosen by inspection. For
most other coding systems, the coder looks at an event, scans the possible
categories, and casts the event into one of them. A vitally important distinctive feature of SASB is that classification is instead determined by the
three-step process just described. To review: Decision 1, about focus,
placed Kenneth in the top third of Figure 4.2. Decision 2, about affiliation,
placed him on the left-hand side of that upper section of the model. Decision 3, about interdependence, placed him in the lower half of the space
identified by decisions 1 and 2.

This three-step dimensional analysis allows SASB to unpack very complex communications, and sometimes to yield multiple categories for a single event. Typically, the multiple categorical descriptions in these complex
contexts bring clarity to what otherwise might seem unfathomable. An
example is the SASB coding of Bateson's "double bind" or Wynne's
"pseudo-mutuality," each of which is defined and dissected into underlying
dimensionality by Humphrey and Benjamin (1986). An introduction to
complex coding is provided in Appendix 4.1.

How Coding Can Be Applied to the Therapy Narrative, Process, and Indirect Process

The case formulation comes largely from codes of the *content* of the stories
the patient tells. For example, Marie described herself as a PROTECTer,
whereas Kenneth's story suggested that his mother mounted a campaign of
BLAME to force his father to return. While coding the content of the narrative, the clinician simultaneously tracks the therapy *process*. For example,

Marie's position in relation to the interviewer was one of friendly dependency (<u>TRUST</u>); Kenneth was quite interested in CONTROL (at one point, he asked that the video camera be turned off, and the interviewer complied). Finally, the therapist can make note of *indirect process*—that is, process in relation to someone who is not present. For example, Kenneth's narrative was saturated with indignation directed at his wife, who was not present. Interviewers who track content, process, and indirect process in terms of SASB dimensionality have an accurate and comprehensive awareness of important interpersonal processes.

How Coding Can Define Red and Green Empathy

Red empathy reflects the dimensionality of the patient's maladaptive statement in pure form. Green empathy would add something else[12] to the message from the core algorithm. Here are SASB-based analyses of some of the examples of Red empathy that might have been given to Kenneth (see Chapter 3):

• "Her lying made you furious." The therapist might have reminded Kenneth of one of the behaviors that Kenneth was angrily trying to change in his wife. It would reflect his hostile, controlling focus.

• "She was a sneak." Hostile control would be represented in process as well as content in this example. The therapist would implicitly[13] have joined Kenneth in angry judgment of his wife

• "Your marital contract was violated."[14] Again, the therapist would both have reflected Kenneth's angry judgment of his wife, and also appeared to agree with him. If the therapist had instead said, "You feel that she violated your marital contract," the therapist would have distanced him- or herself a bit from Kenneth's opinion. In that case, the therapist would merely have reflected Kenneth's view, and not engaged in indirect process toward the wife.

THE CLUSTER MODEL

Overview of the Quadrant, Cluster, and Full SASB Models

The quadrant model is very helpful in codifying the "feel" of an exchange. Greater degrees of resolution are made possible by using the scale markers in Figure 4.1 to create more exactly defined categories. The most extreme level of detail is shown in the full SASB model (Appendix 4.1, Figure 4A.1). According to the full model, possibilities for describing Kenneth's hostile controlling focus on his wife would include **138. Enforce conformity; 137. Intrude, block, restrict; 136. Put down, act superior; 135. Accuse, blame; 134. Delude, divert, mislead; 133. Punish, take revenge; 132.**

Rip off, drain; 131. Approach menacingly. The details of how to generate these full-model categories are presented in Appendix 4.1. They are listed here simply to show that hostile control can be broken up in a variety of ways,[15] each with discernibly different meanings.

The SASB cluster model offers an alternative that is midway in complexity between the full and quadrant models. The cluster model provides enough differentiation among categories to permit more refined understanding, and yet it is relatively simple to use. The cluster version has been applied in an earlier book (Benjamin, 1996a) to provide precise interpersonal descriptions of the DSM-IV personality disorder categories. The present explanation of features of the SASB model is also based on the cluster model. The reader who would prefer to use the quadrant model will find that principles described here for using the cluster model can be generalized directly and easily to the simpler quadrant version.

Brief Description of the Cluster Model

The cluster model appears in Figure 4.3. The three types of print in Figure 4.3 mark the three types of focus shown at the top of Figure 4.1. BOLD print indicates transitive focus on other. UNDERLINED print indicates intransitive focus on self. *ITALICIZED* print indicates transitive focus turned inward upon the self.

As in all SASB versions, the horizontal axis in the cluster model runs from maximal hostility on the left to maximal friendliness on the right. The vertical axis runs from maximal enmeshment at the bottom to maximal differentiation at the top. For example, if there is transitive focus on other, the point for maximal enmeshment is CONTROL. If there is intransitive focus on self, the point for maximal enmeshment is SUBMIT. EMANCIPATE and SEPARATE represent the differentiation poles of the cluster model.

In the cluster model, there are categories that are composed of combinations of the basic underlying dimensions. For example, PROTECT, shown in the lower right-hand part of Figure 4.3, combines CONTROL and ACTIVE LOVE in about equal amounts. Among other things, the analysis of protective behavior in terms of underlying dimensions suggests that those who eschew any form of therapist control might reconsider that assumption. Friendly control is very important in therapy, especially in therapy with nonresponders.

PREDICTIVE PRINCIPLES

The predictive principles specify likely relations among interpersonal and intrapsychic positions. They describe specific possibilities for copy process links.

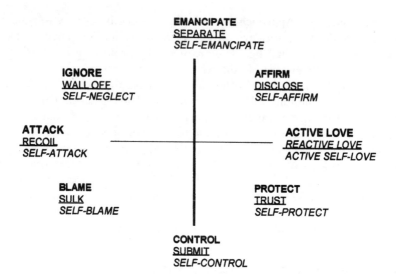

FIGURE 4.3. The simplified cluster version of the SASB model. The horizontal (affiliation) axis runs from maximal hostility on the left to maximal friendliness on the right. Variations in focus affect the nature of the affiliation. If the focus is on other (**BOLD**), the range in this axis is from **ATTACK** to **ACTIVE LOVE**. If focus is on self (<u>UNDERLINED</u>), the range in affiliation is from <u>RECOIL</u> to <u>REACTIVE LOVE</u>. If focus is turned inward (*ITALICIZED*), the range of possibilities is from *SELF-ATTACK* to *ACTIVE SELF-LOVE*. The vertical (interdependence) axis runs from maximal enmeshment to maximal differentiation. In addition to these categories located on the horizontal and vertical poles of the model, there are categories that combine the basic underlying dimensions. For example, the category **PROTECT** combines **CONTROL** and **ACTIVE LOVE** in about equal amounts. Its geometric and psychological opposite, **IGNORE**, combines the underlying opposites, **ATTACK** and **EMANCIPATE**. Other features are discussed in the text. From Benjamin (1996a). Copyright 1996 by The Guilford Press. Reprinted by permission.

Complementarity

Every adjacent pair of **BOLD** and <u>UNDERLINED</u> points in Figure 4.3 is complementary. The pairs are matched exactly on the affiliative and interdependence dimensions, but are complementary in focus. Foci are complementary if a member of a dyad is focused on other, and the partner is focused on self. For example, if Kenneth focused on his wife and his wife focused on herself, then Kenneth and his wife would be focusing on the same person. If two people have complementary focus and are matched exactly on affiliation and interdependence, they are fully complementary.

If Kenneth's wife were to complement his **BLAME**, she would <u>SULK</u>; this lies within the domain of <u>III. Hostile comply</u>, according to the quadrant model (see Figure 4.2). Kenneth's ongoing blaming suggested that he had faith in complementarity. His plan was that his wife would give up her autonomy and submit to his demands that she return and comply with his marital expectations. A slightly less hostile version of Kenneth's plan would be shown by the complementary pair on the cluster model: Kenneth CONTROL, wife SUBMIT.

There are eight sets of complementary behavior shown in Figure 4.3. Pairs in complementary relation are likely to be stable. For example, if a husband BLAMEs and a wife SULKs, they are more likely to stay together than if either of them does something else.

Complementarity has long been recognized intuitively, but was first discussed in the context of interpersonal modeling by Carson (1969). The validity of complementarity has been contested during the past three decades, but the SASB-based definition of it has survived harsh empirical tests (e.g., Gurtman, 2000; Benjamin, 1994).

Introjection

Every *ITALICIZED* point in Figure 4.3 represents introjection. The introject points plot the expected result of turning transitive action upon the self. Consequently, matching[16] BOLD points specify the predicted antecedents. For example, a person who engages in *SELF-BLAME* is predicted to have or to have had an IPIR who engaged in BLAME. A person who takes good care of him- or herself (*SELF-PROTECT*) is predicted to have or to have had an IPIR who engaged in PROTECT. Since correlational predictions go two ways, the figure also shows expected impacts of parental (or therapist) behaviors on the child's (or patient's) self-concept. For example, an inattentive parent (coded IGNORE) enhances the likelihood the child will ignore him- or herself (*SELF-NEGLECT*).

Opposition

Psychological and geometric opposites are shown at 180-degree angles on Figure 4.3. For example, the opposite of BLAME is AFFIRM. Whereas BLAME is saturated with hostile control, AFFIRM is characterized by friendly autonomy giving. With his exclusive focus on blame, Kenneth was as far away from affirming his wife as he could be. Figure 4.3 details 24 pairs of opposites. Two other examples are (1) PROTECT versus IGNORE, and (3) *SELF-AFFIRM* versus *SELF-BLAME*.

Similarity

Two people are similar if they can be coded at the same point on the cluster model. If a husband and wife each have to win and are characterized by BLAME, they are similar. Similar dyads show maximal instability.

Antithesis

An antithesis is the complement of an opposite.[17] This concept is important when trying to maximize the chances of obtaining a behavior that is the opposite of what is at hand. For example, suppose someone WALLS OFF (i.e., is in a state of being [focus on self] that reflects hostile autonomy). The principle of antithesis specifies an optimal stance to encourage a shift from hostile withdrawal to friendly compliance (e.g., TRUST). That would clearly be to PROTECT. To illustrate, a patient who is complementing perceived abandonment (IGNORE) and is off on his or her own too much is likely to become more socialized if given consistent, warm, moderate structure (PROTECT). Kenneth's wife showed angry withdrawal. According to this principle, his "best bet" would be to show loving, caregiving behaviors to her.[18] Kenneth, of course, was angry and focused on justice and control, so this way of behaving was unlikely.

There are eight sets of antithetical interpersonal behaviors shown in Figure 4.3 as opposite BOLD and UNDERLINED points. For example, REACTIVE LOVE is the antithesis of ATTACK. Eight more antithetical sets are shown between *ITALICIZED* self-concept points and opposite BOLD focus-on-other points. For example, if a small boy affirms himself for his nice painting (*SELF-AFFIRM*), but his parent belittles it (BLAME), he is more likely to feel badly about his painting and himself (*SELF-BLAME*).

Predictive Principles as Statements of Probability Only

Any given predictive principle is not always actualized. Without knowledge of an individual's interpersonal habits, it is not possible to be sure which, if any, of the predictive principles he or she will show in a given situation. Nor is it possible to predict which of the principles may foreshadow a child's habits in adulthood. For example, an abused child may find an abusive partner (recapitulate a complementary position), become an abusive parent (identify with the parent's similar position), or neither. It is appropriate to think of the predictive principles as markers of likelihood.

Different characters will have different probabilities in response to a given interpersonal situation (Benjamin, 1996a). For example, a person with Passive–Aggressive Personality Disorder is extremely likely to respond to CONTROL with its antithesis, SEPARATE, or the closely related position of WALL OFF. By contrast, a person with Dependent Personality Disorder would show the principle of complementarity by SUBMITting to CONTROL. A person with Antisocial Personality Disorder might invoke the principle of similarity and meet CONTROL with CONTROL. Each of these representative persons is likely to invoke a different predictive principle in response to CONTROL. Although it is not clear which predictive principle will be invoked when one is meeting an unknown person, once the baseline patterns of personality have been identified, predictions on the basis of a principle can improve greatly.

Using Within-Subject Correlations to Estimate Strength of Predictive Principles

If relationships are assessed by the SASB Intrex questionnaires, within-subject correlations can be used to assess the percentage of variance shared by foci that are predicted to be related.[19] For example, Jessica's rating of her abusive brother's transitive focus on her (her ratings of him on the eight BOLD clusters in Figure 4.3) showed an r of .85 with her view of her intransitive reaction to him (her ratings of herself with him on the eight UNDERLINED clusters in Figure 4.3). Even though the relationship was abusive, she showed a strong tendency to react to his transitive focus as predicted by the principle of complementarity.[20]

Operation of Predictive Principles from Infancy through Adulthood

The validity of the predictive principles offers sensible support for DLL theory. On quick reading, one might conclude that DLL theory proposes that experiences in infancy set the lifetime patterns. This is not the case. Learning continues throughout the life cycle. If it did not, a psychosocial therapy would be impossible. However, patterns that are practiced in infancy and childhood set templates that are likely to be continually practiced and supported via the predictive principles in the years that follow. For example, an infant whose parents IGNORE him or her is likely to WALL OFF. His or her unresponsiveness makes it more likely that new acquaintances likewise will IGNORE him or her, further supporting the position of WALL OFF. To the extent that a child, adolescent, or adult can be frequently exposed to varying important figures (teachers, coaches, neighbors, etc.), the chances of developing new patterns are increased.

Using SASB to Assess Traits, States, and Situations

During his DLL consultative interview, almost every one of Kenneth's statements was coded as BLAME. If that held true in other contexts, Kenneth could be said to have a blaming trait. However, he might not be the same in other situations, and the interviewer did not attempt to assess how he was outside the context of his current preoccupation with his wife's infidelity. Hence, the present discussion of Kenneth as having a blaming trait would need to be confirmed by evidence that he did it in most other contexts. Although Kenneth was remarkably consistent in his stance during the interview, people usually show flexibility in the process and in the content of the narrative in an interview. Most patients describe a variety of relationships and situations, so that SASB coding provides a steady stream of changing information about a person's interpersonal and intrapsychic world. After a while, a set of baseline (i.e., most likely) positions is established. These may be considered to be traits.[21]

Copy Processes and the Predictive Principles

Identification

Identification can be shown by online codes suggesting that the patient is behaving like an IPIR. The SASB principle of similarity corresponds to identification. For example, Patsy's father attacked her viciously, and she attacked her children in a similar way.

Recapitulation

Recapitulation represents continuation of a complementary pattern in a new relationship. For example, Jessica complemented her siblings' IGNORE (full model: **126. Ignore, pretend not there; 125. Neglect interests, needs**) with her own WALL OFF (full model: 226. Busy with own thing; 225. Wall off, nondisclose). In her marriage, she maintained the same sense of disconnectedness with her husband, who like her siblings, was grossly inattentive to her needs and concerns.[22]

This principle frequently describes the tendency to repeat problem patterns in choice of intimate partners. The relationship may begin very differently, but eventually drifts to an old familiar pattern. For example, a man who suffered from parental neglect (IGNORE) may find a loving wife. Eventually his habit of WALL OFF will lead her to quit trying to connect, and she may begin to IGNORE him.

Introjection

Introjection is recorded when a person treats him- or herself as he or she was treated by others. For example, as noted above, Jessica repeatedly experienced her siblings' IGNORE. She showed marked *SELF-NEGLECT* (full model: *326. Fantasy, dream; 325. Neglect own potential*). This particular form of introjection can be summarized as follows: "If nobody cares about me, I don't either."

Antithesis and Opposition

The predictive principles of antithesis and opposition describe variations on simple copy processes. For example, a man may have had a father who engaged heavily in CONTROL, and as a result never sets limits on his own children (EMANCIPATE). In his opposition, he copies his father in negative image. Variations of this sort are discussed further in Chapter 6 (see Table 6.1).

Parentlike Patterns in Children, and Vice Versa

Note that patient patterns can be coded in the parentlike as well as child-like domain even if they were first practiced in childhood. For example, recall that Marie's patterns for adaptation were parentlike. Her mother showed TRUST in her to handle her father's aggression. Marie complemented her mother's childlike behavior with parentlike behavior as she acted to PROTECT her mother and siblings. She was a "parentified" child, and recapitulated that protective stance in adulthood.

THE PARALLEL AFFECT AND COGNITIVE MODELS

Cluster versions of an affect model and of a cognitive model appear in Appendix 4.1. They are designed to parallel the SASB model and along with it, systematically to plot the expected ABCs of any episode. For example, when Kenneth engaged in BLAME, the parallel affect model suggests he will feel **Scorn**, and that his cognitive style would be to **Condemn**, to judge unfavorably. When the predicted parallels are not found, defenses may be operative.[23] Whereas the SASB model itself has passed intensive tests of validity, tests of the affect model have not progressed far. Tests of the model for cognitive style are nonexistent. The SASB-based description of defenses (Benjamin, 1995) likewise is not at all validated. Nonetheless, these early drafts of parallel models are sketched in Appendix 4.1 for readers who might like informally to explore their validity in clinical practice. They do, for example, correspond reasonably well to the suggestions in Chapter 2 for drawing connections between patterns shown in relation to IPIRs (SASB descriptions) and some Axis I symptoms (affective and cognitive parallels).

USING THE SASB MODEL TO DEFINE
NORMALITY AND CLEAR THERAPY GOALS

Many psychodynamically oriented clinicians are reluctant to specify therapy goals. The idea is that each patient will make his or her own choices for how he or she wants to be. The therapy should be value- and culture-free. Behavioral and medical treatments, by contrast, focus sharply on the goal of reducing symptoms. The IRT therapist also strives to reduce symptoms, but the emphasis is on coming to terms with problem internalizations associated with the symptoms. Once the patterns associated with an IPIR are given up, they can more easily be replaced by normative behaviors, cognitions, and affects. As this happens, the symptoms are expected to abate.[24]

The IRT Therapy Goals

Appealing to the SASB model and its underlying emphasis on attachment as fundamental to development and survival, the IRT therapist presents clearly defined therapy goals of baseline friendliness with moderate enmeshment and moderate differentiation. On the SASB model, these patterns are described by the Attachment Group (AG) of behaviors. They include the three clusters on the friendly (right-hand) side of the cluster model (Figure 4.3), all three surfaces. Normal friendly, patterns are accompanied by pleasant affects and effective cognitive styles.[25] A normal friendly adjustment is also characterized by the ability to focus on another person about as often as one focuses on oneself.

By contrast, problem patterns are described on the left-hand side of the SASB cluster model. These are called the Disaffiliative or Detached Group (DAG) of behaviors. They are accompanied by unpleasant affects and maladaptive cognitive styles. Problem patterns also include extremes of enmeshment (too much CONTROL or SUBMIT; too much EMANCIPATE or SEPARATE). Imbalance of focus and inability to respond appropriately to context[26] are additional markers of problem patterns. It is true that normal individuals can show behaviors in DAG space, but the hostility is clearly limited by time and context. For example, a mother whose behaviors are generally in AG space, but who aggressively defends her children from a hostile intruder, would be normal.

The therapy goals, then, are (1) to diminish DAG behaviors and the extremes of enmeshment or differentiation; and (2) to enhance AG behaviors, as well as to achieve balance in focus plus the ability to respond to context. Using everyday terms understandable to the patient, the IRT therapist describes these interpersonal goals and the associated affects and cognitions (see the "goals speech" in Chapter 5, Table 5.1).

Although the therapy goals are set by the therapist and not by the patient, the patient has informed choice about whether to pursue them. For example, Kenneth's goal was to bring his wife to heel. That goal would not be compatible with IRT. Before agreeing to an IRT contract, Kenneth would be helped to understand that the therapist would not work to help him better control his wife. Rather, the goal would be, among other things, to help him learn to be more generally friendly and moderate in his expectations regarding control and submission. The hope would be that his wife might react favorably to this change, but the therapist would acknowledge to Kenneth that she might not. In that case, Kenneth nonetheless might find that these new patterns would serve him well in any future relationship.

The normal AG region of the SASB model also encompasses two types of normal marital/couple relationships: a traditional style and an egalitarian relationship. The traditional way of relating typically shows one partner with friendly control and the other offering trusting deference (lower right-hand side of the AG region in Figure 4.3). Traditional partners may reverse this pattern in different domains—as, for example, in a marriage where the husband is in charge of the money while the wife has more influence on what happens to the children.

The lower part of Figure 4.4 includes this friendly version of an enmeshed relationship. There it is suggested that two enmeshed individuals come together to make a whole. Neither is complete without the other, but one can be larger than the other. It is important to note that enmeshment can be friendly (coded in the lower half of the AG region) or hostile (coded in the lower half of the DAG region). It is common in clinical practice to think of enmeshment as pathological, but the SASB definitions suggest that friendly and moderate versions of enmeshment can be perfectly normal. By contrast, if a pair's enmeshed behaviors are better described on the hostile (DAG) side of the SASB model, enmeshment is pathological.

The upper part of Figure 4.4 includes a friendly version of a differentiated relationship. Here, two distinctly defined individuals choose to overlap to varying degrees. To the extent that their behaviors can be coded in the AG region of Figure 4.3 and represent friendly differentiation, they will show more overlap. If their behaviors are coded in the DAG region of Figure 4.3, they will show little or no overlap. Their relationship can be characterized in terms of hostile differentiation, and will be pathological.

A person can implement the goals of IRT within a large number of cultural traditions. An individual who clearly understands his or her patterns, where they are from, and what they are for has all the advantages of awareness and choice. Since the IRT goals are explicit and clear (see Table 5.1), it would be very unusual for a patient to begin IRT, only later to discover that the therapy model is inconsistent with his or her cultural values.[27]

Rationale for Setting Such Clear Therapy Goals

The rationale for taking such a clear position on what is normal and what are therefore the goals of therapy is based on evolutionary and attachment theories.[28] As suggested in Chapter 2, primates are group animals, and attachment is fundamental to survival. The SASB model presumes to describe interpersonal and intrapsychic behaviors in terms of primary underlying dimensions[29] that serve adaptive purposes. Structure, physiology, chemistry, genes, and so on all relate directly to adaptive behaviors, affects,

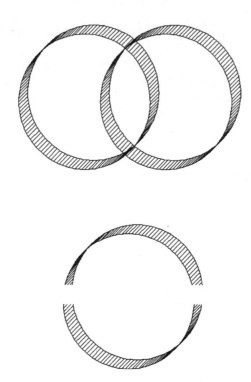

FIGURE 4.4. Two models of marital/couple relationships. At the top, two well-defined individuals choose to overlap to greater or lesser degrees. At the bottom, two enmeshed individuals require each other to be whole. Friendly versions of either pattern are included in the IRT therapy goals, while hostile versions describe problem patterns.

and cogntions. Behaviors shown anywhere on the SASB model can be interpreted as normal if they serve the evolved purposes of helping individuals meet their own needs while also being responsive to the needs of the community.[30] The importance of being able to relate well to others was summarized by Harlow when he said, "A lone monkey is a dead monkey."[31]

THE RELATION BETWEEN THIS
CHAPTER AND APPENDIX 4.1

With this introduction, perhaps the reader can interpret SASB-related footnotes in other chapters. He or she may also have a sense of how SASB technology makes it possible to assess and test hypotheses proposed by DLL theory and by IRT. Ideally, the reader also sees how the SASB model is used to increase the accuracy of therapy communications and to define therapy goals. If the reader wishes to know more about SASB, overviews that include proper acknowledgment of its intellectual history[32] appear in Benjamin (1974, 1984, 1996c). Additional themes are pursued in Appendix 4.1. It includes some uses of SASB that are frequently helpful to IRT; an introduction to complex coding; the full SASB model; and details about the affect and cognitive models that parallel the SASB cluster model.

NOTES

1. Intrex@Psych.utah.edu.
2. A list is provided on the Intrex Web site, which can be located by searching for "Intrex" or "SASB" within the web site for the University of Utah (http://www.utah.edu).
3. Examples include patterns of personality disorder and the likely interpersonal histories, as described in Benjamin (1996a).
4. Suppose the patient is asking for help, but give messages suggesting subtle "defiance." The Passive–Aggressive Personality Disorder diagnosis would become more likely. Hence the clinician would only respond to the request for structure by surrounding any suggestions with caveats and options. If the patient behaviors instead suggested Obsessive–Compulsive Personality Disorder such wishy-washyness would be a problem. In that case, the suggestions would be straightforward.
5. According to the *American Heritage Talking Dictionary* (1997), "transitive" means "Expressing an action that is carried from the subject to the object; requiring a direct object to complete meaning."
6. The common and unfortunate tendency to confuse listening with submission is discussed in Appendix 4.1.
7. According to the *American Heritage Talking Dictionary* (1997), "intransitive" means "Designating a verb or verb construction that does not require or cannot take a direct object, as *run* or *sleep*."
8. Sullivan (1953, pp. 164–171) cautioned against overly simplified descriptions of the origin of the self-system. According to him, the self-system is *in part* formed by incorporation or introjection of the "bad" mother's forbidding gestures that appear as the infant tries to meet his or her "zonal" needs. Introjection is only one of many methods the infant uses to avoid anxiety arising from, as Sullivan says, the need to live with this significant other person. Sullivan's interpersonal emphasis on self-development had a major effect on psychiatric theory. It seemed important to acknowledge his major contribution by using the same word he used to describe parentlike action directed inward. In Appendix 4.1, it is made clear that accurate descriptions of internalizations in terms of SASB require all three types of focus, not just introjection. This is in accord with Sullivan's arguments that the self-system's interpersonal origins involve more than introjection.
9. For example, the clinician may think, "This feels like hostile withdrawal. That

happened right after I said, 'Please give an example.' Perhaps I should ask how he feels about this conversation right now." The simplified cluster model in Figure 4.3 uses **BOLD**, <u>UNDERLINED</u>, and *ITALICIZED* font to distinguish among foci. The other models (e.g., full model; Figure A.1 in Appendix 4.1) do not because foci are distinguished by their location on space. However, to facilitate comparison among models, mention of particular points from any SASB model in the text will apply, the font style of Figure 4.3.

10. Only the three stick figures and the endpoints of the scales shown in Figure 4.1 are used to locate positions on the quadrant model.

11. The sectors of the quadrant model are numbered I, II, III, and IV, as is the custom in plane geometry. The full model is presented in Appendix 4.1.

12. An example would be teaching (cluster model: **PROTECT**; full model: **144. Sensible analysis**) about patterns, as shown in an example of Green empathy in Chapter 3.

13. In the formal coding system, the therapist would be coded in terms of hostile control toward the wife if she were present. If not, then the therapist's hostile control would be called indirect rather than direct. Investigators differ in terms of whether they wish to make a distinction between indirect and direct process. Clinicians need to know that a therapist's indirect process is almost always heard by a patient as if it were direct. For example, Kenneth might have told his wife that the therapist providing such a Red reflection agreed with him.

14. To code the wife as subject (rather than the marital contract), the active voice might have been considered: "Your wife violated your marital contract" rather than "Your marital contract was violated." The passive form would have been a better match for Kenneth's distant, legalistic style.

15. According to relative proportions of controlling and attacking behavior.

16. On affiliation and interdependence.

17. Or the opposite of a complement.

18. On the full model, **142. Provide for, nurture**, which is the opposite of **122. Starve, cut out**.

19. Within-subject correlations are, at most, measures of association. They are not suitable for hypothesis testing.

20. For example, she gave his **CONTROL** high ratings, and her own <u>SUBMIT</u> equally high ratings.

21. The Intrex questionnaires ask the rater to assess a series of relationships (situations) and if, appropriate, in different states (e.g., best and worst). Characterizations are made in terms of traits × situations × states.

22. The additional salient tendency to allow herself to be exploited requires a complex code. Complex codes are discussed in Appendix 4.1.

23. Or the parallel models may be invalid.

24. For example, a dysthymic patient may often <u>SULK</u>. This pattern is predicted to be accompanied by an affect of <u>Agitated</u> and a cognitive style of <u>Secretive</u>. These qualitative descriptors of aspects of depression should abate when the baseline interpersonal position is changed from <u>SULK</u> to behaviors on the friendly side of the SASB model. Figures 4A.2 and 4A.3 suggest that friendly behaviors are accompanied by more pleasant affects and more effective cognitive styles. Note that the parallel-models argument takes no position on directionality. Changes can be initiated by cognition, affect, or behavior.

25. As predicted by the parallel affective and cognitive models, presented in Appendix 4.1.
26. Impaired ability to respond to context can be reflected in rigidity, lability, or psychosis.
27. For example, oppression of others, as in the Ku Klux Klan.
28. It turns out that patients typically embrace with enthusiasm the IRT goals of AG behaviors and their associated pleasant affects and effective cognitive styles.
29. Hypotheses about how these dimensions might be encoded neurologically appear in Benjamin and Friedrich (1991).
30. Anger is not a primary energy that has to be expressed one way or another. Rather, it is an evolved mechanism for implementing control or distance. Both of these purposes are important at times, but they are not adaptive baseline positions. Destruction as a delight, and control as an ideal, are goals that may be adapted by persons whose attachment processes have gone awry.
31. Personal communication, 1958.
32. SASB incorporates the work of Schaefer, Leary, Sullivan, and many others (see Benjamin, 1996d).

Appendix 4.1

Supplementary Information about SASB and the Parallel Models

SOME COMMON DESTRUCTIVE MISCONCEPTIONS CLARIFIED BY SASB

Language reflects cultural understanding. Some common misconceptions about the meanings of words are relevant to psychopathology and psychotherapy. SASB coding can help both clinicians and patients grasp alternative meanings of easily misunderstood statements and make better choices. Here are some examples.

1. *Independence denotes hostility.* Differentiation from problem wishes in relation to IPIRs is a part of the treatment plan in IRT. If a patient believes that separation necessarily means hostility toward and alienation from loved ones, he or she is less likely to agree to work toward this treatment goal. However, a glance at the upper halves of each of the three sections of the quadrant model (see Figure 4.2) makes it clear that there are two types of independence: hostile and friendly. The SASB definition of friendly independence demonstrates that one can be self-defined and still relate in warm ways to others. If shown Figure 4.2, patients can be reassured that they can work toward the therapy goal of being free from old wishes in relation to IPIRs, and still be cordial to family members.

2. *If one is not in control, then one is being controlled.* "You always control everything. I wanted you to stay home and mow the lawn yesterday, and instead you went on a hike." Here the speaker assumes that because her husband did not defer to her, he controlled her. This perception is common among people who see the world in terms of just two positions: "You are the one in control, or you are the one being controlled." This view is likely in families that dwell almost exclusively in enmeshed space.[1]

Differentiation as described by the SASB model can help enmeshed people relate in new and better ways. Demonstrating (e.g., with Figure 4.3) that SEPARATE is not the same is CONTROL is very useful. If one person focuses on him- or herself as a separate person, that is not the same as telling another person what to do. Adding the notion that separation need not be hostile can provide great relief to persons struggling with how to be self-defined and still relate well.

Consider both hostile and friendly versions of the hiking husband who went on a hike instead of mowing the lawn. If he left while his wife was preparing dinner for guests he had invited for the evening, his separation would be hostile. If he was self-absorbed, it would be coded WALL OFF (full model: 226. Busy with own thing). If his leaving was focused on her ("I can't stand being around you"), it would be coded as IGNORE (full model: 121. Angry dismiss, reject). On the other hand, a friendly version of his leaving for the hike might be "I need to go on a hike to recover from work this week, and I will mow the lawn tomorrow." The hike would be coded SEPARATE, while his friendly explanation would be coded DISCLOSE. Performing the dimensional analysis of the hike in various contexts would help narrow the meaning of his taking a hike when his wife asked him to mow the lawn.[2]

3. *To listen amounts to giving in.* "Listen to me" is often used to mean "Do what I say." Children who receive this message will correctly hear it as CONTROL demanding that they SUBMIT. If they continue to believe that listening simply means submitting, they are unlikely to attend carefully to what others say. However, they can be encouraged to do more listening if they see on the SASB model how listening actively differs from submission. Listening is coded AFFIRM (full model: 115. **Friendly listen**) and is different from SUBMIT (e.g., full model: 237. Apathetic compliance). Friendly focus on other that accepts autonomy is not the same as hostile, submissive intransitive focus on self.

4. *Loving someone means doing what he or she wants.* "If you love me, you will do what I want." When people speak this way, ACTIVE LOVE or REACTIVE LOVE and SUBMIT are fused. This belief may cause members of a couple to defer to each other during courtship, believing that deference is a sign of love. Once the relationship is cemented by marriage, or otherwise becomes more routine or long-term, one or both partners may become less willing to defer and there is trouble. The SASB model places these concepts at right angles, which means they are unrelated. People can love without submitting, and can submit without loving. Unhooking these concepts can be very helpful to those who seek both to love and to be self-defined.

5. *Good self-care is "selfish."* Quite a number of depressed people believe that self-care is bad. As a result, they are unable to assert themselves, to plan self-nurturing activities, or even to tolerate good things happening to them as they progress in therapy. These folks' early training that encouraged the idea that self-care detracts from the good of others. The distortion involves confusing *SELF-LOVE* with exploitation, coded ATTACK in Figure 4.3 (full model: 132. **Rip off, drain**). A variation on this theme might be that *SELF-LOVE* means to IGNORE the interests of others (full model: 123: **Abandon, leave in lurch**). In either case, the idea is that taking care of oneself means taking away from others.

Sometimes self-care in fact is fused with exploitation—as it is, for example, by unscrupulous executives who misuse company funds to leave thousands of employees bereft of their retirement savings. However, there are many situations where self-care does not mean harming others, and patients need help learning to see the difference. If people are deeply interested in helping and serving others, it can be good to know that they must take care of themselves first in order to have more strength to serve others.

These examples show how use of the SASB model can help clarify common destructive misunderstandings. The main purpose of such clarifications is to challenge any associated motivations supporting the problem patterns. Again, consider the example of how a simple shift in belief about the meaning of listening can help the person become more collaborative.

COMPLEX CODES

If a message simply contains several components or elements, they are each coded separately and without complication. Consider this example: "You make me mad, and I am out of here." This sentence includes a BLAME and a SEPARATE that are distinct, successive messages. They can be registered separately and are called multiple messages.

Other messages have two or more components that are inextricably combined. They are called "complex messages." Using SASB, the clinician can extract their underlying dimensions to see more clearly what has been said. For example, suppose the therapist says, "I am not sure I can help you if you continue to make these suicide attempts." What is the message to the patient? The therapist's self-description is delivered in a warm and separate way, so it is coded DISCLOSE. But there is more. The patient can also hear autonomy giving and hostility in the focus on him or her. These are coded as IGNORE. So with this warm threat, the therapist is described by this complex code: DISCLOSE plus IGNORE. If the patient complements both components[3] of this complex message, he or she will AFFIRM and WALL OFF from the therapist. Perhaps such a therapist will welcome the affirmation and the break from hearing about suicide, but the therapy results are questionable.[4]

Using the SASB model to recognize the potential danger in giving such complex "warm" messages can help the therapist give cleaner messages. For example, if there are too many suicide attempts, the IRT therapist might say something like this: "Let's look at what is going on here. This is your second attempt in a month. Perhaps we are taking the wrong approach. Are you willing to look at this again and see if we can figure out how to address your needs in a better way?" This message is focused on the patient, is warm, and is controlling. It is coded PROTECT (full model: **143. Protect, back up; 144. Sensible analysis; 145. Constructive stimulate**). It ends with a request for collaboration, coded AFFIRM (full model: **116. Carefully, fairly consider**). This message has two clean components, and therefore is multiple rather than complex. First there is warm structure; then there is a request for collaborative work on the problem.

Complex coding skills are difficult to acquire, but worthwhile. Interested readers might consult Humphrey and Benjamin (1986) for further examples,[5] and the SASB coding manual (Benjamin & Cushing, 2000) for details about the method.

THE FULL SASB MODEL

The full SASB model appears in Figure 4A.1. Although it may look overwhelming at first, the principles are the same as those used to construct the simple quadrant version in Figure 4.2. The three dimensions of Figure 4.1 fully define the full model in Figure 4A.1, as well as the basic quadrant model in Figure 4.2. The only difference between the full model and the other versions (quadrant and cluster) is that the full model has finer degrees of resolution in defining the categories.

In the main text of this chapter, there is a comparison between the potential descriptions of Kenneth in the quadrant and full models. In the quadrant model, his behavior would be classified as **III. Hostile power**. The full model (see Figure 4A.1) offers nine different possible categories that are within that same quadrant of interpersonal space (focus on other with hostile control). The text of this chapter provides several other examples of using the full model to obtain better resolution. These appear in parentheses after the cluster or quadrant model classifications.

The only feature of the full model that has not already been discussed in connection with the cluster and quadrant versions is the numbering system that labels the full model's points. The 100s digits describe focus. Points with numbers beginning with 100 describe focus on other; those with numbers that start with 200 describe focus on self; finally, those with numbers that begin with 300 describe introjections. The 10s digits describe quadrants as labeled in Figure 4.2. They begin with 1 in the upper right-hand quadrant and proceed counterclockwise through 2, 3, and 4. Finally, the units digits describe the subdivision of the quadrant and range from 1 to 8. For example, **123. Abandon, leave in lurch** describes focus on other (100s), second quadrant (20s = hostile autonomy), third subdivision (units = 3, meaning it is three steps away from ATTACK and six steps away from EMANCIPATE). The axes naturally have a units digit of 0. The units digits are handy for tracking predictive principles. Opposite points will have the same units digit. For example, the opposite of **123. Abandon, leave in lurch** is **143. Protect, back up.** Complements are also easy to track via the units digit: The complement of **143. Protect, back up** is **243. Ask, trust, count upon.**

The full model makes the biological bases of the SASB model explicit. The poles are shown as poles, not as arbitrarily designated points on a circle. The polar points describe the "primitive basics" that underlie all other transactions, whether simple or complex. The respective poles are sexuality (110/210), power (140/240), murder (130/230), and separate territory (120/220). By so clearly naming these

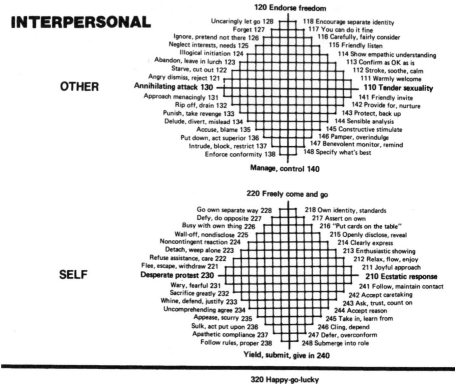

INTERPERSONAL

120 Endorse freedom

Uncaringly let go 128
Forget 127
Ignore, pretend not there 126
Neglect interests, needs 125
Illogical initiation 124
Abandon, leave in lurch 123
Starve, cut out 122
Angry dismiss, reject 121
OTHER   Annihilating attack 130
Approach menacingly 131
Rip off, drain 132
Punish, take revenge 133
Delude, divert, mislead 134
Accuse, blame 135
Put down, act superior 136
Intrude, block, restrict 137
Enforce conformity 138

118 Encourage separate identity
117 You can do it fine
116 Carefully, fairly consider
115 Friendly listen
114 Show empathic understanding
113 Confirm as OK as is
112 Stroke, soothe, calm
111 Warmly welcome
110 Tender sexuality
141 Friendly invite
142 Provide for, nurture
143 Protect, back up
144 Sensible analysis
145 Constructive stimulate
146 Pamper, overindulge
147 Benevolent monitor, remind
148 Specify what's best

Manage, control 140

220 Freely come and go

Go own separate way 228
Defy, do opposite 227
Busy with own thing 226
Wall-off, nondisclose 225
Noncontingent reaction 224
Detach, weep alone 223
Refuse assistance, care 222
Flee, escape, withdraw 221
SELF   Desperate protest 230
Wary, fearful 231
Sacrifice greatly 232
Whine, defend, justify 233
Uncomprehending agree 234
Appease, scurry 235
Sulk, act put upon 236
Apathetic compliance 237
Follow rules, proper 238

218 Own identity, standards
217 Assert on own
216 "Put cards on the table"
215 Openly disclose, reveal
214 Clearly express
213 Enthusiastic showing
212 Relax, flow, enjoy
211 Joyful approach
210 Ecstatic response
241 Follow, maintain contact
242 Accept caretaking
243 Ask, trust, count on
244 Accept reason
245 Take in, learn from
246 Cling, depend
247 Defer, overconform
248 Submerge into role

Yield, submit, give in 240

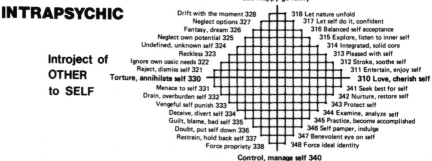

INTRAPSYCHIC

320 Happy-go-lucky

Drift with the moment 328
Neglect options 327
Fantasy, dream 326
Neglect own potential 325
Undefined, unknown self 324
Reckless 323
Introject of   Ignore own oasic needs 322
OTHER   Reject, dismiss self 321
to SELF   Torture, annihilate self 330
Menace to self 331
Drain, overburden self 332
Vengeful self punish 333
Deceive, divert self 334
Guilt, blame, bad self 335
Doubt, put self down 336
Restrain, hold back self 337
Force propriety 338

318 Let nature unfold
317 Let self do it, confident
316 Balanced self acceptance
315 Explore, listen to inner self
314 Integrated, solid core
313 Pleased with self
312 Stroke, soothe self
311 Entertain, enjoy self
310 Love, cherish self
341 Seek best for self
342 Nurture, restore self
343 Protect self
344 Examine, analyze self
345 Practice, become accomplished
346 Self pamper, indulge
347 Benevolent eye on self
348 Force ideal identity

Control, manage self 340

FIGURE 4A.1. Structural Analysis of Social Behavior (SASB): Full model. From Benjamin (1979). Copyright 1979 by the William Alanson White Psychiatric Foundation. Reprinted by permission.

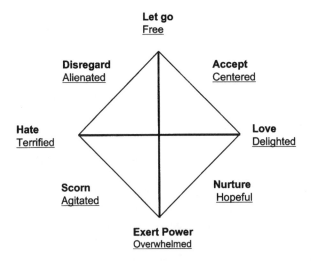

FIGURE 4A.2. Simplified affect model, SAAB.

primitive basics and showing that "higher-level" functions can be seen in terms of these givens, the full model makes explicit the evolutionary assumptions invoked by SASB. Further details about the full model are given in Benjamin (1974, 1979, 1996a).

THREE PARALLEL MODELS

DLL theory assumes that affect, behavior, and cognition evolved together, each serving the others. If so, and if behavior is well described by the SASB model, then it should be possible to construct parallel models for affect and for cognitive style. The first drafts of the parallel models appeared in Benjamin (1986). More recent versions were in Benjamin (1996b). Colleagues have tried empirically to test the structure of the proposed parallel affect and cognitive models.[6] Their good efforts to successfully revise the early drafts have failed to pass the dimensional ratings tests required for validation of SASB-related models (Benjamin, 2000).[7] For her dissertation, JuHui Park plans to test, revise, and empirically validate an affect model that arose from our combined efforts to cull appropriate affective dimensions from the literature in 2001.[8]

Despite the promise of that empirically based effort, I prefer to rely on integrative theory more than on dimensions reported in the empirical literature.[9] Therefore, the affect and cognitive models presented in this chapter attempt to better articulate and cross-compare the affective, cognitive and social dimensions described in Benjamin (1986). The present models have not been tested, but a very small pilot sample suggests they will survive dimensional ratings tests without a large number of revisions.[10]

The SASB model is presented in Figure 4.3. The parallel affective model, called Structural Analysis of Affective Behavior (SAAB), appears in Figure 4A.2. The cognitive model, called Structural Analysis of Cognitive Behavior (SACB), is in Figure 4A.3.[11]

Table 4A.1 presents the basic dimensions shared by the three parallel models; SASB, SAAB, and SACB. Table 4A.2 provides the names of the end points (poles) for the horizontal dimensions on the different models, while Table 4A.3 gives the names of the poles for the vertical dimensions.

Table 4A.1 suggests that when focus is on another person, the horizontal dimension for each model involves some version of **Hate** (left-hand side) or **Love** (right-hand side). The horizontal dimension is named the Affiliation (hate/love) dimension. The vertical dimension involves a position that ranges from **Make it happen** (lower part of the figure) to **Let it happen** (upper part of the figure). The vertical dimension is named the interdependence (Enmeshment/ differentiation) dimension.

Model Points are Defined by the Underlying Dimensions of Affiliation and Interdependence

To see how the underlying dimensions define the model points, consider **Understand** on the cognitive model (upper-right-hand part of Figure 4A.3). The generic dimensional ratings test based on Table 4A.1 would first have the rater judge

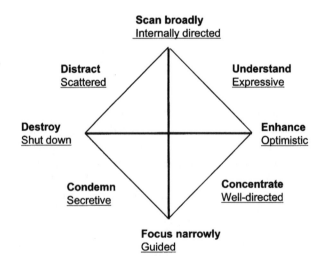

FIGURE 4A.3. Simplified cognitive model, SACB.

TABLE 4A.1. Dimensions Shared by Three Parallel Models

Horizontal dimension	Left-hand pole	Right-hand pole
Focus on other	**Hate**	**Love**
Focus on self	Hate	Love

Vertical dimension	Bottom pole	Top pole
Focus on other	**Make it happen**	**Let it happen**
Focus on self	Expect others to intervene	Do it on one's own

TABLE 4A.2. Horizontal Poles of the Dimensional Models

	Left-hand pole	Right-hand pole
Focus on other		
Affective behavior (A)	**Hate**	**Love**
Social behavior (B	**ATTACK**	**ACTIVE LOVE**
Cognitive behavior (C)	**Destroy**	**Enhance**
Focus on self		
Affective behavior (A)	Terrified	Delighted
Social behavior (B)	RECOIL	REACTIVE LOVE
Cognitive behavior (C)	Shut down	Optimistic

TABLE 4A.3. Vertical Poles of the Dimensional Models

	Lower pole	Upper pole
Focus on other		
Affective behavior (A)	**Exert power**	**Let go**
Social behavior (B)	**CONTROL**	**EMANCIPATE**
Cognitive behavior (C)	**Focus narrowly**	**Scan broadly**
Focus on self		
Affective behavior (A)	Overwhelmed	Free
Social behavior (B)	SUBMIT	SEPARATE
Cognitive behavior (C)	Guided	Internally directed

Understand in terms of the degree to which it invokes **Hate** or **Love** (horizontal dimensional judgment). Many would agree that it involves a moderate amount of **Love**. Next, the rater decides the degree to which **Understand** involves **Make it happen** or **Let it happen** (vertical dimensional judgment). Perhaps the reader agrees that **Understand**ing a person or an issue involves more "letting" than "making." These two judgments place **Understand** about where it is in Figure 4A.3 (in the **Love** direction, and in the **Let it happen** direction). Similar sets of horizontal and vertical judgments on the affect model would place the parallel point, **Accept**, at about the same location. The same result is obtained for AFFIRM, on the SASB model. The social behavior AFFIRM, the affect **Accept**, and the cognitive style **Understand** consist of approximately the same amounts of **Love** and **Let it happen**. The three parallel terms respectively emphasize the social, emotional, and cognitive components of an event that has the general dimensionality of focus on another person that is friendly and permits separateness.

The same procedures apply for the points that describe social behavior, affect, and cognition when the focus is on self. The general dimensions listed in Table 4A.1 for focus on self should apply to all model points for focus on self. For example, the point Centered, on the affect model (Figure 4A.2), should receive moderate ratings on the Love side. On the vertical scale, Centered should receive moderate scores in the direction of *Do it on one's own*. These ratings place *Centered* in the upper-right-hand part of Figure 4A2. Similar dimensional scores should be assigned to the parallel points on the SASB model (DISCLOSE) and on the cognitive model (*Expressive*). These three respective terms represent social behavioral, affective, and cognitive components of a position that is focused on self, basically friendly, and moderately differentiated.

A Given Word Can Apply to More than One Domain

There is substantial overlap among the domains of affect, behavior and cognition. For example, the word "love" has social, affective, and cognitive domains. Yet, if one thinks about "love," it is not difficult to associate it with specific social behavioral events, specific feelings, and specific thoughts. It is expected there are different neurological, neurochemical, and neurophysioloical events for these different facets. The construction of parallel models to codify these different aspects of a given episode is useful in therapy. For example, such explicit recognition of parallelism frees the therapist from having to subscribe to a given school of thought that may emphasize one domain (e.g., affect is favored in psychodynamic therapy) more than another (e.g., cognition is favored in cognitive-behavioral therapy).

Poles of the Model Should Define Axes Oriented at Right Angles

When the horizontal poles are given very high ratings on the horizontal dimensions in Table 4A.1, and low ratings on the vertical dimensions, the horizontal axis will be properly oriented. Then, if poles on the vertical dimension receive very high scores for the vertical, with low scores for the horizontal, the vertical axis will be upright and at right angles to the horizontal. For example, the point Terrified, located on the left hand-pole of the affect model, should receive very high ratings on **Hate** and negligible ratings on Expect others to intervene or Do it on one's own.[12] By contrast, Overwhelmed on the affective model should receive very high ratings on Expect others to intervene, and rather small ratings on **Hate** or **Love**.[13]

For another example, CONTROL on the SASB model should receive very high ratings on **Make it happen** and very low ratings on either **Hate** or **Love**. Understanding CONTROL in this way helps raters separate it conceptually from **Hate**. Adolescents, young adults, and individuals with Passive–Aggressive Personality Disorder are especially likely to see interpersonal control as hostile. Yet the models make it clear that CONTROL is neutral with respect to the **Love/Hate** dimension. A good example of neutral CONTROL is the societal agreement to create and obey traffic signals. Stop lights are obeyed for the common good, and few healthy people feel oppressed by them. CONTROL can even be loving, as in the highly structured directions given by Mission Control to astronauts under life-threatening difficulties on a mission in space. Nobody could doubt that the controllers in that situation care greatly about the people they are directing.

Such great variability in the potential uses of CONTROL relative to **Love** and **Hate** means that there is no necessary link between CONTROL and the **Love/Hate** axis. Of course, with a given individual or personality type, there definitely can be strong links between CONTROL and either **Hate** or **Love**. Individuals with Obsessive–Compulsive Personality Disorder, for example, are frequently very angry about the failure of others to comply. Some inordinately controlling mothers deeply believe their efforts are out of love. The fact that such correlations between hostility and CONTROL are easy to find does not prove that they are connected by definition.[14]

Midpoints are Defined by Model Points as Well as by Underlying Dimensions

Model points midway between the axes need to be rated relative to the poles that surround them, as well as by the basic dimensions of Table A4.1. For example, **Condemn** on the cognitive model consists, as required by Table 4A.1, of **Hate** and **Make it happen**. **Condemn** should be placed in the lower-left-hand corner of the cognitive model when rated by the polar points that surround it. It should be judged to lie in the direction of **Focus narrowly**, and in the direction of **Destroy** (Table 4A.3 and Figure 4A.2).

The Predictive Principles Apply to All Three Models

In addition to following dimensional rules just discussed, the affective and cognitive models should conform to the same predictive principles described for the SASB model. For example, a person confronted with ATTACK would be predicted by the SASB model to complement it with behavioral RECOIL Complements can be observed between models. If a feeling of terror arises in the victim, that complements the aggressor's ATTACK. The complementary cognitive style of Shut down (freezing, blanking out) also is frequently reported by individuals who survive life-threatening attack.

A scan of Figures 4A.1 and 4A.2 shows that the principle of opposition applies to them too. Examples from the cognitive model include **Destroy** and **Enhance** as conceptual opposites. **Focus narrowly** and **Scan broadly** also clearly are opposites. In the affect model, **Exert Power** and **Let go** seem opposed, as do, for example, Hopeful and Alienated. All points located at 180 degrees on any of the three models are conceptual opposites. The independent dimensional ratings tests by naïve judges will be the arbiters of this claim.[15]

Complex Codes are Appropriate for SAAB and SACB as Well as for SASB

The SAAB and SACB models can be used to describe complex affective or cognitive codes that complement complex SASB codes. For example, consider the affect predicted for the patient who gets the complex therapist message discussed in the section of Chapter 4 headed "Complex Codes": "I am not sure I can help you if you continue to make these suicide attempts." Recall this is coded in the SASB model as DISCLOSE plus IGNORE. SASB complementarity theory predicted the patient would respond with AFFIRM plus WALL OFF. The expected parallel affects for the patient (Figure 4A.2) should be **Accept** the therapist plus be Alienated from him or her. And the parallel cognitive model suggests the patient must **Understand** the therapist even as he or she is Scattered him- or herself. If this analysis is correct, it is even easier to see why the therapist's pseudo-niceness in dealing with the suicidality is destructive to the patient. As he or she is confronted with the complex job of affirming the therapist, while feeling alienated, collaboration is likely to be weakened.[16] No wonder complex codes are often associated with poor outcome. The clinician who masters complex coding is more likely to be able to give "clean" messages, even in a situation where his or her own feelings are quite complex.

NOTES

1. The perspective is so common that widely used versions of an interpersonal circle (Leary, 1957; Wiggins, 1982; Kiesler, 1983) include only enmeshed space. These models do not include differentiation in their underlying dimensionality, although some have an isolated segment that puts separation in hostile space.
2. The wife's approach to the lawn-mowing problem was unskilled. The example was chosen to introduce the topic of fusion of control and separation.
3. A clinician who carefully tracks clinical narrative will often see complex codes complemented component for component, as in this example.
4. Henry, Schacht, and Strupp (1992) have reported that therapists who use more complex codes have poorer therapy outcomes. In IRT, as in some versions of family therapy (Watzkawick, Beavin, & Jackson, 1967), carefully chosen complex messages can block maladaptive behaviors. Examples will be given in upcoming workbooks for IRT.
5. The IRT therapist learns to deliver complex codes that are therapeutic. Constructive use of constructive paradoxical therapist interventions is illustrated in Chapter 7.
6. Paul Crits-Christoph and Amy Demorest worked on the affect model, and John Paddock

worked on the cognitive model. It is clear that the drafts described in Benjamin (1986) were not adequate.

7. The dimensional ratings test asks for ratings of each item in terms of the hypothesized underlying components. The picture that results from many such judgments should agree closely with the theoretical model. Examples are provided later in this chapter.

8. JuHui Park completed an extensive search of the literature, and served as a rater of items and dimensions I selected from the material she gathered. She is coauthor on that version of the affect model.

9. A encouraging precedent is the fact that the SASB model deviated significantly from the models extant in the literature when it was first published. SASB's robust ability to survive many subsequent validity tests (sketched in Benjamin, 1996) suggests that it can be rewarding to let theory and reason have a dominant role at first, later subjecting those results to empirical test.

10. The reader can explore this claim by conducting his or her own dimensional ratings tests as illustrated in the discussion of the figures and tables below.

11. Some readers may notice that all three model names end with the word "behavior." Elsewhere in this book, ABC refers to affect, behavior, and cognition as distinct domains. In the ABC algorithm, "behavior" refers to interpersonal and intrapsychic behavior that can be coded by the SASB model. That very specific meaning of behavior is a narrow subset of events marked by general usage of the word "behavior" in Psychology. *The American Heritage Talking Dictionary* (1997) describes psychological usage for this word as: "The actions or reactions of persons or things in response to external or internal stimuli." This definition permits cognitive behavioral psychologists to deal with mental events called cognitive "behavior." Likewise, psychologists who study affect are permitted to use the term affective "behavior," even though affective events are not always observable. The reader likewise is asked to accommodate to the general dictionary definition of behavior when using the parallel models. The SASB, SAAB, and SACB models describe social, affective and cognitive "behaviors." When using the ABC algorithm, the referent of "behavior" is specifically restricted to interpersonal and intrapsychic events that can be described by the SASB model.

12. Perhaps the reader can see that the idea of being terrified in reaction to **Attack** could involve much or little of either Expect others to intervene or Do it on one's own. That variability, which will depend on situation as well as person, means that there is no clear association between Terrified and the vertical dimension. Such indeterminacy defines independence, and is shown geometrically by placing axes or vectors at right angles.

13. There can be semantic confusion from the thought "But if the position involves expectations of others, how can the focus be on self?" The answer lies in the formal definition of focus on self, namely, concern about what is to be done to, for or about the self. Here, expectations of others are specific to what will happen to, for, or about the self.

14. The complex topic of links among the many forms of hostility described by the three parallel models and wishes for control or distance will be discussed elsewhere (Benjamin, in preparation).

15. I am unaware of any other so-called circumplex model that uses dimensional ratings tests. Other modelers (see comparisons in Benjamin, 1996d) use factor analysis of self-ratings to extract underlying dimensions, and then reconstruct models based on factor loadings. SASB also has been tested by that method and does yield circumplex order, but not at perfect 45-degree angles. The dimensional ratings method has priority for SASB because it examines the dimensions of items, not self-described behaviors in people. The factor analyses of self-ratings contain more cultural contaminations, as, for example, when control is correlated with hostility in young American college students, but perhaps not in selected Asian cultures.

16. Complex codes within the affect model can account for affect words that seem to be missing. For example, "surprise" is a word that frequently appears in affective models. Surprise is a complex event that has different dimensions depending on the nature of the surprise and on the condition of the person before the surprise occurs. For example, suppose a depressed person is Alienated and Disorganized over the departure of a loved one. Suppose the loved one reappears unexpectedly. The surprise, then, is a combination of Delighted and Alienated, since the depressed person likely will continue to suffering from a certain degree of mistrust over the departure. It is not possible to locate "surprise" at a single point on the SAAB or SACB models. As usual, context matters.

5

Step 1: Collaboration

A primary function of the therapy relationship[1] is to enhance the patient's willingness actively to work at strengthening the Growth Collaborator (Green) relative to the Regressive Loyalist (Red). This is the optimal form of collaboration in Interpersonal Reconstructive Therapy (IRT). The therapy relationship also facilitates the development of a circumscribed attachment between patient and therapist, and this provides a secure base for exploring new, more adaptive patterns. This attachment encourages internalization of the IRT rules and values that the patient shall treat him- or herself and others in a fundamentally friendly, moderately enmeshed, moderately differentiated way. Drawing from the security provided by the therapy relationship, the patient develops the courage and ability to "defy" Red and implement Green (normative) behaviors in his or her relations with others. This results in greater success in ongoing relationships outside therapy.[2] As those relationships become more benign, their internalizations also begin to support normal patterns of behaviors, affects, and cognitions.

In this chapter, these principles about the role of the therapy relationship in therapy change are explored, starting with a careful examination of the role of attachment in collaboration in particular and the process of IRT in general.

ATTACHMENT IN IRT

Attachment has central roles in the Developmental Learning and Loving (DLL) theory of pathology and in IRT itself. In the first place, attachments that organize the problem behaviors are a main focus of the treatment. In the second place, enhanced attachments to others are among the explicit goals of IRT. Finally, as this chapter's opening paragraph suggests, attachment within the therapy relationship is an important part of the change process in IRT. Before discussing the roles of attachment in IRT, however, there will be a review of the research findings on the relationship between the therapy alliance and outcome.

Empirical Literature on the Therapy Alliance and Outcome

One of the more robust results in the therapy research literature is that a good alliance between patient and therapist is associated with a good therapy outcome (Horvath & Symonds, 1991; Martin, Garske, & Davis, 2000). Definitions of the therapy alliance vary. Most are consistent with Horvath's (1994b) conclusion that an alliance that facilitates good outcome involves a useful positive relationship between therapist and patient. The patient agrees to engage in therapy tasks and collaborate in setting realistic goals. Some investigators include the idea that when the outcome is good, the patient is confident in and hopeful about the therapy process (Hatcher & Barends, 1996; Frank & Frank, 1993). Interestingly, the patient's ability to disagree with the therapist also correlates positively with good outcome (Hatcher & Barends, 1996). Lists of additional patient characteristics that enhance or interfere with the alliance are long.[3] There are also some studies of therapist characteristics and the alliance.[4] The robust effect of the therapy alliance appears to be independent of the theoretical orientation of the therapy itself and is sometimes called a common factor.

The common-factors effect has been used as evidence of the power of psychotherapy (Norcross, 2002). It has also been cited in devastating criticisms of psychotherapy. For instance, Donald Klein (1996) reviewed the results of the National Institute of Mental Health (NIMH) collaborative study of depression (Elkin et al., 1989), which contrasted four treatment groups respectively receiving imipramine, a placebo, cognitive-behavioral therapy (CBT), and interpersonal psychotherapy (IPT):

> These findings (tentative and unreplicated as they are) are inexplicable on the basis of the therapeutic action theories propounded by the creators of IPT and CBT. However, they are entirely compatible with the hypothesis (championed by Jerome Frank; see Frank & Frank, 1993) that therapies are not doing anything specific; rather, they are nonspecifically beneficial to the final common pathway of demoralization, to the degree that they are effective at all. Presumably, this antidemoralization effect is initiated by having a strong, knowledgeable, professional ally who therapeutically provides the patient with emotional support, usable coping skills, and success experiences and helps reframe life experiences so as to heighten self-esteem. (Klein, 1995, p. 82)

In this and other versions of the controversy about psychotherapy versus psychopharmacological treatments of depression, there has been a tendency for each side to preach to its own choir. For an interpersonal approach like IRT, it is important to attend to the allegation that psychotherapy offers little more than what can be had if a friendly authority listens, gives good advice, and cheerleads.

One of many reanalyses of the NIMH collaborative study of depression noted incidentally that an alliance effect was observed even within the group that was given placebo medication (Krupnik et al., 1996). It should be noted that none of the treatments, including imipramine, was found to be superior to placebo,[5] and that over 40% of the placebo group showed clinically significant improvement (Ogles, Lambert, & Sawyer, 1995; Benjamin, 1997). These observations on the power of placebo, plus the finding that there was a significant association between alliance and outcome within the placebo group, are very interesting. Clearly something good happens within placebo groups, and it is related to the therapy alliance. One could ask: Is an alliance effect "only" a placebo effect, or is the placebo effect a result of interpersonal process inherent in a helping relationship?[6] And even if that process is a "hope and faith" effect, how and why does it work?

These observations about the effectiveness of placebo notwithstanding, a meta-analytic study of the research literature has established that the effects of psychotherapy generally surpass whatever is accomplished within groups receiving placebo alone (Grissom, 1996). In other words, therapy effects are usually larger than placebo effects. The accepted fact that no one psychotherapy treatment is better than any other (Luborsky, Singer, & Luborsky, 1975) does not vitiate that conclusion.[7] Clearly there remains a need to better detail and document the effects and interactions among placebo, alliance and therapy technique. In any effort to separate the effects of IRT (or any other) technique from the alliance, and/or placebo factors, there will need to be appropriate control groups,[8] along with measures of alliance that include the hope and faith perceptions.[9]

The Importance of Both Alliance and Technique to IRT

The working assumption in IRT is that a strong alliance, including any placebo or hope and faith effects, is a necessary but not sufficient condition for change. According to DLL theory, the attachment "circuits"[10] of patients with treatment-refractory disorders have been preoccupied with following the rules and values of Important Persons and their Internalized Representations (IPIRs). It is assumed, given the record of these so-called nonresponders that no new acquaintance (charismatic therapist or not) is going to outweigh these attachments in the long haul. To affect the internalizations constructively, well-focused technical interventions (as pictured in Chapter 3, Figures 3.1, 3.2, 3.3, and 3.4) are needed. Alliance or hope and faith in the therapy alone cannot release nonresponders from their old loyalties. On the other hand, these factors are surely components of collaboration, which is required to implement the IRT techniques.

How and Why Attachment Facilitates Change in IRT

Brief Summary of the Functions of Attachment in IRT

The alliance, including any placebo effect, helps the patient engage with hope and faith in the worth of IRT tasks. It helps the patient become increasingly active in implementing the core algorithm.

Alliance may also include a bonding component, which involves some version of attachment. In a longer-term treatment, an attachment has time to develop. When this happens, the therapist can provide a secure base from which the patient is more likely to be able to deal with the fear of changing and trying new ways of being. The patient will choose to follow the new rules and values discussed and modeled by the therapist, not only because they make sense, but also because implementing them meets with affirmation from the therapist.[11] Eventually this process yields internalization of and psychic proximity to the therapist. As the patient tries behaviors that are modeled, discussed, and supported in these ways, he or she succeeds in creating better relationships outside of therapy.[12] Then the new ways of relating are sustained on their own merits. This sequence replicates the process of normative socialization. When copy processes initiate normative ways of being, these friendly patterns are constantly supported by satisfying interpersonal interactions and need not be sustained by a fantasy relationship with an internalization.[13]

This brief summary of the vital role of the therapy relationship in IRT includes propositions about attachment that may raise questions in the mind of the reader. It is important to be unambiguous about what is and what is not being proposed. To help clarify these points, the subsections that follow provide precise definitions of attachment, plus relevant clinical observations and references from the literature.

Formal Definitions of Attachment

Cassidy (1999) explains that attachment *behavior* facilitates proximity to the attachment figure, while an attachment *bond* is an internalized "bond that one individual has to another individual who is perceived as stronger and wiser. A person can be attached to a person who is not in turn attached to him or her" (p. 12).

The *American Heritage Talking Dictionary* (1997) definition of attachment is quite intense: "The condition of being closely tied to another by affection or faith: love, bond, tie, loyalty, affection, devotion, fondness." Many patients in dynamically oriented psychotherapy do say that it is an intimate, highly personal, very intense experience.

Differences between Therapy and a Love Relationship

Although therapy and a love relationship can be equally intense at times, the therapist and patient should take great care not to confuse the two. Some patients will attempt to turn therapy into a love relationship for reasons based on their templates. In pursuing this Red goal, such a patient may appeal to a therapist's wish to be seen as a loving person. The therapist should be aware that being a kind and tolerant person[14] is appropriate in IRT. However, being a loving person[15] is not part of the therapist's baseline position. Most especially, therapy relationships are not and should not be intimate in the sexual sense.[16] Present ethical constraints appropriately prohibit that.

Nonetheless, many of the other dictionary descriptors of intimacy do apply to the therapy relationship. For example, familiarity is implicit in the discussion of deepest inner thoughts and feelings. The relationship is private, and the therapist, among other things, is a confidant. Many patients naturally develop feelings of affection for their therapists simply because of this intimacy, which is facilitated by the therapists' attentive and caring manner. A connection between intimacy and attachment seems natural. Despite these resemblances, the differences between therapy and a love relationship are significant and extend beyond the prohibition against sexuality:

• The therapy relationship is severely constrained by controls on time and space. In a normal love relationship, the partners' relatively free accessibility to each other is important.
• The therapist focuses exclusively on the patient and not on him or herself, except as that might facilitate the patient's development. In a normal love relationship, the focus goes both ways: Each focuses on the other, and on him- or herself in about equal amounts.
• The patient pays the therapist a fee. The fee meets the therapist's major needs, and the service meets the patient's major needs. The patient is expected to pay the bill, and the therapist is expected to provide helpful and meaningful service. In a normal love relationship or close friendship, the exchanges are more flexible and usually balanced in kind. Nothing is "expected" or "deserved," as is the case in a therapy contract.

If these remarks do not suffice to establish that therapy is not a love relationship, consider how unfair it would be to think of it that way. The patient only knows the therapist in the role of therapist. He or she is quite uninformed about the therapist as a person outside of the therapy context.[17] For example, how does the therapist behave when his or her dearest beliefs or feelings are being challenged? In therapy, it is inappropriate for the therapist to speak of such concerns. In a normal relationship, it is often inappropriate not to speak of them. What about the therapist's ability to take personal risk and disclose some of his or her vulnerabilities? In therapy, it is rarely appropriate to do that. In a normal and viable intimate relationship, it is inappropriate not to do that. In these and many other ways, there are important discrepancies between a therapist's behavior in therapy and the therapist's behavior in everyday life. There should be.[18] So the patient who loves the therapist as a potential romantic partner "knows not whereof he [or she] speaks." The attachment appropriate to IRT follows a very different model.

Internalization of the Therapist

Although rarely discussed in the literature (outside of psychoanalysis), the process of internalizing the therapy relationship is easily observed in ongoing therapy. As the patient begins to handle situations differently, he or she deliberately recalls discussions of these problems in therapy and uses what was learned there as guidelines for new patterns. It is not unusual to learn that change was accomplished by self-talk that goes like this: "I wonder what [therapist's name] would say now." The memory of the therapist's words and ways of looking at things serves as a concrete model that helps the Growth Collaborator prevail.

Therapists are not the only people to be internalized during therapy. The wisdom and ways of lovers, close friends, teachers, and others are incorporated too. Internalization probably occurs throughout the life cycle, but it may be more potent early in the developmental cycle than in adulthood. Like language learning, internalization is probably faster and more firmly encoded in early childhood. In adulthood, more practice is needed, and the new habits are more easily forgotten unless nurtured by frequent reactivation. Although I know of no studies of internalization during adulthood, I believe that influence and warmth (the benevolent teacher's position) facilitate it.[19]

Initial Support for New Behaviors via the Wish to Please the Therapist

The therapist serves as an effective advocate for the patient's Growth Collaborator. When the Regressive Loyalist "acts up," the attachment to the therapist can help the patient resist the wish to behave in old ways. Suppose the patient is struggling (self-management; see Figure 3.1) not to lose his or her temper, or not to engage in self-cutting, or not to get drunk. If he or she feels the therapist's advocacy and caring, and also is concerned about what the therapist thinks, it will be easier to resist the call of the Regressive Loyalist. Wanting the affirmation of the therapist is one reason it can be important for a patient to discuss any "backsliding" in great detail in the next therapy session. The discomfort in having to share the episode with someone the patient cares about can serve as a deterrent next time. Of course, discussing the episode should also facilitate learning about triggers to and consequences of engaging in unwanted behaviors.

The Therapist's Role in Encouraging Normative Behaviors

An intense, well-focused, longer-term relationship can start the process of forming better relationships in several ways. First, the therapist encourages and supports positive exchanges in the patient's ongoing relationships. In addition, the therapist's own behavior provides a model for friendly focus on another person. Unless new behaviors are matched to a reasonable degree by other people in the patient's world,[20] they may fade as the old ways reemerge. Realistic support for positive change in the patient's current relationships is very helpful in the effort to transform the old templates in relation to earlier IPIRs.

Does Attachment to the Therapist Facilitate Destructive Dependency?

The fear that attachment to the therapist may create crippling dependency is warranted only if a therapist actually does encourage it. In that case, the therapist is facilitating the Regressive Loyalist and is not IRT-adherent. By contrast, a therapist who supports the Growth Collaborator celebrates strength and independence in every possible way. Developmental data and theory assure that a healthy attachment is one that fosters independence and personal strength.

Independence from the therapy attachment is facilitated by the clear definition of the therapy tasks and goals (see later discussion). It is also facilitated by the formal structure of and constraints on the therapy relationship; by the unambivalent recognition on the part of both participants that this is not a love or familial relationship; and by the fact that independence from therapy is expected and obviously appropriate.

Testing Hypotheses about the Role of Attachment in Therapy Outcome

Therapy improvement, then, is partly implemented through a clearly constrained version of attachment to the therapist and the associated therapy rules and values. It is consolidated, maintained, and expanded by better experiences that follow in the patient's life. These hypotheses about connections between the therapy relationship and change could and should be checked. An initial study might debrief patients to see whether (and, if so, how) they attribute any behavior changes to the therapy. If they no longer cut or burn themselves, lose their temper, miss work, and so on, they may be able to describe their present mental processes and any associated changes in relation to internalizations of early IPIRs. For example, such a patient may say, "I know that my suicidal attacks always are set off by reminders of rejection by my siblings. Now I usually can stop the wish to die by thinking about its connection to their hatred of me."

A patient who remains more attached to destructive internalizations than to the therapist and his or her advocacy for the Growth Collaborator may say instead, "When I start to feel suicidal, I know [therapist's name] would want me to look at what happened and how I felt. He [or she] would ask me to look at how it might relate to my relationship with my father. But I really think my father was right. I am worthless."[21] Presumably, patients who continue to talk this way show less symptomatic improvement. These are only a few examples that illustrate how the IRT concepts are amenable to testing and refutation by careful analysis of the highly specific case formulation and its clear implications for therapy process.

The Psychoanalytic Perspective on Attachment in Therapy

Blatt and Behrends (1987) reviewed the history of psychoanalytic thought on attachment to the therapist. Although the subject is controversial, some psychoanalysts argue that introjection of the therapist is essential for therapeutic change. Blatt and Behrends (1987, p. 283) concluded that the therapy relationship is essential in this way, but they added that interpretation—a principal tool for intervention in psychoanalysis—is also required. These reviewers explicitly compared the therapy relationship and the normal developmental trajectory between mother and child. First there is attachment, and then there is differentiation. Examination of the theoretical differences between the DLL view and the psychoanalytic view of mechanisms for internalization is beyond the present book's scope. The point here is that some psychoanalysts have long emphasized of the role of attachment in therapy.

COLLABORATING IN IRT TO ACHIEVE CLEAR THERAPY GOALS

Therapy goals are made explicit early in treatment. After helping to shape the case formulation, the patient understands what is Red, and agrees to diminish it and to increase Green. Red is defined in terms of copy process links between problem patterns and IPIRs. Green is defined by the absolute norms developed in Chapter 4, which can be summarized as having a friendly baseline with moderate degrees of enmeshment and differentiation. Focus on self and other is equally distributed, unless therapy roles require an imbalance—as when the therapist focuses mostly on the patient. In addition, hostile behaviors, or extremes of enmeshment or differentiation, may be appropriate in limited contexts (as explained in the section on IRT goals in Chapter 4).

Table 5.1 provides a "goals speech" that details Green behaviors along with the expected parallel affects and cognitions.[22] These, like the copy process, gift-of-love, and learning speeches discussed in Chapter 2, are prototypes. They summarize the ideas that the clinician weaves into a narrative specific to each individual. Table 5.2 details the behaviors, affects, and cognitions that characterize Red functioning. It is recommended that the goals in therapy as described in Tables 5.1 and 5.2 be discussed while the patient is completing the IRT therapy contract (see the sample contract in Appendix 3.1). The form of this discussion is up to the therapist and should be based on his or her judgment about what might be easiest for the patient to understand. Many patients like to have a copy of Figure 1.1, which depicts the constant Red–Green conflict. Some may want to have copies of Table 5.1 and 5.2.[23] Just as the case formulation is specific to each patient, the discussion of Tables 5.1 and 5.2 should be tailored to each patient's needs and abilities.

For example, a conversation with Jessica about goals might indicate that the goals would be for her to become less walled off, self-attacking, and self-blaming; less likely to disregard and distract from her self-interests; and to be less troubled by her condemning voices. Instead, she would try to learn, along with everything else in Table 5.1,[24] to be more centered, hopeful, and self-loving; more optimistic; and better directed. Again, examples specific to Jessica would enrich the meaning of the speech for her. For example, the therapist could mention she might become less likely to

TABLE 5.1. Goals Speech: A Description of Green Behaviors, Feelings, and Ways of Thinking

"The goal of this therapy is to help you learn to relate to yourself and others in friendly and balanced ways that are neither too controlling nor too compliant nor too disconnected. Examples of goal behaviors are these: Affirm others and yourself. Disclose honestly to yourself and loved ones. Love others and accept love from them. Love yourself too. Protect loved ones and yourself. Trust.

"The goal ways of relating tend to be associated with feeling that you can: accept, love, and nurture. You can be: centered, delighted, and hopeful.

"The goal ways of relating tend to be associated with thinking that you can: understand, enhance, and concentrate. You can be: expressive, optimistic, and well directed."

TABLE 5.2. Supplement to the Goals Speech: A Description of Red Behaviors, Feelings, and Ways of Thinking That Are Expected to Diminish or Disappear If IRT Is Successful

The goal is that the following behaviors, if present, should become less likely: Ignoring the interests and well-being of others or self; walling off from others; attacking others or self; recoiling from others; blaming others or self; sulking; extreme tendencies to control, to submit, or to distance from others.

To the extent that these behaviors change, associated feelings should diminish: These include tendencies to: disregard, hate, or scorn others. To be: alienated, terrified, or agitated.

To the extent that these behaviors change, associated ways of thinking should diminish. These include tendencies to: distract, destroy, or condemn others. To be: scattered, shut down, or secretive.

believe she should disappear, and more likely to be fairer and kinder to herself. To assure collaboration on goals, the clinician says, "Does this sound like something you would like to work toward?" If Jessica disagreed, the conversation would continue until a goal acceptable to both Jessica and the therapist could be defined. This is not always possible.[25]

The Need for Consistency between the Patient's Goals and the IRT Definition of Normality

The overarching goal of IRT is clearly described: The patient will learn to function in Green ways. IRT is not appropriate for those who do not want to work toward that goal. As indicated in Chapter 4, IRT is not appropriate for individuals, families, or cultures that value baseline positions of absolute dominance of some people over others, aggression as a virtue, shunning as desirable, and so on. To illustrate, an IRT therapist usually will not accept for treatment[26] a wife who is depressed in reaction to culturally sanctioned beatings her husband frequently administers for her failure to perform to his exacting standards.

Example of a Person Who Was Willing to Change Her Goals to Those Suggested in IRT

Identification of cultural clashes with the goals of IRT is relatively easy. It is somewhat harder to deal with personal goals that may be common, but nonetheless are incompatible with the normative goals of IRT. Here is an example. A depressed elderly woman was seen by a student therapist skilled at supportive listening. The patient's sessions were dominated by stories about how unappreciative and neglectful her adult children and grandchildren were. When she was asked for further details, it became clear that the patient wanted her adult children to be with her all or most of the time and to include her in most of their social activities. She had no social life of her own and was painfully lonely when not with them. She let everyone know about this, and the children felt very guilty whenever they were not taking care of her. In short, this woman's ideal—her "treatment plan"—was wholly incompatible with the IRT norm that she could develop her Green and relate to her children in a less coercive, better-differentiated, and more friendly way.

A therapy that facilitated expression of her anger at her children would support her plan that she should be taken into the next generation's household. Her Regressive Loyalist would be in command of the plan to force her children to take care of her. IRT held that she needed instead to work on friendly differentiation and good self-care. She was not disabled in any discernible way, other than her presenting depression about her negligent children. She did tend to think about suicide as a way to let them know how seriously she needed their attention. A discussion of therapy goals and ways of achieving them was vital before treatment could begin.

The student IRT therapist was able to help the patient connect her expectations and disappointments to her experience with her own mother. She recalled how she had felt about her mother's demanding dependency, and then begin to consider developing her own social network so that she would not do the same to her children. She responded well to the therapist's offer to discuss how she might find peer group activities to help her begin to develop her own identity and ways of having fun with peers, independently of her children. It was expected that her ability to play with peers would relieve the pressure on the children, and that relations with them would improve greatly. The student therapist's academic term ended after 3 months of treatment, and so the therapy was terminated over the summer. When the student therapist was again available in the autumn semester, the patient said that she was better and did not need to return to therapy. It is not known whether she was able to sustain this new adaptation.

An Example of a Person Who Would Not Agree to Collaborate

Even if there are no cultural clashes between patient values and the IRT Green goal, patients are not always willing to consider changing their given preferences, and work toward the IRT goal of balanced friendliness. Here is an example where no such agreement could be negotiated, despite a 10-week trial of IRT. A husband wanted his wife treated for her rages. She rated herself highly on the Symptom Checklist 90—Revised Hostility Scale, but she saw no problem with her anger. She had always been seen in the family as the bright but difficult one who had a temperament like her father's. She remembered one time when her father broke all the living room furniture, including the TV, because she had behaved so badly. The father often had such rages. The family consensus was that the father's rages were the fault of the patient, and she was comfortable with that perspective. She dismissed therapy exploration of the idea that her rages might not be inevitable, and that maybe they had to do with her relationship with her father. There was no change in her raging in the marriage. She left therapy after a short while, correctly declaring that it was not doing any good. Because collaboration never was established, IRT could not begin.[27]

IRT STEP 1: COLLABORATING TO MAXIMIZE THE GREEN AND MINIMIZE THE RED

The preceding discussion suggests that collaboration in general includes forging an alliance that facilitates willingness to participate in therapy procedures aimed at achieving the Green goal. It may also include a placebo or "hope and faith" effect. In addition, collaboration invokes a limited version of attachment, which helps provide a secure base for change, and which facilitates new internalizations. Additionally, collaboration within therapy can provide a useful model for how to relate to others in friendly, moderately differentiated,[28] and moderately enmeshed[29] ways.

To some, it might make little sense apparently to speak of collaborating with the (growth) collaborator. Readers confused by that may find it helpful to consider three points.

1. In IRT, the Red (Regressive Loyalist) refers to a set of very specific behaviors, affects and cognitions described by the case formulation. The Green (Growth Collaborator) refers to a set of very specific behaviors, affects, and cognitions that are defined by the Green goals in Table 5.1. There is a conflict between the Red and Green, and the therapist tries to help the patient choose Green. The chooser, the patient's will, is neither Red nor Green.

2. In psychotherapy research, the meaning of the term collaborate is very broad. There is not universal agreement about its meaning, but at a minimum, collaboration includes willingness to work on the therapy task plus a relevant bond between patient and therapist.

3. It is quite possible to collaborate as it is generally meant in the literature, and not support choices to diminish the Red or enhance the Green. All that is required to fail to minimize Red and maximize Green, even while collaborating, is to have a different definition of the nature of the therapy task and of the therapy bond. For example, consider collaboration in Rogers's (1951) therapy, which proposes that unconditional acceptance, empathy, and positive regard are sufficient conditions for therapeutic change. It is possible to collaborate in those three therapy tasks, but

support Red rather than Green if the patient is discussing Red wishes and behaviors. Hence, collaboration in its general sense is not automatically Green. An IRT-adherent therapist tries consistently to collaborate in ways that enhance the patient's Green, but cannot achieve this all of the time.

Collaborative (step 1) therapy activities are listed in the first row of Figure 3.1, a summary of tasks related to the five steps of IRT. According to Figure 3.1, the main collaborative activity under the heading of self-discovery is "Disclose and listen to self." The main collaborative activity in the category of self-management is to engage Growth Collaborator. The core algorithm is used at every step of IRT, whether the activity is classified as self-discovery or self-management. The first three elements of the core algorithm are especially important in creating collaboration. These are as follows: (1) Work from a baseline of accurate empathy; (2) support the Green more than the Red whenever possible; and (3) relate every intervention to the case formulation.

Self-Discovery Activities

Using the Patient's Unconscious to Provide the Initiative

Whatever is on the patient's mind for the day directs the therapy session, and the therapist tries to follow along collaboratively. The therapist's job is to pick up the theme for the day and efficiently relate it to the case formulation and the treatment plan.

For example, Jill reported being exploited and criticized by her boyfriend. She felt inadequate and stupid in the relationship. At first, the IRT student therapist let Jill's resentment and anger about that dictate the flow of the session. Jill explained that the day before, her boyfriend had asked her to do a large number of errands. Although she too had a job, she did many of them. That night, he made no comment about her helpfulness, but only complained about the things that had not yet been completed. Jill declared that no matter how hard she tried to please him, something was always wrong. By empathizing and then asking for associations to previous familiar situations, the student therapist helped her link this pattern to her relationship with her older brother.[30] He too always expected favors to be completed and then criticized her for alleged shortfall. The student therapist asked Jill how she felt about this; she commented, "It convinces me that I am destined to be stupid, and that I am completely unable to do anything."[31]

Sharpening the Patient's Images

The self-criticism suggested that Jill needed to stop being loyal to her brother's rules and trying to "make it" with her internalized representation of him. Merely seeing the similarity did not engage Jill's collaboration to block Red and build Green. A more explicit connection, sharply reframed, might help her go beyond her Red condition. The therapist might say,

> "Sounds like you agree with your brother. He taught that you didn't do enough, and what you did was all wrong anyway. Now [name of boyfriend] says similar things. Sounds like even though you spent 2 hours of time on your boyfriend's errands yesterday, you buy his accusation that you did not do enough. I guess you agree that he was right and fair, and you get down on yourself for allegedly not doing enough for him, just as you used to agree with your brother. Is that right?"

The not-so-subtle phrasings here would help force a different perspective.[32] Consider the phrasing "I guess you agree that he was *right and fair.*" Fairness would be introduced to stimulate a more balanced perspective. Jill was getting down on herself for *allegedly* not doing enough. The added words would convey that the boyfriend's opinion was only an opinion, and not a fair one at that. The outrageously clear summary would make it very difficult for Jill to agree with her self-criticism. Sharing the therapist's perspective on her own story could enhance collaboration. A statement like this from Jill would be evidence of emerging collaboration: "Well, no. It wasn't fair. He had a lunch break and could have done some of it. And he never does stuff like that for me." This would create an opening for Jill to develop a more realistic perspective on her patterns with her boyfriend. That discovery might help her decide to change her devotion to her old rules.

Encouraging the Patient to Take Maximum Initiative for Self-Exploration and Management

The descriptions of IRT show that it is active and planful. This might suggest that the IRT therapist is controlling and directive, and does a lot "to" rather than "with" the patient. That impression would be inaccurate. The emphasis on the core algorithm, and the marking of the need for explaining and getting permission (see below), illustrate how this active and focused approach nonetheless emphasizes the patient's experiencing and choice. In reality, the IRT therapist is silent for a significant proportion of most sessions. He or she can be quite active when implementing the flow diagrams, especially in times of crisis. The rest of the time, the IRT therapist mostly reflects the narrative in ways that help keep the focus on the underlying Red attachments and support the work of the Green. An IRT therapist typically encourages the patient to take the active role. This is done by giving the patient time and space to proceed, once the overall structure of the therapy process is understood. The reason for this is simple: Active learning is far more effective than passive learning. However, if the therapy process starts to stray, the therapist nudges the process back onto the core algorithm, much as a canoeist might feather a paddle when drifting downstream.

Self-Management Activities

Asking Permission and Explaining

In the flow charts for coming to terms and exploring blockers to change (Figures 3.2 and 3.3), there is continual reference to the therapist's need to ask permission and to explain why something is being done. Asking permission and explaining are very important parts of collaboration. The IRT therapist does not confront or press on despite a patient's protest, as is characteristic of some brief therapies (e.g., Sifneos, 1979; Malan, 1976). If therapy is a learning process analogous to learning to swim, practitioners sing the more confrontive, anxiety-arousing approaches would seem to advocate that the best thing is to throw the patient in and let him or her discover that survival is possible.[33] The more collaborative orientation of IRT would hold that the patient needs to be coaxed to enter the water gradually, and to develop emotional as well as cognitive and behavioral understanding about what is dangerous and what is not. The patient also needs to be able to choose when to go to the next step. The collaborative perspective is implemented by asking for the patient's understanding and consent before changing the direction of the narrative in a big way. When the patient chooses to do so, that is an act of self-management.

Implicitly Training the Patient in IRT Procedures

Suppose a patient spends the first 15 minutes of the session on a minor concern after having stumbled onto a major but painful theme at the end of the previous session. The therapist might say, "Are you content with the way you are spending today's time?" That small inquiry is very likely to help the collaborating patient choose to go back to work on the troublesome theme of the previous session. Through repetition, patients become "trained" to implement the core algorithm, and to follow the flow charts in Chapter 3.

Consider this simple example: It is not unusual for patients participating in the DLL inpatient interview to stop and say in a playful way after the first half hour, "I know. You want an example." By then, they have been asked so many times for a concrete example that they already know rule 4 of the core algorithm (seeking details about input, response, and impact on self). This same sort of learning happens with the more complex aspects of IRT, like the flow charts in Chapter 3. I was reminded of how dramatic this change can be when some supervisees asked to see an outpatient therapy tape of mine. After securing permission from the patient for this specific use, I "randomly" selected a therapy tape and gave it to the trainees, with the usual warnings about when, where, and how the tapes could be viewed. The case had been described as difficult, and five previous treatments had proven unsuccessful for this patient. Of course, I did not tell the students about this history. Earlier in this therapy, there had been narratives of other incompetent therapists and occasional threats to commit suicide, to trash my office, and so on. This patient had been fiercely alienated from society in general, but by 3 years into therapy had made some good friends and had gone back to school to finish her degree. She did stay in therapy for almost a decade altogether (coming monthly for the last several years). She ultimately became successful professionally and enjoyed her marriage and friends.

Not knowing any of this, the students returned the tape the next week and said it was a great session with a very cooperative, high-level patient. They asked whether they could now see a therapy tape with a "hard" case. They observed that this patient, unlike theirs, was doing all the work. In short, the difficult patient had learned about good therapy process and was collaborating fully. I had done relatively little other than nod and reflect carefully throughout the session on the tape they had. The students were disappointed to see collaboration in action with a difficult patient. And I had not realized how dramatic the change had been.

Occasionally "Cozying Up to" the Red

Some patients agree generally to the therapy goal of being more friendly and loving, but still will not participate in treatment if the Red cannot control the process. They may discuss the past as well as the present, but may be reluctant to accept any accurate description of their current problem patterns. If they do not acknowledge their present patterns, it is not possible to discuss a case formulation that accounts for them. Some of these motivated individuals can use a brief trial of several sessions to try to engage the IRT process. They may be able to use largely Red sessions progressively seasoned with more Green to decide to acknowledge current problems, develop a case formulation, and work on coming to terms.

For example, consider the case of Carol, a secretary who brought her husband, John, a welder, for marital therapy to correct his many flaws. Carol qualified for the label Obsessive–Compulsive Personality Disorder, and her plan was to have John work toward her idea of perfection in relationship; she felt that this would result in a more loving relationship. John, whose mother also was controlling and blaming, came for two sessions, which he felt were not helpful. He refused to attend any more. John qualified for the label Passive–Aggressive Personality

Disorder. Carol and John represent the "demand–withdraw" pattern that is frequently seen in couples seeking treatment (e.g., Heavey, Layne, & Christensen, 1993).

After John refused to work in conjoint therapy, Carol then wanted to enter individual therapy to decide what to do. Ironically, she wanted more love, but her angry demands for it precluded success. Control repelled John, especially if it was hostile. Carol resisted the idea that her own patterns contributed to the marital difficulty. An IRT therapist does not necessarily confront such resistance.[34] Resistance after initial tentative attempts to switch the focus to the patient suggests that the Red psyche is dominant. In that case, there might be only a general allusion to the need to strengthen the patient's Growth Collaborator. If the procedures for developing a case formulation (Chapter 2) could gradually be implemented, Carol might begin to see correspondences between her behavior in her marriage and that of early figures.

For example, it was possible that she identified with a demanding woman who "stole" her beloved father and destroyed her mother and the family. Carol's identification with the demanding behaviors that seemed to get "the other woman" exactly what she wanted might have seemed like a good idea. It would take a while in individual therapy for her to begin to trust the therapist, and become secure enough to reconsider her ways of relating to her husband and others.

At that point, the therapist and patient might be better able to agree on the description of presenting problems and on what needs to change and why. Carol's Red plan was to use angry control to try to force her husband to be more loving. He reacted to this by passive resistance and withdrawal. This new description of problem patterns for individual therapy would relate directly to the issues she brought to therapy (marital difficulty), and the goal would be the same (having a loving relationship). However, the patient rather than the husband would be the focus of her individual therapy. When the time comes, here is one way to broach that topic of working on oneself more than on one's partner.

THERAPIST: I realize that you feel comfortable with where you are, and that changing your husband would be your first preference. However, the point of individual therapy now is to figure out how to help you consider whether there are changes you would like to make within yourself. Such changes could help in your marriage—or in a new relationship, if you decide you want to pursue divorce.

CAROL: What do you mean by that?

THERAPIST: That therapy is a learning experience. It can help you learn about your patterns, where they came from, and what they are for. Then you might choose to learn some new ones. So the focus in your individual therapy will be on your patterns and what they are all about. Maybe you would decide to change some things. If your husband did the same, changes in each of you could make things much better.[35]

CAROL: Well, I've done all that in my other therapies.

THERAPIST: So there is nothing more that you might work on?

CAROL: Not that I know of. I just need more validation and support.

THERAPIST: I can see the sense in that. But in addition, I think you might find it useful to understand more about how you relate to your husband.

CAROL: Like what?

THERAPIST: Well, this pattern of being angry at him because he does not support you enough. Is that a pattern you have experienced before?

CAROL: No.

THERAPIST: Does the pattern of telling somebody they are letting you down, and they'd better figure out how to do better, seem at all familiar to you?

CAROL: Oh, yeah. That's just like my father's girlfriend. I saw her do that all the time. I could never understand why he put up with it.

THERAPIST: So you might have learned something about that way of relating from her?

CAROL: I hate her.

If the therapy relationship was strong enough at this point, Carol would acknowledge her copy processes, her despair over the breakup of her family, her chronic aloneness and pain, and her decision to keep things under control (as did the "victor" over her mother). Gradually, as Carol became more comfortable, a fully reconstructive therapy as sketched in Figure 3.2 could follow.

COMMON DILEMMAS IN COLLABORATION

Many frequently discussed therapy impasses typically interfere with collaboration. A few illustrative dilemmas are discussed here, with the hope that the general style of thinking about them will generalize easily to similar other situations.

Responding to Long Silence

A patient's silence needs to be understood in context. Sometimes the silence is pregnant, and the best and only response is to wait quietly. Sometimes the silence is resistant and needs to be discussed, or the session will be wasted or worse. The best initial response is to wait for a while to see what happens. Silences in therapy are longer and more frequent than in ordinary social intercourse. The context of the silence and familiarity with the patient's style will help the clinician know whether it is a "working silence," an indication of blocked process, a matter of the patient's cognitive style, or something else.

Working silences usually end at the patient's initiative with a step forward. Typically, such productive silences follow an important statement by the patient or the therapist. Sometimes working silences come because the patient is deeply engaged with his or her thoughts and feelings. At other times, a patient may habitually function with deliberation and slowness. If the clinician notices that long silences are usually ended by an important and relevant remark, the clinician knows to allow extra time for this patient to process therapy events.

On the other hand, long silences can be markers of some kind of problem in the therapy process. If the therapist is unsure, it is usually appropriate to ask, "Are you willing to say what you have just been thinking about?" The response here will tell the therapist whether the silence was fruitful, part of blocked process, or something else.

Examples of a working silence and of a problem silence for Jill, the woman with the overly demanding boyfriend, follow.

Example of a Working Silence

Suppose Jill were to be silent and then say, "I was just thinking about how much my boyfriend is like my brother." Here an "um-hmm" and more silence from the therapist would be a good idea. In this case, Jill would be actively working on understanding her patterns (step 2), and the more she did, the more likely she would be to want to change them (step 4).

Example of a Blocking Silence

An example of a blocking silence for Jill might be this: "I don't know what to say now. I don't know what you want." This comment would mark a serious problem in the therapy relationship, and it would have to be discussed.

THERAPIST: You are trying to give me what I want?

JILL: Yes.

THERAPIST: So you come to therapy to get some help for yourself, and you end up trying to take care of me?

JILL: Well, I need to do what you want to get better.

THERAPIST: I see the sense in that idea, but I want to remind you of what this therapy offers. It's a chance to learn about your patterns, where they came from, and what they are for. So it seems to me that we have a pattern right here. This is supposed to be for you, and suddenly you are shaping it to please me. Am I making sense?

JILL: Yes. It feels the same here as with my boyfriend.

THERAPIST: Anybody else?

JILL: Yes. With lots of people.

THERAPIST: How far back in time can you go back and still find it?

JILL: With my mother.

THERAPIST: (*Silence*)

JILL: It's always that way.

THERAPIST: Well, if I understand this well enough, I would like you to know that it's the other way around. Here [i.e., in therapy], I am trying to give you what you want and need—and to help you learn how to make it more likely that others will be more respectful of your needs. It is not your job to please me. It's your job to get something from this therapy experience that helps you feel and do better.

Responding to the Patient's "What Should I Talk About Today?"

The question "What should I talk about today?" comes up often early in therapy. The IRT therapist responds with the typical "Whatever is on your mind," but accompanies it with an explanation and an alternative. The explanation is that whatever concerns the patient now is probably related to the underlying issues.[36] However, if that does not suffice to start the session, the therapist offers an alternative. He or she tries to avoid starting a passive–aggressive war to the effect that "I can wait longer than you can."

Here is an example. Jill's therapist might say, "Well, it would be best if we work with whatever is on your mind right now. If you can't or don't want to talk about that, or aren't clear about what to do, I could try to help you get started." Much of the time, this simple summary functions as permission to talk about what is on a patient's mind, even though the patient thinks it is probably not important. On the other hand, suppose Jill were to say:

JILL: I'd rather have you start.

THERAPIST: Well, let's see. We spent last session comparing your brother and your boyfriend. We explored whether you are ready to take better care of yourself by looking for more fairness and balance. How did you feel about that session?

Such a brief but pointed summary of a recent key issue is highly likely to get the session off to a good start. The practice of giving pointed summaries is a wonderful way to reengage collaboration in many contexts. It helps consolidate gains and presents the "What next?" dilemma. The therapist orients the process and makes it easier for the patient to take the next step.

If that fails, and a patient stays stuck and persists with statements like "Well, you are the doctor. If I knew what to say, I wouldn't be here," some of the interventions discussed in connection with Figure 3.3 (the flow chart for exploring blockers to progress) are appropriate responses to that protest. Handling things when they become this challenging is discussed further in Chapter 7, "Blocking Maladaptive Patterns."

Responding to Pointed Questions with Disciplined Personal Disclosure

Some patients will ask questions that might seem invasive to the therapist. However, because a therapist asks patients to disclose much about themselves, it seems only fair to be directly responsive. In general, the therapist tries to understand the meaning of the personal question in the light of the case formulation. He or she also gives a direct answer framed within the limits specified by the core algorithm. Answering personal questions is a different problem from spontaneously offering personal stories to facilitate therapy at a critical moment. The discussion that follows is only about answering patient-initiated personal questions.

Questions about Marital Status

Patients frequently ask questions about the therapist's personal life. The "classical " response is to reflect the question back upon the patient who asked it, and explore the motivation behind it. Within traditional psychodynamic therapy, all personal contact and expression of opinion is labeled inappropriate. In IRT, it's not so clear. In fact, because the therapy relationship is real,[37] responses to such questions are also real. Normal social courtesy is in order, but responses must also be appropriate to the therapy context. Demographic questions about the therapist can be answered in a straightforward manner, while taking care to understand the reason for each question and the response to the answer. Consider Charles, a particularly confrontational person.

CHARLES: Are you married? Do you have children?

THERAPIST: May I ask why you ask?

CHARLES: I just wondered.

THERAPIST: We may need to talk more about the reasons you ask this question. But the straightforward answer is that I am divorced. I have two children and three grandchildren. Can you say how you feel about that?

Almost always people say something like "Fine." If not, the therapist can continue, "Should we spend a little time on why you ask?" If the answer is no, then the matter can be dropped unless there is evidence that it might be relevant to the therapy relationship and process. If the patient continues with focus on the therapist, it is important to restore the proper focus.

CHARLES: Why did you get divorced?

THERAPIST: Lots of reasons. But all of that is not the point of your therapy. Shall we get back to what's going on in your life today?

If the patient persists, the therapist continues to explain the need to maintain focus on the patient, without becoming attacking or dismissive.

CHARLES: I really want to know. Maybe if you got divorced, you can't help me.

THERAPIST: Well, I would hope that is not true. I guess you will need to be the judge of that. Therapy is a learning experience. My job is to help you learn about your patterns, where they came from, and what they are for. Once you see that, you may decide you want to learn new ones. My patterns and learning experiences are different from yours, and going into all of that is not the point of your therapy. I will share with you that I think that having made it through some hard things can sometimes help therapists better appreciate the struggles of others.

I have never had such a conversation go beyond this point. Patients usually understand it and appreciate the honesty. If someone were to press on with the theme, I would again comment that the patient needs to decide whether this therapy is helpful or not, and if it is not, I would suggest some names of other therapists with whom the patient might be more comfortable. Indeed, if the patient is not comfortable even after being given a chance to understand the procedures and its reasons, IRT is not going to be helpful to him or her.

The rationale for this rather unusual recommendation is (as mentioned above) that the therapy relationship is real, except for the one-way focus and the constraints on intensity. Although the focus is supposed to be exclusively on the patient, it is normal and natural for patients to want to know basic facts about the therapist as a person. It seems rude to completely refuse to answer such basic questions. If such information can be given in a matter-of-fact manner, without deflecting the therapy focus from the patient, it makes sense to do so.

Questions about Religion

Sometimes questions about religion represent vital interests, not just personal curiosity. Suppose the question is about my religion, and the patient is committed to a specific religion that has specific views about therapy. After making sure I understand the patient's concern about this, I will make a brief statement about my own religious orientation and its possible relevance to this therapy process. It is important to express the fact that the therapist respects the patient's religious choice, even if different from his or hers. Then the therapist should inquire about whether the patient is still worried that the therapy will interfere with his or her religion. Because IRT leans heavily on the therapy relationship, and because spirituality is a major part of a person, it is probably dishonest to declare that the therapist's religion is irrelevant to the therapy process.

The role of spirituality in therapy is a controversial, important, and (until recently) forbidden topic. An excellent, data-based review of this subject has been offered by Bergin (1991). In IRT, a patient's inquiry about a therapist's religious orientation is seen as reasonable, and as deserving a straightforward response. It should be obvious from everything else that has been said about IRT that a therapist would never, under any conditions, seek to "convert" a patient to a different religious view.[38]

Questions about Beliefs about Sexuality

Another common example of legitimate patient inquiry is questioning about the therapist's attitude toward sexual orientation. The first response is to acknowledge that many people believe that homosexuality is inherited and the individual has no choice about it. I add my own view that I agree with Freud (1908/1959) that bisexuality is the more universal tendency.[39] However, society provides such harsh sanctions for deviation from heterosexuality that choice of the homosexual lifestyle introduces stress, to say the least. For those who can choose, making the homosexual choice in the face of severe social punishment could become a therapy topic if the patient wanted it to be. The issue of how much is genetic and how much is learned—how much is choice and how much is not—is not important, simply because sexual orientation itself is not relevant to the goals of IRT. The IRT goals of a balanced, friendly baseline, with moderate differentiation, moderate enmeshment, and balanced focus, have nothing to do with specific sexual practices.

On the other hand, interpersonally destructive patterns are a focus in IRT, whether they be homosexual, heterosexual, or autoerotic. Sexual practices that involve non-normative interpersonal patterns do need discussion. For example, if the patient has eroticized fantasies involving fear and degradation, and comes to therapy to deal with those very problems, "something is wrong with this picture." The patient will need to choose to reprogram the interactive patterns in his or her fantasies if he or she wishes to succeed in adopting a more benign interpersonal baseline.[40]

In sum, a therapist can give simple, factual answers to personal questions, while remaining alert to the possible meanings of the questions and impacts of the response in the light of the case formulation. Whatever unfolds from exchanges in response to personal questions, the discussion should end with a comment like this: "If you find yourself becoming concerned about this in ways that are affecting your therapy, let's always take the time to talk about it. OK?"

Inappropriate Personal Disclosures

Disclosures are inappropriate if they fail to relate directly and constructively to the treatment plan based on the core algorithm. I once heard from a divorcing patient that her husband was sharing notes on the divorce process with his therapist. The therapist was also in the midst of divorce, and they started discussing the details of their divorces. According to the focus rule here, such therapist disclosure would be inappropriate, because the focus would be switching too much to the therapist. The two alienated husbands in this case might have "bonded" over this, but the likelihood that the therapist was concentrating on the patient's needs and not his own was considerably diminished.

Responding to Questions about Therapy

It is common—in fact, recommended—that patients ask, "What is your therapy approach?" This can be answered in varying degrees of detail. The simplest answer is to say, "IRT is a developmental social learning approach. Therapy is a matter of learning what your patterns are, where they are from, and what they are for. Once you understand all of that, you might be in a position to decide to change and to learn new patterns that work better for you." This, of course, is a version of the learning speech (see Table 2.5). As therapy goes along, the collaborative therapist discusses the case formulation and the treatment plans, and the patient has no doubt about the nature of the approach. However, he or she may have doubts about whether to participate. Having to give up old hopes and wishes is not attractive or easy.

Another fairly common question about therapy is "Am I making progress?" Responses to this sort of question should begin with an assessment of the patient's perspective. The therapist asks, "Can you say whether you feel like you are making progress?" Usually the answer to that starts the therapy work, and there is no need to return to the question. The patient answers it for him- or herself. However, if the question is asked by a patient who is not collaborating, the response may be different. Consider Lilly:

LILLY: I think this is a big waste of time.

THERAPIST: So you feel like you are not getting what you need and want?

LILLY: No, not really.

THERAPIST: What is it that you are missing?

LILLY: Well, I've come to therapy several times now, and I just don't feel better. That's all.

THERAPIST: You are waiting to feel better?

LILLY: Yes. Isn't that the point of all this?

THERAPIST: Well, sure. You would feel better after a therapy that works. But I need to explain again how it goes here. Therapy is nothing more or less than a learning experience. We can study your patterns, where they came from, and what they are for. If you decide to change them, we can then turn to learning new patterns. Hopefully, you will feel better with those new patterns.

LILLY: Well, I don't want to do any learning. I just want to feel better.

THERAPIST: I can understand that wish, but I am sorry that I can't help you with it.

LILLY: So what am I supposed to do?

THERAPIST: Well, we could try to learn something from this discussion right here. You could see if what we learn makes sense, and then you could decide whether you can make progress with this approach.

LILLY: Like what?

THERAPIST: Like being disappointed when you go to get help. Is that something that has happened to you before?

LILLY: Are you kidding? It is the story of my life.

THERAPIST: So disappointment is an old pattern for you.

LILLY: Yeah. So what?

THERAPIST: If we can go back to the beginning of your disappointments, we might understand it better, and we might begin to find ways you could relate differently so things would go better for you.

LILLY: What could I do differently?

THERAPIST: Let's talk about this conversation. You are giving me all of the initiative. If I drop the ball here, you are going to be disappointed again. If I don't come through with something different, you'll be hurt. You have given all the power to me.

LILLY: I have?

THERAPIST: Seems like it.[41] The pattern might be "Ask and expect to be disappointed." That sounds painful. But if you became more active and decided to work here on your own behalf, you might be pleased with your ability to have a bigger effect on how things go.

And so on. A case this difficult will require a lot of such cheerleading and much use of the therapy relationship to gain the patient's collaboration in helping with self-discovery and working toward more constructive self-management. The patient will have to resist the temptation to cling to the familiar hostile enmeshment stemming from loyalty to IPIRs.

Sometimes the question about progress is "clean," and the patient really wants to know. In that case, it is appropriate to detail what has been going well—for example, "We have identified some things to work on [list them], but we need to find a way together to start learning more about some of your other patterns [list a problem or two]."

In sum, a question like "Am I making progress?" can mean many different things. As usual, the therapist assesses the meaning of the statement in the light of the case formulation, and then tries to implement the core algorithm.

Responding to a Patient's Request for Social Contact during or after Therapy

If a patient requests social contact with the therapist either during the course of therapy or after its termination, this is politely declined. Again, there is an explanation:

> "Therapy is not a social relationship, because the focus is mostly one way—me to you. If you start to worry about making it a social relationship either now or later, the focus shifts in my direction, and your therapy work probably will be blocked. It's too bad, but the two ways of relating—therapy and social relationships—are incompatible."

One minor exception I make to this rule is that if the patient is a coprofessional, and there is a likelihood of meeting outside the therapy context, I am comfortable with developing a case of "split brain." When encounters occur independently of therapy, I relate in a normal social manner appropriate for relationships with peers.[42]

Responding to a Patient's Request for Therapist Participation in Legal Disputes

Collaboration can be compromised if the therapist has to participate in legal disputes involving the patient. If at all possible, it is recommended that an independent consultant perform the evaluative function. The reason is that the IRT therapist is a strong advocate for the patient's Green. In therapy, episodes of Red are treated with tolerance, understanding, and an attitude of "Let's move past this now." By contrast, legal disputes, which may involve patient behaviors in the past or present that are Red, are more likely to be "absolute." The judgmental thinking in legal contests is, quite simply, incompatible with the IRT orientation that understands and accepts the extant Red–Green conflict.

If absolutely required to provide such documentation or testimony, the IRT therapist tries to respond to the situation honestly, framing the report as much as possible to help the patient's Green.

METHODS TO REPAIR COLLABORATION

Addressing Fears about Therapy

Fear of therapy may be conscious, as in some preceding examples wherein fears are related to incompatibility of goals. Patients may worry that the therapist will challenge their religion, sexuality, lifestyle, and so on. As illustrated above, such concerns can be addressed by explanations of the therapy process and by relevant therapist disclosures. Patients then can give informed consent for the therapy process to go forward—or not.

More subtle or unconscious fears come from the Regressive Loyalist, which is appropriately threatened by IRT. These fears become increasingly powerful as therapy gets underway. The part of the patient that wants to remain loyal to old and familiar ways most certainly does not want to be "treated." At some level, the patient knows that if he or she seriously engages with the IRT process, many beloved values, rules, and wishes will have to abandoned. These fears can be addressed by identifying and discussing them in a collaborative way. Asking permission, explaining the process in general, and clarifying the purpose of specific interventions can be very helpful. Examples of this style have appeared already, and are repeated in the chapters on each of the successive therapy steps. Chapter 8 focuses most directly on the problem of reluctance to change.

After a few sessions of IRT, some nonresponder patients whose Red is large will honestly say that they are "not ready to deal with this yet." They are to be affirmed for their candor, and invited to return if they change their minds. Others abruptly terminate or simply disappear. Treating this patient population is "no picnic." The success rate is a fair distance below 100%—but it also is quite a distance above TAU. My impression is that failure in IRT is most often due either to inability to engage the Growth Collaborator at step 1, or to running out of time before the five steps can be completed.

Addressing Negative Feelings about the Therapist or the Therapy

In IRT, there is rarely reason to let transference distortions (irrational views of the therapist that are based on patterns learned in relation to IPIRs) bloom. The challenge is to "get on the same page," as the patient—in other words, to collaborate, as rapidly and as often as possible. By being personally palpable within the therapy process, the IRT therapist lets the patient know how he or she is trying to help. The point is for the patient to learn about patterns and to practice being free of them. Letting problem patterns fester unexamined in the therapy relationship itself can interfere with collaboration.

Good ways to approach negative feelings about the therapist include the following:

- Clearly reflect the negative view (or a suspected negative view).
- Show understanding of why the person may have reached that conclusion.
- Review the therapy model (i.e., give the learning speech).
- Consider the relevance of the case formulation.
- Disclose the original intention of an "offending" remark.
- Apologize or rephrase (if necessary).
- Invite further discussion.

Using one or more elements from this sequence almost always restores the collaboration. Consider this example of Constance, a patient who had been suicidal for years, including several hospitalizations. After she started IRT, her hospitalizations ceased and her suicidal ideation had diminished somewhat.

CONSTANCE: I was mad at you last week. I felt like you told me I was wallowing in my depression. Then at work . . . [describes an unrelated event at work].

THERAPIST: Let's go back to your being mad at me.

CONSTANCE: I felt like you criticized me for being sick. You said I was acting in old ways and seemed comfortable with the old pattern. It bothered me that I should have been able to make it different.

THERAPIST: Talking about that pattern sounded like a scolding?

CONSTANCE: Yeah. If only I would try hard enough, I would not be suicidal.

THERAPIST: Is there a reason you did not tell me about those feelings last week?

CONSTANCE: I didn't know I was at the time. I just felt hurt.

THERAPIST: Can you say more about that?

CONSTANCE: I don't mean you shouldn't tell me those things. I get hurt too easily.

THERAPIST: Let's stay with your feelings of being uncomfortable with me.

CONSTANCE: I often am. I can't explain it.

THERAPIST: Let's try to figure out what this is about. Let's go back to last week.

CONSTANCE: I know I came out of my suicidal spiral. You blew the whistle, and I obeyed and came out of it.

THERAPIST: You are saying that you don't like that?

CONSTANCE: There is a comfort I have with being very upset and tearful and distressed.

THERAPIST: Thank you for being so very honest.

CONSTANCE: But I have this feeling that I can never get rid of that feeling by blocking it. I remember how angry I was when [former therapist] told me I needed corrective thinking. My view of reality is not real. I must change how I am.

THERAPIST: If you are suicidal, you preserve your own reality.

CONSTANCE: I refuse to listen to reason because it is your reason. (Becomes very tearful) As long as I refuse to be me, I can't feel better.

THERAPIST: You can't have your reality, your suicidality.

CONSTANCE: I am confused. I know my reality is distorted. . . . I have to acknowledge it may be really very true. As long as everybody says this to me, I can't be me. The person I think I am. I can't hold to my values and ideas. I can't do that and be me and be happy. . . . It sounds like I am not doing this right. I am being a bad girl. I try very hard to do it right. I do know that you like me. I know we have done well.

THERAPIST: I agree. But I really want to understand this feeling you have right now.

CONSTANCE: Something is blocked. I think I want to get rid of the *reason* I feel so bad. To stop valuing sad feelings is reasonable. But I feel like I have to give up all of what I have believed.

From here, the discussion went on to the copy processes from the patient's highly controlling and critical IPIRs; her sense of being disliked by everyone; her feeling of being responsible for everything that went wrong; and her view that she deserved punishment. Constance struggled to be able to give up those old "values" of being hyperresponsible and self-critical. The passage illustrates her struggle with the Regressive Loyalist. There were signs of strength from the Growth Collaborator, and those were acknowledged.

The steadfast adherence to the unresolved theme of anger at the therapist, who was being seen as like the patient's parents and previous therapists, was very important in this session. In the end, Constance began genuinely to question her devotion to self-attack. Collaboration in the therapy relationship helped make this possible.

Sometimes anger at the therapist is not just transference; sometimes it is justified. In that case, the therapist's error should be acknowledged. Consider Tilly:

TILLY: I am really mad at you for suggesting last week that I was giving my son the burden of making me feel better about myself. I try hard to see what I do, and I can see my depression should not be his problem. I try hard not to attribute my problems to anyone.

THERAPIST: And it seems to me that you do it very well.

TILLY: I thought you were saying, "What is she doing with that child?"

THERAPIST: You thought I was condemning you to protect him?

TILLY: Yes.

Next, the conversation went to Tilly's distrust of me and of people in general—especially those who "pretended" to be kind. She noted that patients have no idea what therapists really think, because they are trained in what to say and they work under controlled conditions. She returned to the theme of feeling criticized and condemned by me last time. I replied,

> "I can see how you might have felt that way about it. I was trying to help you get free of the burden of worrying so much about him, but I said it poorly. I think I said something like 'He need not feel responsible for assuring you that you are doing well.' Logically, that does include the idea that you had asked for such reassurance, and so I can see how you might have felt 'accused.' The important point now is that you do know in your heart that you do not wish to, and do not actually, make him feel responsible for lifting your depression. Perhaps we should talk about ways to help him know that better. I am sorry I was not clearer about that."

I believe that in this case there was also transference distortion. Tilly's view of me as "accusing" her of burdening her son was close to her view of her mother. However, the fact was that I had been unclear and not careful in a very touchy area. To focus on the patient's readiness to distort in this instance would not have helped her experience the trust that very much needed strengthening. Trust, or collaboration, belongs to step 1 and has priority over learning about patterns (e.g., transference distortions), which belongs to step 2.

Establishing Responsibility

Patients and therapists frequently have collaboration difficulties over who is responsible for what. Some therapists tell patients that what to talk about in therapy is their choice, their responsibility. To probe, to give advice, or to make suggestions would rob them of their own sense of empowerment. These therapists are careful to convey that they care a lot about the patients, and want to provide a nonjudgmental, truly accepting environment. Ideally, the resulting milieu provides a setting in which the patient can heal him- or herself (Rogers, 1951).

The preceding discussions and examples should make it clear that IRT embraces many of these ideas from Rogers. It involves much understanding and caring. But the approach is not *laissez-faire*, and acceptance is not extended unconditionally. The Red is not supported any more than necessary to maintain the working connection. IRT calls for the therapist to direct the therapy process if it is not going well.

IRT offers clear definitions of psychopathology, concrete descriptions of correct therapy process, and a nonrelativistic statement of therapy goals. Demands on the patient are equally firm. The patient is to learn about his or her patterns, where they came from, and what they are for. Then he or she can decide whether he or she wants to learn new ones, and go ahead and learn them. The new patterns will be consistent with the definition of normal Green. In IRT, the therapist works hard to facilitate this learning, but learning and the choosing to learn are the patient's responsibility.

In sum, the therapist is responsible to facilitate learning (affective, behavioral, and cognitive). The patient is responsible to choose to learn and to do it. Although the therapist gives the therapy process clear direction, its content is up to the patient. For example, the therapist supports patterns of interaction that are friendly, moderately enmeshed, moderately differentiated, and balanced in focus. But the therapist does not have anything to do with decisions about the persons with whom such patterns will be manifested, other than to be sure they are contextually appropriate.

Dealing with Occasions When the Therapist Disappoints the Patient

The clear perspectives on the nature of psychopathology, therapy process, and therapy goals in IRT allow easy resolution of a common dilemma that stymies therapists who offer a simpler "caring and acceptance" model. A rather large number of patients come to therapy hoping at some level to be loved and supported, and therefore to feel better. They inevitably are disappointed. Here is an extreme version of that dilemma, as posed by a recent attendee at one of my workshops. The workshop participant played the part of the patient, and I played the part of the IRT therapist.

PATIENT: If you care about me, why do you send a bill?

THERAPIST: Therapy is a learning experience for you, and the bill is for my work in trying to help you learn about your patterns, where they came from, and what they are for. I also can help you learn new ones when you want to.

PATIENT: Come on. You know nobody loves me, and you are the only one who can give it. That's what I need. How can you say you care if you charge money?

THERAPIST: I care about your learning to have a better life. It bothers me to see the potential you have wasted. I would love to see you get free of all this.

PATIENT: But what I need is love.

THERAPIST: Well, part of the learning here can be about that. I'll try to teach you to find love.

PATIENT: Huh?

THERAPIST: The idea is that if I would give you love, you would be loved for a day. If I teach you to love and to find love, you will be loved for a lifetime.

The Biblical[43] reference is not disguised. Its wisdom is transcendent.

COUNTERTRANSFERENCE

Countertransference traditionally refers to a therapist's personal reactions to a patient that arise from his or her own unresolved conflicts. Naturally, it can interfere with the therapy process. The implication is that therapists should have had their own treatment, so that countertransference is minimized. Successful resolution of a therapist's own inner conflict should assure that he or she can maintain a neutral and nonjudgmental stance. Sullivan's (1954/1970, pp. 18–25, 50–55) concept of participant observer spells out how the therapist can be highly interactive, and yet clearly focused on the patient's interest rather than on his or her own concerns.

In the 1950s, analysts began to believe that rather than reflecting a therapist's pathology, the therapist's feelings about a patient were an excellent barometer of the patient's impact on others (Thoma & Kaechele, 1987, pp. 86–97). It was argued that a patient creates an analyst's countertransference. This led to the suggestion that analysts ought to report their feelings about their patients to them. The rationale, according to Toma and Kaechele (1987) was that the " 'analyst indirectly ruins his credibility by putting himself beyond good and evil.' . . . We therefore consider it vital to let the patient participate in the analyst's reflections, including those about the context and background of interpretations, in order to facilitate his identifications" (p. 97).

From the perspective of IRT, the practice of reporting feelings to patients may be either therapeutic or iatrogenic, depending on the case formulation and the disclosure's consistency with the core algorithm. For example, suppose that the patient shows a pattern of dependency, which makes the therapist angry. Suppose also that the therapist's wife is dependent and he is burned out with trying to meet her needs. His mother was the same way. Now, according to the idea that countertransference provides important information about the patient, suppose that the analyst tells the patient, "Your dependency is annoying me. I appreciate your strength, and I wish you would tap into it."

The patient may be able to use this comment well if she has a history of coping, but has recently become dependent because her new husband seems to demand that she appeal to him before every little move. She may come to her senses, and regain her strength, and begin to work toward better balance in her marriage (among other things). However, she may be devastated and sent down into a depressive spiral if she has a history of being harshly overcontrolled and has been taught that she is incompetent, unworthy, and altogether unable to function on her own. Her therapist has turned out to be just like all the others. She may conclude that they all must be right. Once again, according to IRT, a "technique" can be good or bad, depending on the case formulation and the relation of the intervention to the core algorithm.

On the basis of years of supervising therapists, I think one of the more common manifestations of countertransference is frustration or anger. The therapist is likely to respond to his or her angry feelings by escalating directives until there is a crisis, probably suicidal. Then the typical response is to withdraw. The therapist becomes quieter and begins to dread the patient's sessions. If unable to refer the patient elsewhere, the therapist may become passive–aggressive and "forget" appointments or become seriously distracted during sessions.

According to SASB theory, anger is best interpreted as a wish to control or a wish to distance. Therefore, when discovering feelings of frustration or anger, the therapist should ask, "What am I wishing I could control here?" or "What am I trying to distance from?" Expressing the anger is out of the question until and if these questions have been answered and it is clear how such an expression would fit the core algorithm. Normally there is little need for therapist anger; patients usually have had massive doses of it already. Here is an example of Shirley, a patient who expected anger:

SHIRLEY: You must be frustrated with me.

THERAPIST: Why would I be frustrated with you?

SHIRLEY: Because you are trying to help me change, and here I go doing the "same old, same old" again. I don't think I can do this therapy thing.

THERAPIST: You feel that I am going to be frustrated and angry if you don't succeed in changing?

SHIRLEY: Well, yes. Won't you?

THERAPIST: Not angry. And I am not frustrated. Those words suggest that I am trying to make you do something, and you are not cooperating. But I am only trying to help you make things better for yourself. If you can't or won't, that is sad. It is a loss. It is a loss for you, and I would feel grief about the continuation of pain and all the lost opportunities. Right now, it makes me sad to see you hurt yourself this way. I wish we could find a way to make this be the last time this problem comes up.

Such a conversation makes it clear that the therapist is working for the patient, and not vice versa. People with problems in self-definition often arrive in therapy quite confused on this point. It is not the therapist's job to make the patient change. It is not the patient's job to please the therapist. Again, it is the therapist's job to provide optimal conditions for change, and the patient's job is to choose to change or not. This perspective relieves the therapist of the impossible assignment to "make" the patient change, and its likely correlates of anger and frustration.

Therapist frustration in the service of distance is also handled by clear thinking about boundaries and responsibilities. It is important for therapists to know how to get adequate distance from their work when they are not in the office. I prefer the defense of isolation in time and place. This basically amounts to telling myself something like this: "That is really bad, but right now, I am not dealing with it. I will—at the next session."[44] At different times in one's life, one has different personal vulnerabilities. It is important to recognize these, and not attempt to treat people who exacerbate sensitive areas when they are tender. Such personal sensibilities are too likely to divert the therapist from the main job: constructive focus on the patient. These potential diversions represent the main problem with countertransference.

In other words, countertransference exists in IRT in the classical sense. It can be a problem if the therapist is affected by distortions based on his or her own IPIRs. The IRT therapist is expected to have identified these and to be able to manage them—either by avoiding cases that touch on them, or by coming to terms with them (see Figure 3.2).

SUMMARY AND CONCLUSIONS

Collaboration specific to IRT occurs when the therapist and the patient work together to enhance the patient's Growth Collaborator and diminish his or her Regressive Loyalist. Green functioning is the overarching therapy goal, and Green behaviors, affects, and cognitions are clearly explained to the patient in the terms specified in Table 5.1. Without collaboration to work toward Green therapy goals, there is no IRT. Every other level of the five-step therapy hierarchy (see Figure 3.1) depends on step 1.

Collaboration in IRT is implemented largely via the first three elements of the core algorithm: (1) Work from a baseline of accurate empathy; (2) support the Green more than the Red whenever possible; and (3) relate every intervention to the case formulation. The therapy relationship is central to collaboration and also has a direct role in therapy change. Contributions of the therapy relationship to therapy change include enhancement of willingness to participate in therapy procedures; inspiration of hope and faith in the approach; development of a circumscribed attachment that provides a secure base for exploring new patterns; internalization of the therapy learning; and determination of Green goals that support new patterns. These are subsequently sustained by the patient's greater success in ongoing relationships outside of therapy.

Many other longer-term therapy approaches probably inspire change by similar mechanisms. What may be unique about IRT is its relentless focus on underlying motivation represented by the Red–Green conflict, and its unusual and constant explicitness about the case formulation, therapy process, and therapy goals.

NOTES

1. A good relationship can also increase hope and faith in the approach—a powerful effect that should not be ignored. Hope and faith will not survive long

unless there is substance to the therapy experience, and unless the patient can see that the process is actually helping.

2. According to SASB predictive principles of complementarity and similarity.

3. For example, Pavio and Bahr (1998) reported associations between outcome and personality types, severity of interpersonal problems, and more.

4. For example, Dunkel and Friedlander (1996) reported that a therapist's hostility toward him- or herself was negatively correlated with outcome.

5. This result held true until the sample was divided according to severity, at which time the imipramine was superior to placebo for the more severely depressed subjects, while CBT and IPT were not (Elkin et al., 1995). However, this revised finding failed upon replication by Schulberg, Pilkonis, and Houck (1998).

6. Using SASB codes of the doctor–patient relationship in treatment and placebo groups could begin to explore this possibility. Of especial interest would be any distinctive features of the relationship for individuals in the placebo group who show improvement.

7. If results are the same for both modes, it does not follow that neither is effective. If I travel by plane or train to a city 200 miles away, the fact that I arrive at the same place at the same time does not prove that my mode of travel was ineffective.

8. At first pass, it will make sense to have a treatment as usual (TAU) control group, composed of professional therapists practicing state-of-the-art therapy as they see it.

9. Beyond the early sessions of therapy, this will not be easy to assess. Hope and faith are probably affected by results that do or do not emerge as the therapy continues. Groups subjected to an effective technique are likely to maintain or increase hope and faith because they see good results. Hence a correlation between hope and faith and outcome would not necessarily indicate that technique was irrelevant. Analyses of hope and faith and of symptom change will need to be tracked and cross-lagged over time.

10. Chapter 2 has included a discussion of developmental neurology and attachment. This reference to "circuits" has no technical or empirical basis.

11. When and how the therapist shows empathy can affect what happens next (Pugh, 1999).

12. Mostly through complementarity principles. For example, AFFIRM rather than BLAME yields DISCLOSE rather than SULK.

13. That is, by wishes in relation to early IPIRs.

14. PROTECT, AFFIRM.

15. ACTIVE LOVE.

16. The most recent version of the American Psychological Association (APA, 2002) code of ethics states: "10.05 . . . Psychologists do not engage in sexual intimacies with current therapy clients/patients. 10.06 . . . Psychologists do not engage in sexual intimacies with individuals they know to be close relatives, guardians, or significant others of current clients/patients. Psychologists do not terminate therapy to circumvent this standard. 10.07 . . . Psychologists do not accept as therapy clients/patients persons with whom they have engaged in sexual intimacies. 10.08 . . . (a) Psychologists do not engage in sexual intimacies with former clients/patients for at least two years after cessation or

termination of therapy. (b) Psychologists do not engage in sexual intimacies with former clients/patients even after a two-year interval except in the most unusual circumstances. Psychologists who engage in such activity after the two years following cessation or termination of therapy and of having no sexual contact with the former client/patient bear the burden of demonstrating that there has been no exploitation, in light of all relevant factors, including (1) the amount of time that has passed since therapy terminated, (2) the nature, duration, and intensity of the therapy, (3) the circumstances of termination, (4) the client's/patient's personal history, (5) the client's/patient's current mental status, (6) the likelihood of adverse impact on the client/patient, and (7) any statements or actions made by the therapist during the course of therapy suggesting or inviting the possibility of a post-termination sexual or romantic relationship with the client/patient. (See also Standard 3.05, Multiple Relationships.)"

17. Some patients devote considerable energy to finding out as much as they can. This information is necessarily secondhand and therefore likely to be inaccurate.

18. I frequently advise therapists in training not to try to act like therapists in their personal relationships. If they function like therapists with their spouses/partners and friends, they soon will be surrounded by "patients," and they will be on a fast track for total burnout.

19. The biological rationale for believing this has been mentioned in Chapter 2: Attachment facilitates staying with the mother and the primate troop, which in turn facilitates individual survival. Deference to the dominant group leader facilitates group survival. Hard-wiring to copy dominant and warm figures makes sense at both the individual and the group levels.

20. Through complementarity principles. For example, if the patient becomes more friendly, it is better if people in his or her everyday life also become more friendly.

21. This statement would be SASB-coded as SELF BLAME plus <u>SUBMIT</u> to the father internalization.

22. The goals are based on the SASB model and its parallel models for affect and cognition, discussed in Chapter 4 and Appendix 4.1.

23. Some appreciate having an illustration of the SASB model with their own problem patterns and the connections to IPIR patterns clearly marked. The goals region of the model, discussed in Chapter 4, also seems clear to this group.

24. Here the emphasis is on the exact behaviors, affects, and cognitions associated with one aspect of Jessica's problem patterns. Details are provided by the SASB, SAAB model and by the affect and cognitive models. This extreme specificity is a refinement that is not necessarily required of therapists unfamiliar with the three models. It should, however, be a target in any research assessments of validity of DLL and IRT.

25. When therapists are required by health maintenance organizations to define therapy goals, presenting problems can be translated into DSM terms if needed. For example, <u>SULK</u> (hostile compliance) has a lot in common with dysthymia. When the therapist is describing goals, terms from Tables 5.1 and 5.2 that relate most directly to the presenting problems can be chosen. For

many versions of dysthymia, for example, reasonable goals suggested by Figures 4A.2, 4A.3, and 4.3 would be to become less agitated and more centered; less secretive and more expressive of feeling; less sulky and more willing to disclose his or her views.

26. Without some sort of "special dispensation" from credible, relevant figures within the culture.

27. Ideally, an IRT therapist would successfully request to work with the family, to see whether discussions with the father could help the patient differentiate herself from him—either by getting "permission" from him to be different, or by helping her more clearly see the total picture, reflect upon it, and decide to take a different path. In this case, the father refused.

28. Behaviors coded as **AFFIRM**, <u>DISCLOSE</u>, and *SELF-AFFIRM* in the SASB cluster model.

29. Behaviors coded as **PROTECT**, <u>TRUST</u>, and *SELF-PROTECT*.

30. The therapist did this by asking her if she had ever felt this way before the current relationship.

31. In response to complaints like this, an rational–emotive therapist (Ellis, 1973) or a CBT therapist (Beck, Rush, Shaw, & Emery, 1979) might try various well-known methods of helping the patient see that her response was irrational. An IPT therapist (Weissman, Markowitz, & Klerman, 2000) might encourage her to become more assertive. The IRT perspective would be that once she had grieved for the loss of hopes to reconcile with the internalized representation of her brother, she could use CBT, IPT, or other approaches to learn more rational and adaptive patterns in love relationships.

32. It should be noted that if a patient is near-psychotic, this tactic of paraphrasing the perception of the IPIR at its worst will not work. A dominant Regressive Loyalist like Jessica's would simply agree that her brother was right and fair, and possibly see the therapist as agreeing to boot. This present example of a reflection designed to heighten the Red for contemplation is only appropriate if a patient has enough Green available to become able to consider the picture from a Green perspective.

33. Some recent research (e.g., Lambert, Hawkins, & Hatfield, 2002) surveys deterioration effects in therapy and suggests that therapy casualties are more likely with more confrontive, aggressive approaches.

34. Blatt and Behrends (1987, p. 280) observed, "Freud (1913, p. 139) himself had noted that 'it remains the first aim of the treatment to attach . . . the patient to it and to the person of the doctor'. Freud cautioned that success could be forfeited if the analyst adopts any other stance but 'sympathetic understanding' before the attachment occurs (1913, p. 140)."

35. This is the learning speech.

36. This has been illustrated in the earlier discussion of the value of letting whatever is on the patient's mind direct the process of discovery.

37. Within clearly defined professional and ethical constraints in professional codes, and as discussed in different contexts throughout this book.

38. Conversion is not in the therapy contract and would not conform to the IRT core algorithm or the flow charts.

39. "Generally speaking, every human being oscillates all through his life between heterosexual and homosexual feelings, and any frustration or disappointment

in the one direction is apt to drive him into the other" (Freud, 1911/1951, pp. 429–430).

40. This problem is discussed briefly in Chapter 8, where it is described as the *Klute* syndrome.

41. The patient is likely to be one of the types discussed in Chapter 4 who confuses SEPARATE with CONTROL.

42. It is appropriate that the current APA (2002) code of ethics forbids therapy with a colleague with whom one has any actual or potential administrative connection. This essentially rules out people in the same administrative unit as the therapist (e.g., department, division, partnership), as well as their families.

43. A popular version of this perspective is: "Give me a fish and I eat for a day. Teach me to fish and I eat for a lifetime." That saying has always seemed Biblical to me because of its message that satisfying immediate needs is less important than working on higher long-range goals (Luke 12:15-34; John 14:23-27).

44. Of course, if the situation involves psychiatric emergency, the therapist does not use the defense of isolation until the emergency has been addressed satisfactorily.

6

Step 2: Learning about Patterns,
Where They Are From,
and What They Are For

"Oh, my God, I can't believe I have done that! I've been suicidal just to show her she can't win. What a stupid reason to kill myself. You are right—I am trying to win by losing. I guess I won't be doing that again!"

These are the words of a psychiatric inpatient, Martha, who was participating in a Developmental Learning and Loving (DLL) consultative interview. After following the trail from presenting problem through current social stresses and relevant developmental learning, Martha saw the organizing theme that explained her irrational, self-destructive behavior. Her mother had seemingly micromanaged every detail of her life. She would, for example, call Martha's boss and declare what assignments would and would not be appropriate for her daughter. The same overcontrol was attempted in relation to her daughter's choice of friends and social activities. In the face of all this monitoring and management, Martha felt unable to lay claim to her own identity and life. She had chosen suicidality to prove that there was something her mother could not control.

With this insight, Martha resolved to abandon the suicidal strategy and find her own more constructive ways of being. In the weeks following discharge, until she left the city to resume her business career, Martha consolidated this new perspective during therapy with a graduate student in the Interpersonal Reconstructive Therapy (IRT) practicum. There were threatening moments as she wavered in reaction to her mother's declarations that her new assertiveness was a manifestation of a brain disorder caused by a chemical imbalance. While acknowledging that she might have inherited a vulnerability to negative affect, Martha was also able to understand the priority of her need for friendly differentiation from her devoted mother. Following the brief therapy, Martha moved on without further self-destructive thinking or behavior. Suicidality and rehospitalization were no longer issues.

Martha had presented as chronically depressed and unresponsive to any therapy or medications over several years. The key to change was her discovery of the motivation for her suicidality and her failure to perform. Both the suddenness and the relative stability of her constructive change following this insight were unusual.

Learning about patterns, where they are from, and what they are for is the essence of insight in IRT. Once the patient understands the case formulation, insight has been achieved. Although Martha made dramatic changes after understanding her case formulation, insight usually does not result so rapidly in such lasting constructive change. In most therapies, understanding of the case formulation marks the beginning, not the end, of the change process. Indeed, Martha's response to insight was so extraordinary that it is necessary to explain why she was able to change so rapidly while others are not. A hypothesis is sketched in the section below on how insight works in IRT. Overall, this chapter provides a brief review of related literature, defines insight in IRT, considers its role in change, describes a number of ways to facilitate the development of insight, and mentions a few common errors in the pursuit of insight.

PERSPECTIVES FROM THE RESEARCH LITERATURE

Definitions

Within the psychodynamic literature, insight is believed to help patients by bringing forbidden or otherwise frightening thoughts and feelings to awareness. Awareness facilitates resolution of conflicts associated with these hidden feelings and any defenses against them. This psychoanalytic perspective drives the popular belief that remembering childhood traumatic experiences is vital to successful treatment.

An important review of research related to this traditional view of insight was offered by Luborsky, Barber, and Crits-Christoph (1990). As they addressed insight and other major tenets of psychoanalysis, these authors described the function of insight in therapy as follows: " . . . knowledge is added to the ego through greater awareness of the forces of the id. It is a generally accepted tenet of technique in dynamic therapy that the therapist should strive to help the patient gain an understanding of what had been only partly or entirely unconscious, especially aspects of the transference pattern . . . " (Luborsky et al., 1990, p. 281).

In their review of the general research literature on insight, Elliott et al. (1994) concluded that insight is likely to have four major elements: "internal seeing," linking, suddenness, and newness. Their own definition, which resulted from component analyses of insightful moments in two cases, suggested that insight is accompanied by contextual priming; therapist presentation of novel information, usually in the form of an interpretation; client initial reaction with what they call distantiated processing; and then insightful connection or reconnection that includes an observable emotional expression of surprise. Finally, there is elaboration, which indicates that the insight is not merely intellectual. Theirs is a reasonable summary of what many clinicians mean when they speak of insight.

Research on the Relation between Insight and Outcome

Although much has been written about the theory of insight and the practice of interpretation that facilitates insight, well-designed research on the connection between insight and outcome is not plentiful. Elliott et al. (1994) concluded that at the time of their writing, no large-scale studies clearly established a connection between insight and outcome. A more recent study of time-limited psychoanalytic counseling has continued the practice of modest sample size (Kivlighan, Multon, & Patton, 2000). These investigators asked judges to rate 12 cases on an Insight Rating Scale, and reported that greater insight was associated with greater symptom reduction.

Judges' opinions about the nature and degrees of insight are interesting, but the ability objectively and specifically to describe underlying conflict is a precursor to definitive study of insight. Promising available methods for research study have translated conflict into interpersonal terms, as suggested by Sullivan (1953). One of the more widely used of these interpersonal approaches is Luborsky's Core Conflict Relational Themes (CCRT) assessment method.[1] The CCRT method measures three potential components of conflict that are manifested in any identified relationship episode: (1) the patient's wishes or needs in interpersonal situations; (2) the perceived responses of others toward the patient; and (3) the consequent responses of the patient. Each component is coded in terms of interpersonal and affective categories.[2]

An important application of the CCRT method specific to the study of insight-related outcome is the degree to which therapists accurately discuss the conflictual relationship themes being assessed. Using a sample of 28 therapists treating one or two patients each, Crits-Christoph, Cooper, and Luborsky (1988) established that therapist accuracy[3] is significantly related to treatment outcome even after effects of the therapeutic alliance are controlled for. Further analyses based on the CCRT method suggest that insight assists the alliance, but also makes its own independent contribution to outcome.[4] Similar studies of patient awareness and outcome will be of vital interest. A newly validated measure called Self-Understanding of Interpersonal Patterns (Connolly et al., 1999) is likely to enhance much-needed study of patient awareness of patterns[5] and outcome.

In conclusion, the research literature provides modest support for the idea that insight enhances outcome. From the perspective of IRT, assessment approaches are more convincing if they specifically define the conflict and/or problem patterns rather than if they gather judges' opinions on the degree to which unspecified types of insight are present. Studies using the CCRT method to precisely define patterns and conflict suggest that therapies facilitating accurate recognition of specific interpersonal patterns and wishes do have better outcomes.

DEFINITION OF INSIGHT IN IRT

In IRT, insight is said to have been achieved if the patient understands and acknowledges the accuracy and completeness of the case formulation. This means that he or she can identify (1) a problem pattern in terms of input, response, and impact on the self; (2) copy process links between a problem pattern and one or more Important Persons and their Internalized Representations (IPIRs); and (3) wishes in relation to the IPIRs that support the problem pattern. When insight is well developed, these three forms of pattern recognition (description, links, wishes) are accurate and are expressed in all three domains: affect, behavior, and cognition.

Identifying Patterns in Green Ways

When developing the case formulation, the clinician can identify patterns and their copy process links to IPIRs by using the procedures described in Chapter 2 (see the flow charts there).[6] No matter which flow chart is invoked, the core algorithm is always implemented to the maximum possible degree. For example, suppose Richard were to complain to his therapist about his parents, who apparently criticize his every move. In turn, he is very critical of them. Let us assume that this is a long-standing pattern for everyone in the family. After eliciting detail and ABCs of the latest struggle with the parents, the therapist could say many things. He or she might be empathic and say, (1) "It must be really hard for you to endure their constant harping." Or the therapist could say (2) "It is important for you to keep letting them know how angry you are," (3) "You are repeating an old pattern again," or (4) "It sounds like you are again disappointed that they do not approve of your decisions."

Alternative 1 would be most helpful early in therapy, during consolidation of the relationship. Expressing empathy for Richard's position would follow the principle of giving enough support to Red to maintain the relationship before pressing on to Green.[7] Later on, however, such support for the blaming and suffering position could be seen as enabling Red. Alternative 2 not only would support the basic pattern of angry recrimination, but would actually inflame it. Although alternative 3 would refer to a "pattern" (as specified by IRT), Richard—already too familiar with hostile enmeshment—would be very likely to experience it as hostile control. The therapist would probably be seen as the accusatory parent, and the old pattern thereby would be played out in the therapy relationship. The resulting "negative transference" would bloom. If given in a context of warm understanding, alternative 4 would focus on the underlying wishes and facilitate a tiny step in the direction of recognizing the gift of love. Consequently, alternative 4 would be the Greenest, most IRT-adherent[8] of these possibilities.

Identifying Gifts of Love

After the patterns and their copy process links are identified, the patient has completed two important tasks: learning what his or her patterns are, and where they are from. The third task, learning what they are *for*, is somewhat more difficult to accomplish. Yet this last learning task is necessary for change. The gifts of love that constitute the underlying motivation for the problem patterns must be identified if the patient is to decide to give them up and go on to learn more adaptive ways of being. To help the clinician know what to look for, various examples of gifts of love and their associated copy processes are presented in Table 6.1. A few examples follow to illustrate how the table applies to cases.

Martha's pattern was to recapitulate (continue) her oppositional pattern with her mother. Her wish would be described by line 2B in Table 6.1: " I will do the opposite of what you want from me until you admit I am right and you are wrong. I want you to accept me on my own terms. Please love me 'as is.' " In her DLL interview, described at the beginning of this chapter, Martha saw that this wish was costing her dearly; she immediately decided it was a poor strategy.

Marie, by contrast, directly recapitulated her childhood pattern in adulthood as she continued the role of rescuing others. Her gift to her parents and her siblings appears in line 2A: "Your rules and views are my rules and views. I will hold faithfully to them now and forever. When you see how powerfully you have affected me, you will love me more."

Patsy, whose violent patterns of discipline reflected her own experience, illustrated the type of gift shown in line 1A: "I am like you. This means I love and forgive you. We are birds of a feather. See how I provide testimony to you. Please love me for it." Kenneth also gave this gift, as he identified with his mother in his "courtroom" approach to marriage.

A helpful key in identifying gifts is to attend carefully to whether the links represent identification, recapitulation, and/or introjection. The gifts associated with these different links can be found in Table 6.1. Identifica-

TABLE 6.1. Examples of Copy Processes and Gifts of Love

Copy process	Gift-of-love message
1A Identification—same	"I am like you. This means I love and forgive you. We are birds of a feather. See how I provide testimony to you. Please love me for it."
1B Identification—opposite	"I am the exact opposite of you. I devote my life to being everything you are not, and I want you to know it. Admit you were wrong, and make it up to me. Love me after all."
2A Recapitulation—same	"Your rules and views are my rules and views. I will hold faithfully to them now and forever. When you see how powerfully you have affected me, you will love me more."
2B Recapitulation—opposite	"I will do the opposite of what you want from me until you admit I am right and you are wrong. I want you to accept me on my own terms. Please love me 'as is.' "
3A Introjection—same	"I treat myself as you treated me. I agree with you about me. Love me for agreeing with you."
3B Introjection—opposite	Not observed except in triangles—for example, "Dad hated me; Mom adored me; I hate me = opposite of Mom." But the pattern also represents agreement with Dad.

tion is presented in line 1A, recapitulation in line 2A, and introjection in line 3A. Possible negative images (as in Martha's case) of these particular gifts are presented in lines 1B, 2B, and 3B, respectively.

Linking copy processes to lines in Table 6.1 can help clinicians construct hypotheses about the gift of love. Here are illustrations of how to do that. Martha was recapitulating an oppositional pattern; go to line 2B to find the generic form for her wish. Marie was recapitulating an old adaptation; go to line 2A to find a prototype for her wish. Patsy and Kenneth were identifying with an IPIR; go to line 1A to see a sketch of their likely wishes. All gifts of love seek love in return. Clinician readers might accelerate their learning about different versions of gifts by discussing several different cases in professional peer groups.[9]

HOW INSIGHT WORKS IN IRT

Insight as an Enhancer of the Will to Change

The principal purpose of insight in IRT is to set the stage for enabling the will to change. When the patient sees that his or her current problem patterns are echoes of old relationships and associated wishes, he or she may become more willing to let go of those values and rules and accept the costs. Discussions of the past have no other purpose in IRT. There is no energy to be "released," no revenge to be wreaked, no rite of passage to be negotiated. Although awareness of copy processes and gifts enhances the will to change, it is rarely a sufficient condition for change.

Insight and the Case Formulation as Works in Progress

According to Figure 3.1, therapy activities in step 2 that facilitate self-discovery include Tell the stories and be heard. Discover, and Reexperience feelings safely. Most therapy activities classified in step 2 have to do with self-discovery. However, self-discovery requires the patient to Be honest about thoughts, acts, and feelings, as reflected in the self-management column of Figure 3.1.

Learning about patterns in step 2 begins relatively early and continues throughout the therapy. New perspectives on old themes continually emerge. For example, a patient discovers that he talks to colleagues in the same tone as his father used to talk to him. No wonder they think he is condescending. Next session, he sees that this is happening with his wife too. He understands her response to him better and considers other ways of relating. In another session, he notes he does not use this tone with the therapist, where he is still "the child." Why not? Later, he spends a session on how this works with his son. And so on. The patient's grasp of the case formulation—the insight—becomes richer as it is appreciated in these different contexts and in different ways, all fully explored in terms of the ABCs.

A practical if somewhat arbitrary marker for the achievement of insight might be this: The patient understands the case formulation well enough that he or she is motivated to keep trying to break the link between problem patterns and IPIRs and consistently practice goal patterns. For example, consider George, who observed, " I see I have my parents' habits. I have to shake this off, big time. But I can't rise above it. I can't get beyond it. Something is holding me back." George had insight. He had not yet gone to the next step marked by the learning speech: deciding to let go. However, George had enough insight to know that he wanted to press on to actual change (IRT steps 3, 4, and 5).

Requirements for Change versus Insight

People may fully understand the copy process links and the associated wishes, but may still be vulnerable to reacting in the same old ways. According to DLL theory, the "something" that was holding back George (and others like him) was his gift of love to his IPIRs. George's familial modeling mostly offered absence, explosive violence, humiliation, and broken promises. It was daunting to think of giving up the strategies that had helped him survive up to now.

Developmental data show that the quality of attachment is affected by the quality of interactions over time. Internal working models reflect the quality of experienced relationships, whether they occur in childhood or adulthood. Normal people have secure attachments and internal working models that offer internal security. Nonresponders like George have deficient models, impaired attachments, and poor internal security. To change, they require time to learn about and develop security, which is facilitated by the therapy relationship. The relationship both models and encourages the development of new and better relationships.[10]

Although the therapy relationship in IRT is vital to change, it is important that the therapist resist every pull to become a substitute fantasy figure—a source of "interpersonal methadone,"[11] The most common manifestation of this very Red pattern occurs when patients are attached to a powerful IPIR who is supposed to take care of them, but who is also seen as needing them to be dependent and inadequate. The therapist is a prime candidate to "replace" that IPIR. The IRT therapist who consistently attends to the case formulation is less likely to become a Red enabler in this or in any other way.

In sum, implementation of the insight depends on a secure base.[12] Building a secure base requires extensive experiential learning and practice over time. Once acquired, security helps the patient muster the courage to let go of old fantasies, and to face the task of learning to relate in better ways in their contemporary situations.[13]

Explanation of Why Martha Could Apply Her Insight So Rapidly

Martha's extraordinary ability to put her insight into action immediately provides a preliminary test of the hypothesis that internal security is required to support the decision to give up the problem wishes in relation to IPIRs. She had long known that she was angry about her mother's overcontrol, but remained suicidal and seriously withdrawn, despite a variety of pharmacological and psychosocial treatments. In the DLL interview, it became clear that Martha felt that her mother wanted her to be a marionette. Her suicidal behavior was driven by the unconscious agenda to reverse the definition of who was the puppeteer, rather than simply to cut the strings. Martha's insight was that her efforts to "win" had guaranteed that she would "lose." True, suicide would tell her mother that she could not control everything, but what a Pyrrhic victory! Martha's affect, when she became aware of this pattern was one of surprise and dismay. She became energized, focused, and determined to change. Expression of anger about her mother's excessive monitoring was not changing her suicidal wishes. The case formulation made it clear that her new task was to figure out how to take charge of her life, whether or not her decisions agreed with her mother.

The hypothesis to account for her dramatic response to insight is that Martha already had the basic security needed to give up old wishes and fantasies.[14] Somebody important had managed to communicate consistent, loving support for Martha's own separate well-being. Perhaps this was her mother's underlying intention, even if her concept of good parenting was ill advised. Because of her underlying security, Martha could dare to take a different position once she accurately understood the nature of her choices. When she saw how maladaptive her method of self-definition had been, Martha could go ahead and start taking better care of herself.

A patient with good security is likely to be called a "higher-level"[15] patient by many clinicians. Martha would qualify for this label under that standard. This is somewhat surprising, since she had spent many of the preceding years in therapy and in hospitals. Keeping her in the category of Borderline Personality Disorder (BPD), or just "borderline"—a term that is frequently misused to describe repeatedly suicidal and apparently untreatable cases—would have been tragic. Her nonresponder status was the result of application of models that did not fit her. She had no basic need to "get out her anger." She did not have a major brain disorder. She had not responded to anger management programs, because "being nice" to her mother would have caused her to lose, as she saw it. She did not particularly need instruction in self-regulation, either. What Martha needed most was insight so that she could make better choices. Martha also needed some instruction in how to interact outside the mode of "You are either one up or one down." She needed to learn how to define herself without being confrontational. Martha was secure enough in her relationship with her mother to choose immediately to end the war and learn these new and better ways of relating.

During the brief follow-up course of outpatient IRT, Martha's mother behaved in ways supporting the hypothesis that Martha had good internal security. After a shaky start, her mother ultimately became affirmative and appropriately flexible in response to Martha's new ways of asserting herself.[16] For example, Martha noticed that when she asserted clearly but without attack, her mother would be responsive to her opinions and wishes. Martha then spontaneously coached her brother in how to react to the mother's control with benign assertion. Even though he was highly suspicious of this new advice, he tried the method of simple disclosure. Their mother reacted with appropriate affirmation and autonomy giving to the brother. Martha's insight and lessons in assertion thus reverberated helpfully throughout the family.

ACTIVITIES THAT FACILITATE INSIGHT

The Relevance of Specificity to Accurate Pattern Recognition

In earlier decades, one of the most robust research findings about effective therapy was that specificity is associated with good outcome (Garfield & Bergin, 1986). Eliciting details assures that the therapist accurately understands what is being said.[17] Accuracy facilitates collaboration and outcome.

For example, suppose a patient were to say, "My mother did not love me." The patient's meaning might be a long way from the interviewer's interpretation. The patient might mean only "She did not always give me what I wanted," but the interviewer might be interpreting it as "She beat me every day." No part of the core algorithm can be implemented when there is such gross misunderstanding between a patient and therapist. By contrast, if the therapist were to say, "Can you give me an example that illustrates how you know that she did not love you?", clarity could emerge. The patient then might say, "She never paid any attention to me." Since the interviewer cannot code "not attend," the next question might be "What would be an example of her not paying attention?" The patient might reply, "She missed one of my important football games." Then the interviewer might ask, "Why was that?" Answer: "I don't know. I guess she had to take my sister to the doctor."[18] This detail would suggest that the patient is inordinately sensitive about not having had the mother's prime focus. On the other hand, the patient initially might have answered, "She worked at night and slept all day. I had to take care of the house and the other kids."[19] Still another picture would emerge if the patient's initial response had been "She beat me every day, and I never knew what for or why."[20]

The importance of specificity is best appreciated by considering an example of a patient perception that seems wholly illogical to an ordinary listener. For example, Jerry firmly declared that his dad really loved him.[21] The DLL interviewer asked for examples. It became clear that the dad was rarely home, and that when he was, he had little to do with Jerry. When asked to provided an example of something that let him know his father loved him, Jerry explained that he and his dad once took a little private vacation together. The trip, it turns out, was to a city where there was an antique auto show, and Jerry reported that his father had wanted for years to go to that show. The mother did not want to go, so the father and son had a "private trip." Aside from this episode (which served the father's own interests), Jerry's stories established that his father was essentially absent. It is astonishing that he said his father loved him. Readers not familiar with severe psychopathology may think there has been a misprint. However, the inborn propensity for attachment[22] is so overwhelming that severely abused and neglected people will indeed declare they were loved. They support their claim with wholly inadequate documentation. "My mother loved me," said a profoundly neglected little girl. "She gave me a cookie once." Jerry and the cookie girl show that specificity greatly enhances accuracy, especially when the patient's world is so very different from the therapist's.

Specificity of understanding can be facilitated by carefully choosing to use the patient's own words. Consider Paula, who had been raised in a family where there was chronic and severe abuse of all the children:

PAULA: Saying bad things about my mother was a way to get beat up. Only my father could call her stupid. The rest of us had to show respect. If he heard you insult his wife, then for sure, you were going to get it. I really wish I had provoked them more. Though I was trying to stay out of the way.

THERAPIST: Provoked them?

PAULA: I was way too easy on them. I wish I had been more of a terrorist. This is the only weapon I have. I should have used it. I don't usually admire terrorists very much. But I really wish my parents had been in a position where they had to decide whether to go ahead and kill me. I wish that would have been the only way to really shut me up. The consequences for them of my not shutting up would have been really bad. It would have been good to push it to its limits, even though there was no hope of rescue from the outside world. Instead, the point would have been to put pressure on so that people were forced to show their true colors. Everyone was operating on false hypotheses, so obviously the *reductio ad absurdum* argument needed to be pushed to its limits. The truth would then be apparent, and everyone would start putting on their energy into fixing the situation instead of pretending that it did not exist. You couldn't stand over the battered dead body of your daughter, and still claim to be a loving parent in charge of a safe haven from the hostile world. Who would believe you then?

Paula said she realized that plan would not work. The abuse went on over the years with predictable devastating results. Paula was the only one who made it out, and that was via stunning brilliance that was apparent in school. The therapist's simple reflection of her very unusual word "provoked" elicited an intense explanation of how she had felt. It contributed a lot to the therapist's understanding of the severity of her situation, and a bit to Paula's own insight about the reasons for her fury and her depression.

Examining the Therapy Process

Interpersonal therapies in general and IRT in particular predict that problem patterns will appear at any time in the therapy relationship itself. Since the therapy relationship is central to IRT, it is naturally vulnerable to mischief from the Regressive Loyalist. The Red part of the patient seeks to sustain problem patterns, and so the therapy relationship provides a firsthand opportunity to see the Red in action. The IRT therapist can recognize the problem patterns, understand the draws for complementarity,[23] resist them, and provide corrective experiences.

The Omnipresence of Patterns

Patterns can be seen in unexpected places. Pattern recognition can begin with the opening words in a session even if they seem to be casual remarks. The struggle between the Red and the Green can be engaged by the simple act of keeping a therapy appointment. For example, Larry offhandedly remarked at the outset of a session that his mother wanted a family conference soon, but he did not want one. He then began to discuss his difficulties with his girlfriend. Inquiry about the family conference led Larry directly to the theme of his mother's micromanagement of his life, and his desperate, self-destructive attempts to define himself. Larry's difficulty with self-definition was also relevant to his relationship with his girlfriend. The opening comment marked a major theme in his life.

The Potential for Patterns to Lead the Therapist Astray

It can be very natural for a therapist to respond to patient patterns with Red-enabling behaviors.[24] For example, an IRT practicum student worked with Jeffrey, a paranoid man who took excessive measures to monitor his wife's alleged infidelity. Jeffrey was determined to "discover the truth" about his wife. By the time he had been in the hospital a few days, "seeking the truth" meant determining whether his wife had been unfaithful or whether it was "all in his head." The student therapist felt a very strong pull to help him figure that out. She listened to his lengthy recounting of "evidence," and agreed that a conference with his wife might help him elicit a confession if one were due. From an interpersonal perspective, the student now was in the same position his wife had previously occupied.[25] The student therapist was to take care of Jeffrey by complying with his demands. The treatment began to move in a better direction when the student explained that playing detective was not possible in therapy, but that focusing on his patterns (including ABCs) in relation to his loss of control of his wife could be helpful. With only two more sessions before discharge, it was not possible to progress very far with this approach, even though Jeffrey and his wife showed substantial interest in it.[26]

The therapy process as well as the narrative can reflect the case formulation. Consideration of patterns that emerge in the therapy process can help the therapist consistently support Green more than Red. Discussion of them can contribute to the patient's insight.

The Associative Method

A very helpful way to discover links between problem patterns and IPIRs is to review a current episode in terms of input, response, and impact on self along with the ABCs. After the episode is clearly in mind, the therapist can ask, "Has this happened before?" or "Have you felt like this before?" If the present episode has been clearly detailed, the answer is likely to be "Yes." If the request for associations fails to yield the connections, then the clinician needs sooner or later to ask about the past in general. For example, the therapist can say, "Let's talk a bit now about what it was like for you growing up. The idea would be to see if what you learned when you were little has anything to do with what is going on now."[27] There are many ways patients decline to do this. Some will say, "I cannot remember. That was a long time ago." Others will say, "Fine. I had a happy childhood." Still others will say, "It was not good, and I don't want to talk about it."

All of these ways of avoiding the task can be handled within the same general framework—that is, to remind the patient that the IRT approach is concerned with the possible relevance of early learning to the current presenting problems, and so it could be helpful to check this out. If the patient is willing to proceed, then the therapist tries to elicit specific examples that can be expanded in terms of input, response, and impact on self, and described in terms of the ABCs. The combination of a supportive context, an agreed-upon agenda to learn about patterns and what they are for, and implementation of the core algorithm can rapidly elicit important memories.

For example, Bryan, a securities analyst, had a respectable record—but he always served as the "#2 person," the workman behind the scenes. Although he was smart and wise, he simply could not accept invitations to move into positions where his excellent performance would be "his." In therapy, a current example of this with his employer was reviewed in terms of input, response, and impact on self. There was a big job he was doing for his boss, who depended on his services, but who also diminished and degraded his work. Bryan could see the good results from his efforts, but doubted his worth. As he spoke, he was anxious (energetic, he said) but sad.

In response to the question about whether this situation and these feelings were familiar, Bryan associated to his family of origin. His father, he declared, "needed a kid to be superior to." His mother was bitterly disappointed in her marriage and had "placed her bets" on one of the other siblings. He could not surpass that sibling or his father; otherwise, both parents would lose their bearings.[28] As he developed this theme, he stopped pacing the room and sobbed hard. He said, "As I talk about this, it seems crazy. Irrational. It refers to things I don't remember. I did not know I needed to make my family feel good by doing this. And there is anxiety about it."

A Verbal Walk through a Typical Day

If heightening a specific situation and asking for associations do not work, then other devices might be tried. Here is another way to help the patient become specific: "Let's go back to when you were age 6 or 7. Can you remember the place you lived in? Let's go through a typical day. Who woke you up and how? What was breakfast like? How did you get to school? What was school like? Where did you get lunch?" The questions should continue through the day. In just a few episodes, details usually emerge that help the patterns become clear.[29]

Consider the different pathways that may come from a variety of dinnertime scenarios: Father may lose his temper when he dislikes dinner and throw the food against the wall. Dinner is served at 6:10, whether anybody is there to eat it or not. Little is said, and every plate must be cleaned up. Dinner is never served, and so everyone fends for him- or herself. The different themes of overcontrol, unmodulated anger, abandonment, exploitation, and more are present in these different basic descriptions of a typical dinner at home. The different dinnertime scenarios result in very different patterns of relating to loved ones. Because of the interest in the underlying structure[30] of the narrative, the IRT therapist finds that almost no scenario is "irrelevant."

Using Interpersonal Dimensions to Measure the Copy Processes That Matter Most

It is not unusual for a patient to believe that he or she is totally different from a parent, but actually to be an exact copy. For example, a woman with BPD, who had progressed beyond self-mutilation and overdosing, nonetheless had a severe regression during a fight with her boyfriend. During an argument about his upcoming long trip away from home, they stopped by the roadside to eat lunch. The rest stop happened to be near the edge of a cliff overlooking a lake. The patient impulsively ran at him and tried to push him over the edge. Luckily he saw her coming at the last minute and was able to defend himself.

As we discussed this unacceptable behavior, I reminded the patient that this episode "had to make sense." Previous discussions had made it clear that her father was capable of murderous rage. After a long, thoughtful interval, she said, "I just hate that I am like my father. I thought I was so different. He is politically active, and I am not; he is has a regular job, and I do not; he has plenty of money, and I do not. I am everything that he hates. But I see I am just like him." The treatment then returned to the familiar theme of her need to differentiate herself from the internalization of her father and find her own new identity.

This example clearly demonstrates that copying of symbolic, socially obvious attributes does not necessarily matter much in therapy. The copying that does matter is copying shown in the interpersonal and intrapsychic structure of the personality. By consistently considering interpersonal and intrapsychic structure to find patients' copy processes, clinicians are less likely to be misled by any irrelevant "differences" from the IPIRs.

Dream Analysis

The study of dreams is a time-tested method of identifying patterns and the motives that support them. In IRT, the traditional ways of using dreams to develop insight are often useful. The dreamer reports the story, and the therapist notes each component in sequence. The patient is asked what the dream means, and whatever he or she offers as an explanation is pursued in depth. If the patient has no idea what it means, then the therapist can present each component and ask for free associations. The process is very much like reviewing a Rorschach response, piece by piece. Patterns are noted and related to the case formulation in the same way that any other material is processed in IRT.

Not surprisingly, this method frequently catalyzes discussions of key conflicts. Usually dreams center on feelings and thoughts that are not welcomed by either the Red or the Green. Sometimes the Red inspires a dream about forbidden wishes, or generates a nightmare that is sure to deter the patient from any thoughts about changing things for the better. Analysis of dreams is a topic that deserves a whole chapter, but for now, one example is offered.

Mandy's presenting problem was a very long-lasting depression, accompanied by fury about being female in a society that objectifies and degrades women. She lived with a man who was a good companion, but she otherwise found little reason to participate in life. She felt consigned to a painful existence in the shadows. She had ignored her substantial talent, and had become resigned to living in anger and fear. She saw no hope for reconciliation or recovery. Here is the dream that foreshadowed a turn for the better:

"I had a vivid dream. I keep wanting to reach out and touch it. I was sitting at a dinner table having a meal with others. I saw a spider on a thread coming down to above my plate. I pulled back. It looked as if honey was running down the thread over the spider. It looked more ball-like, with stuff dripping off of it. I thought, 'Now this will get on my food.' It was getting bigger, and it kept descending. When it reached the surface, it had grown and metamorphosed. Now it was a ball with drippy mess all over it. It uncurled itself, a little animal. It was all so messy. It went scooting across the table, leaving a mess behind it. Out the door it went, and I was glad it was going. Outside, there was a swimming pool that somebody was uncovering. Somebody thought it should clean up in the pool, and opened the gate and let it go in. Then, instead of a horrible spider, it was something like an otter. It was bigger now. It was nice, a nice creature, playing in the water. I was thinking what a mistake I had been making to be horrified at it before. I have had spider dreams all my life. This is the first time the spider turned into something really nice."

We spent the whole session on this dream, associating to each part in sequence. Associations to the word "messy" revealed that the patient was working on a project at home, and there were papers all over the apartment. Each failed page had been crumpled into a ball and thrown. The place was a huge mess, with balls of paper all over. The patient had felt overwhelmed by the project and was sure she would fail. As a child, she had repeatedly been called "messy." That link led to the idea that she was the messy critter. I summarized the progress so far: "We have the messy critter going out the door, and somebody invites her into the pool." Mandy replied,

"Yeah. But I did not clean up. Maybe this is a want. Yeah, the dream is the way I wanted it to be, not the way it was. I used to dream about being back in California, where life was nice and playful. I really wanted strongly out of that messy problem. All those panics were just testing the waters to see if I could just stop doing this. Just quit. I thought, 'No, I don't want to panic and give up now. I want to finish.' "

Mandy then talked about what a mess her apartment was as she let everything go to finish this project. She was determined not to give up. I asked whether she wanted to talk about the paper balls. She said, "What are we going to do with you?" These were her mother's words—words she had heard many times. As we talked more about the problem of reducing the mass of material and organizing it, it became clear that Mandy had found a way of completing the project that she liked. I reflected: "So something nice came out of the mess?" Mandy agreed that this made sense, but she worried that she had had the dream before she figured out how she was going to write the paper. I wondered whether the dream reflected her confidence that she could solve the problem. I also asked whether the dream could mean that she was becoming more pleased with herself. She laughed and said, "Possibly." Then there was an extremely rare moment of feeling affectionate toward her mother, with whom she was negatively identified (line 1B, Table 6.1).

Wonderful change did slowly unfold in the next 3 years. The dream was evidence that step 4, enabling the will to change and appreciate herself, had finally started.[31] It probably was important to the success of the therapy that this early sign of change from self-hatred to self-appreciation was identified, consolidated, and affirmed.

Use of the Therapist's Unconscious

Once the therapist has learned to immerse him- or herself in the patient's phenomenology, the therapist's own free associations, fantasies, and musical or artistic associations can provide useful clues to patterns. Almost every day, I notice that a melody that has been hanging in the back of my mind is relevant to what is going on.[32]

For example, a patient was discussing a dream about going to a famous restaurant where the waiters were too busy and the food was bad. She had no idea what the dream could mean, but she knew that it made her very anxious and angry. In recent sessions, she had been considering her husband's extraordinary professional success and ineptitude as a housemate. In my mind, I "heard the hymn 'A Mighty Fortress Is Our God.' " This captured both the patient's strong religious upbringing and the central question in her dream: Do trustworthy love and protection exist? We then related the dream to her distrust of her husband and of the therapy. My musical association "understood" the central theme of the dream; I had only to listen to it. Such messages from the unconscious can provide extra data to help identify themes.[33]

Here is an example of the use of therapist fantasy. A patient was discussing her mother's latest unreasonable demand. I shared with her my fantasy of her mother as a baby, lying in a crib. The patient sobbed deeply for quite a while; then we discussed her pattern of taking care of her mother, and her wishes that she could finally be dependent on somebody. She concluded with "I just have to grow up and accept that time is past." With this remark, the patient tagged the central issue for herself, and began the final stage of letting go of the organizing wish.

Interpretation

Interpretation in IRT usually involves no more or less than sharp mirroring of some aspect of the case formulation. I call this interpretive reflection.[34]

Consider Beth, a highly skilled and incredibly hard-working emergency room (ER) nurse. She was feeling depressed and empty.

BETH: Just being is not enough for me. Just being to be helpful is not enough for me. Being because I am skillful and can accomplish a lot is not enough for me either.

THERAPIST: What would your mother say if she heard this?[35]

BETH: I don't know. Well, she would say, "You think too much. That is your problem. I can't help you with that."

THERAPIST: But you were not asking for help at all.

BETH: I know.

THERAPIST: So you express a need and she feels demanded of?

BETH: Yes. She feels inadequate if she cannot fix it. I don't know if I could accept love if it ever came my way, anyway. I think I would just reject it.

The conversation then turned to Beth's amazement at, and disapproval of, a colleague who successfully insisted that the ER team's next meeting be held at the colleague's convenience. Next, the discussion focused on a mother of a child who had ignored the seriousness of his illness and failed to avert the crisis that resulted in an ER visit.

THERAPIST: You were upset by a parent who did not recognize the needs of her child. Is that familiar?

BETH: Yeah, she does remind me of my mother.

THERAPIST: So the theme of parents who don't listen to the child's need is in your history and your heart.

Beth's severe deficiency in self-care was related by these "reflections" to the lesson from her mother: "Do not have needs, because then I will be compelled to fix them, and if I cannot, I will feel inadequate (and be angry at you)."[36] The episode helped Beth understand and accept that there were good reasons for her despair and her conflict about any nurturance for herself. If she asked for care, she threatened her mother's competence. The lesson clearly implied that she needed practice in accepting nurturance with promising current significant other people. This was facilitated by IRT homework assignments. At least once a week, she was to ask for and accept help from people able to give it. Beth was successful in implementing the homework generated by this insight.

With constructive new experiences, and with the understanding that what happened to her was not appropriate, she eventually was able to distance herself from her mother's rule. Beth conquered her fear of accepting support, and also began to do much better at self-care. Her rage and despair diminished greatly. The insight was not an "epiphany." But it did set the agenda for intrapsychic change in relation to the mother IPIR, and it did suggest clear current homework assignments that provided corrective social learning experiences.

Memorabilia

Another good way to clarify patterns or motivations is to have the patient free-associate to photographs from childhood or other memorabilia. The patient shows the photos to the therapist, and the discussion about them proceeds much like the analysis of dreams, described above. Free associations to the components of the pictures can lead to patterns and motives— provided, of course, that the therapy language remains interpersonal and specific.[37] For example, "Mother was pretty" is not interpersonally informed. By contrast, "She seemed more worried about how she looked than about what happened to us" opens up the possibility of exploring important interpersonal patterns. This method, like all others, is focused by the case formulation and by the interpersonal orientation of IRT.

Here is an example of a therapy discussion by Matthew, an executive in his 40s, who for the first time read some letters that had been stored in the attic of the family home. He found one from his mother, who had died when he was just a toddler. The letter was to her mother, his grandmother, written on her honeymoon.

MATTHEW: She was a picture of contentment and happiness.

THERAPIST: How did you feel as you read that?

MATTHEW: I was sorry I missed her. I would like to have known her. I missed not having her. I am sure she was remarkable. I would love to have her share my life, to know me.

THERAPIST: What would you like her to know about you?

MATTHEW: She would have liked me. What I became. She would be proud. I don't know if I would have been different if she had lived.

Matthew showed here, at the later stages of therapy, that he was now content with himself. At this point, he was consolidating his gains and realized that he not only had resolved his depression, but also had mastered his fear of loss so that he could make a deep commitment to a relationship.

Tape of a Family Conference

A highly effective way of discovering key patterns, copy processes, and connections to underlying wishes is to listen to a tape of a family conference that was designed to elicit various family members' perspective on the

patient. Such a conference begins with affirmation of the family's importance to the patient and a thank-you for helping with the process of trying
to enhance the patient's adjustment. "Are you willing to say how you feel
about [patient's name]?" is about all the therapist needs to do to get this
going. From then on, the job is (1) to clarify emerging patterns, and (2) to
blow the whistle if the meeting degenerates into exchanges of accusations.
Blaming may be appropriate to a justice model, but there is little place for
it in IRT, which is about learning and choosing.

An audiotape[38] of the family members relating to the patient, and vice
versa, is then available for later study. Listening to the tape can help the patient develop perspective on the patterns and wishes in ways that have not
been possible by simply telling stories in therapy. This topic needs a separate chapter, but only a brief illustration is given here. In this example, Karen was listening to a tape of her mother telling her, in effect, what a terrible daughter she was.

KAREN: That negates not just what I said, but it negates me altogether. She
does that a lot.

THERAPIST: I thought you handled it with a great deal of respect and balance.

KAREN: I had no idea I said those things so well.

THERAPIST: What do you think about this?

KAREN: I think that trying to deal rationally with Mother is futile. Our
world is defined by her parameters. She takes her ball and goes home
if she does not like the way you play. It makes me feel very frustrated
and angry. She is just not able to listen. She does not have to agree. I
just want her to accept that there is another point of view. I do not feel
optimistic about what we have to work with in the future.

Listening to the tape made the situation crystal-clear. That objective evidence helped convince Karen to let go of her hope for something different
from her mother. Listening to this type of family tape may be analogous to
viewing the body at a funeral. The procedure serves the purpose of clearly
saying, "It is over. There is to be no more. The cherished wishes and hopes
are not ever to be realized. This is very sad, but it is what it is." The ABCs
in relation to the tape are explored in depth, and as the patterns become
totally clear, it becomes easier to complete the process sketched in Figure
3.2—coming to terms.

The Two-Chair Technique

In the two-chair technique, the patient plays the role of a significant other
person in one chair, and then changes chairs and responds. The clinician

selects a key issue to be discussed in the two-chair exercise. It can be very helpful to ask the patient to "discuss" the conflict between the Red and the Green. As therapy progresses, the Green can prevail when the patient is changing chairs to respond to the Red. Using the two chairs in this way helps concretize aspects of the patient's relationship with an IPIR. Paivio and Greenberg (1995) empirically demonstrated the effectiveness of the two-chair technique during therapy.

The experience threatens to be so real for the patient that often he or she does not want to do it. The idea of role-playing a parent or important sibling can be every bit as threatening as asking this person actually to come to a session. This fear can dominate even if the person to be role-played is deceased. Among other things, role playing of this sort is compelling evidence of the massive power of the IPIR.

Recognizing and Dealing with Defenses

Experimental Data on the Existence of Defenses

The concept of defenses (e.g., projection, repression) has led some to believe that psychodynamic therapy is not amenable to scientific study. Mischel (1973, p. 336) criticized psychoanalysis on these grounds as well as others. Since Mischel's challenge to the concept of defenses, there have been studies providing objective evidence that defenses do exist. For example, Newman, Duff, and Bandmaster (1997) offered clear evidence for the defense of projection in a series of six laboratory studies of normal subjects. They showed that "those people who both avoid thinking about having threatening personality traits and deny possessing them (repressors) also readily infer those traits from others' behavior" (p. 980). The experimental series does not directly establish why there is projection, but it does make it clear that projection exists.

The defense of forgetting unwanted personal memories (i.e., repression) has also been documented. For example, 38% of women who had been brought to hospital emergency rooms for treatment of sexual assault as children did not remember (or chose not to report) the experience 17 years later (Williams, 1994). Forgetting these documented assaults was most likely for younger children and for children who had been molested by someone they knew.

The topic of repression of sexual abuse experiences has been highly controversial. It is not uncommon to talk to patients who report that earlier therapists have described their failure to remember as evidence that they have been sexually abused. Such arguments are not logically sound. Repression implies forgetting, but forgetting does not imply repression. Moreover, there is the possibility that there was no abuse to forget. Attempting to define repression is well beyond the present scope. The general idea is that the individual has forgotten one or more traumatic personal events. Repression can apply to many themes, not just to sexual trauma, as Loftus, Gary, and Feldman (1994, p. 1178) note:

> For example, people (over one quarter of those interviewed) have failed to recall automobile accidents 9 to 12 months after their occurrence, although someone else in the car had been injured (Cash & Moss, 1972 ; see also Loftus, 1982). People (over 20%) who, when they were 4 years old had a family member die have failed to recall a single detail about the death (Usher & Neisser, 1993). People (over 15%) have failed to recall a hospitalization approximately 9 months after discharge (National Center for Health Statistics, 1965; see also Loftus, 1982). Patients have failed to recall visits to a health maintenance organization (HMO) that they made within the previous year for something that was serious or even very serious (Means & Loftus, 1991).

Relevance of Defenses in IRT

In IRT, defenses such as repression or projection can interfere with recognition of patterns, links, and underlying wishes. Most importantly, they can interfere with the willingness to give up the old wishes. The observations cited above that document repression of traumatic experiences[39] buttress the assumption that uncovering forgotten traumatic events can be an important part of pattern recognition during therapy.[40]

For example, consider Jane, who had been incestuously abused in fundamentally pleasurable ways by a socially crippled, very controlling father. She learned from that experience that she was helpless, and yet that she also was very special and powerful. She learned that she could maintain this central and important identity if she was essentially nonfunctional. Jane was very likely to maintain patient status for many years, as well as to be primed for repetition of sexual abuse. In IRT, she would have to confront these most extremely unwelcome truths if she were to master step 4 and enable the will to change. She would have to surmount the defenses of repression and denial (and probably more) if she ever were to have a chance to realize that her choice was between continuing the maladaptive patterns, or functioning well and claiming her share of normal happiness. The IRT therapist would need to recognize her defenses in this situation and provide the support that would help her face the facts and choose differently.

Specific Defenses Applied in IRT

An IRT-relevant classification of defensive strategies has been described elsewhere (Benjamin, 1995). Extended discussion of that perspective is deferred for another time. Briefly, it is proposed that defenses protect the gift of love and can be classified (Benjamin, 1995, p. 67) according to whether they distort (1) input, (2) response, or (3) awareness (impact on the self). Traditional defenses (e.g., repression, denial, projection, reaction formation) can be classified according to these three purposes. The most important differences between this perspective and the original psychoanalytic descriptions of defenses [41] are as follows: (1) Conflict is defined in terms of Red and Green. (2) Defenses serve the purpose of protecting the relationship with the IPIRs; they interfere with the decision to let go of underlying organizing wishes and to give up the gift of love.

For example, Jane's version of BPD involved the use of repression and denial to protect her attachment to her father. In her mind, she could continue existing only if she could remain a chronic patient.[42] Her defenses involved far higher stakes than protecting family secrets. Instead of being the center of concern for being disabled, she would have to change to working on developing instrumental, interpersonal, and emotional competence, including especially the ability to take care of herself. This was likely to be both difficult and boring. It also would be very threatening, because it would include both perceived loss of and abandonment by her father. As defenses fall and patterns are fully appreciated, the many patients like Jane, can become as undefined and vulnerable as a newly fertilized egg without a shell or womb.

Adaptive Aspects of Defenses

It should also be noted that defenses are not always bad or pathological. Sometimes, for example, it can be very helpful to teach patients in crisis how to isolate and how to intellectualize. I have summarized the idea that defenses can be adaptive as "Good defenses make good neighbors" (Benjamin, 1994b), and this is developed further in Chapter 7.

Defenses That Do Not Enhance the Self-Presentation

In some versions of psychoanalytic and social-psychological theories, it is assumed that everyone tries to present him- or herself in the best light. Given this assumption, defenses make the subject look good. Blame avoidance is assumed to be universal. However, these assumptions often do not hold in work with severely disturbed patients. Some distort reality in a direction that is highly unfavorable to themselves. I recall that when I was on my internship, there was a never-solved murder of a female student on campus. After the murder was reported in the press, two psychotic men independently came to the ER "confessing" they had done it. Police established that their claims could not possibly be true, but each of the patients remained convinced he was guilty.[43] In other words, normal assumptions about defenses are "off" when one is dealing with the severely disturbed population.

Such bizarre patterns, of course, are driven by attachment to IPIRs who fostered corresponding values and rules. Examples include telling children outrageous stories about their involvement in adult difficulties. An angry father might "explain" that the overload caused by the patient's birth pushed the mother over the edge of sanity. A furious mother might repeatedly claim that the father was so unhappy to be trapped in marriage by the patient's existence that he had to leave. A parent might declare that a child "is driving me crazy." When such messages are severely discordant with obvious facts, children have little faith in their version of reality, and are prone to dwell at the edge of craziness. Given the right disposition, they can cross over to psychosis. In dealing with these near-psychotic distortions of self, it is sometimes helpful to use a variant of rational–emotive therapy (Ellis, 1973) that leads to the gift of love. Consider this exchange with Harry, a patient with unreasonable self-blame that often led to suicidal thoughts.

HARRY: You are sympathetic, but just because you only have information coming from me.

THERAPIST: OK. Let's look at the facts. The accountant found a bookkeeping error that had nothing to do with you, Right?

HARRY: Right.

THERAPIST: There has been 100% turnover in the secretarial staff in an organization of 30-some people during the past year. Right?

HARRY: Right.

THERAPIST: A consultant came and affirmed a number of your perceptions. Right?

HARRY: Right.

THERAPIST: I invite you to challenge your filter. You may be right that you distort the facts. I believe, though, that the distortion is when the facts are friendly. I do not see that you could or would present a case on your own behalf—even when the facts support your position.

HARRY: OK. I have not distorted those facts. And they do seem to show there is something wrong there besides me.

THERAPIST: So our biggest problem right now is your preference to grab the blame and threaten your life with it.

Notice that the therapist tagged the pattern—blame seeking—and directed attention to the reasons for it. There was only indirect interest in finding out who was "right." The process of distorting, and its relation to the case formulation, were far more important. The insight about blame grabbing could help enable the Growth Collaborator to choose to trump the plans of the Regressive Loyalist.

Validity of Memories

Changes in Memories throughout Therapy

As patients reflect on themselves and others, their perspectives change. Parents, siblings, and others who were seen as loving may now be seen as negligent or punitive. Parents who were seen as monsters may now be seen with compassion and understanding. Sometimes the views of how things were and are comes full circle. Maybe at the beginning of therapy, parents were idealized; at midtherapy, perhaps they were vilified; at the end, they are loved for what they were and are, regardless of what they were not. Ultimately, the patient in IRT should be able to face facts about self and others honestly, and with broadly based compassion and acceptance, as he or she seeks to grow more loving and useful.

Accuracy of Recall

Quite often, psychiatry residents, medical students, and others ask whether patients' stories are "real" when they see the DLL consultative interviews. They ask, "How do we know that patients are telling the truth? How can we base a case formulation on information that comes from a patient only?" It is true that communications from patients (and others) will be affected by defenses, including outright lying. The clinician needs to remain aware of such potential difficulties in obtaining valid data.

Insistence on details that are translated directly into interpersonal patterns helps keep the narrative relevant and accurate.[44] It is hard for the patient to send a false signal to the IRT clinician who listens for consistency in the underlying dimensionality of stories and therapy process. For example, suppose a patient wishes to make the point that her family is mean and bad, and that she has been egregiously wronged. Furthermore, suppose the patient makes up abuse stories to support the position. Suppose this patient were to say, "My father sexually abused me," when he did not. In such a "false-memory" case, the clinician would probably note that the patient's narratives are saturated with blaming and sulking interpersonal process. These patterns would be present in other stories too (e.g., doctors, bosses, teachers, and others would also be reported to have engaged in abuse, negligence, or other forms of bad faith). Soon the patterns of Passive–Aggressive Personality Disorder would be established via the patient's phenomenology and process. The IRT clinician always considers the possibility that any given story is false, and looks for consistency among stories. If a story appears to be false, the challenge becomes to develop a case formulation that accounts for why the patient would make up such a story. The example of passive–aggressive patterns just given illustrates one way the clinician could identify a true "false memory."

The Role of Informants

In addition to relying on the overall coherence of specific patterns to establish a valid case formulation, the IRT clinician recognizes that informants can be quite useful. However, it is also good to remember that informants have their own defensive systems.[45] Although the IRT therapist rarely excludes the patient from discussions of him or her, any informant reports about life-threatening situations are taken seriously. One does not know ahead of time whether reports are accurate or distorted by the informant's own defenses. If someone takes the trouble to call the therapist of a family member, friend, or associate, it is usually optimal, if possible, to invite the informant to the next session (on an emergency basis, if necessary) to gain necessary clarity.

For example, a husband called to report that his wife, a new patient, was regularly yelling and screaming like a banshee at home. Sometimes it was about suicide. The therapist was well aware of and concerned about her suicidality, but not about this form of expressing it. The husband was asked to come to therapy with his wife to discuss this problem. At that session, the patient acknowledged the pattern. She shared her belief that she would have to go psychotic or to die. The yelling and screaming were markers of her desperation. The husband was very helpful in developing a plan for negotiating this period safely (using interventions described in Chapter 7). It was not irrelevant that his behavior had contributed to her despair-laden perceptions. Fortunately, he was not only supportive of her, but also quite willing and able to work on modifying his own behaviors. He only needed awareness of the issues and of better alternatives. Therapy with the wife soon stabilized, and her desperate behaviors abated.

COMMON ERRORS IN PURSUING INSIGHT

Paralysis Associated with Indecision about the "Right" Intervention

The fact that IRT offers a clear model of psychopathology and therapy means that errors can be defined. If an intervention does not conform to the core algorithm, it probably qualifies as an error. However, students sometimes are so worried about implementing the core algorithm that they fear to say or do anything. This is a normal response to any new, complex learning assignment. The "cure" is to start at a very simple level, trying to master only one or two components at a time.

For example, start with working from a baseline of accurate empathy and asking for details about input and response. Other components can be added gradually. Impact on the self, and exploring the ABCs could follow. It is important to know that the therapist does not compulsively explore every component of the core algorithm in a specific order. Some parts, like input and response, flow more easily than others. Others, like impact on the self, are more difficult to obtain, and can be delayed until later after interpersonal patterns are better understood. Once the interpersonal nature of the patterns and their affective and cognitive correlates has become clear, attending to the case formulation and the Red and Green balance can be emphasized more.

Finally, if the many examples in this book have not made the style of an IRT interview apparent, let it be said here that the IRT therapist mindfully attends to the core algorithm, but he or she is not robotic. Usually the patient's unconscious directs the flow of the session, and the therapist rides along, guiding the process unobtrusively. Therapists learning IRT should use lighter rather than heavier hands, expect to make mistakes, and seek to recognize and acknowledge them. They should be patient, and not be surprised if much practice is needed.

Therapist Denial

Once past the barrier of fear of making a mistake, the clinician faces a second common inhibitor: the fact that the patient is going to need to talk about things the therapist does not want to hear. If the patient alludes to current suicide potential or negative feelings about the therapist, it is natural for the therapist to attend to "something else." It is easy to avoid looking at the approaching menace. However, subtle expressions of patterns that are central to the case formulation should be brought to light, no matter how much the therapist wishes they did not exist. For example, suppose a patient says, "I didn't want to come today because I did not use my time well last session." If the therapist begins to reassure, or explain that progress is not always apparent, there is a high risk of overlooking negative feelings about the therapist or the therapy. "Tell me more about that" is probably a better response to such a potentially loaded general remark. Careful listening and thoughtful reflection on therapy process and underlying patterns might follow.

The best way out of an ugly exchange is to go straight to its center and come out the other side with a new perspective in the light of the case formulation. *Dive in!* Throughout this book, there are examples of such difficult discussions of unwelcome messages. Ideally, the clinician reader will become appropriately desensitized after a number of such examples. A certain toughness is needed to work with nonresponders, who sometimes are willing to defy normal social niceties and expose therapists to major interpersonal toxins. Being prepared to be the target of problem patterns and to understand them is an excellent way to enhance the likelihood of being helpful.

Forgetting the Case Formulation

Forgetting the case formulation is a very common error for beginning IRT therapists. It is incredibly easy to provide empathic understanding that goes too far beyond the initial need to make a connection by "cozying up to" the Red (discussed in Chapter 5). For example, a therapist was doing very well at helping his patient, Karl, explore input, and response, in specific terms and at developing the ABCs. He was empathic and supportive, and Karl appreciated the sessions. The discussions frequently centered on his wife's impossible demands and her apparent inability to consider his own perspective. Karl was strongly supported emotionally by the therapist. However, Karl remained, as he said, frustrated with his wife.

To become IRT-adherent, this empathic therapist would need to think of Karl's situation with his wife in relation to a case formulation. Karl's life struggle had always been with an abusive older brother, and it sounded very much as if he had married an interpersonal replica of his brother.[46] In that light, it would be important for Karl to link his feelings about his wife to his feelings about his brother. Ongoing description of the flaws in his wife would change nothing in his life. Karl might do better to begin challenging his apparent assumption that "it is as it was and ever more must be so." Here is a possible shortcut that would work if Karl were basically secure and flexible. First, the therapist would explain complementarity theory[47] and explore whether Karl would be interested in trying some new responses to his wife.[48] A brief role play, wherein Karl played the part of his wife and the therapist modeled alternative responses, might get him started. His subsequent experience and feelings as he tried the new ways of responding with his wife might be a topic for the next session. Some less impaired patients can jump ahead with this kind of structure. Unfortunately, most nonresponders must take the longer route of coming to terms by repeatedly engaging in the activities outlined in Figures 3.2 and 3.3.

"Telling"

"Telling" can be appropriate in a one-time consultative interview, and sometimes during crisis.[49] However, in a growth-oriented, ongoing outpatient psychotherapy, "telling" rarely fits the core algorithm. The validity of the DLL hypothesis is better tested, and the learning is more compelling, if insight emerges out of the therapy narrative. For insight to serve as the prelude to change, the patient must fully experience (in terms of ABCs) the meaning of links between the presenting problems and IPIRs. Active learning is more effective than passive learning. Examples throughout this book attempt to illustrate how recommended interventions evolve in an empathic context, with the patient taking as much initiative as possible.

Timing

Patients and novice therapists are very likely to bring up difficult topics right at the end of the session. A therapist should try hard to avoid this error. If the therapist decides to focus on a new or difficult aspect of a problem, it is good to bring it up when there is time to discuss it. It is most unwise to send the patient out the door with a new, perhaps startling thought without immediate options to explore it further.

For example, a student therapist noticed that a woman was repeatedly getting in debt and her father would have to bail her out. At the end of a session, the student said, "I wonder who you are punishing with your spending?" It was quite clear that this was the patient's father. Bringing up this hypothesis early in the session would have been better. Moreover, the interpretation would be more effective if elicited from the patient rather than imposed by the therapist. For example, early in a session during which money was the topic, the therapist might ask, "Do you have any idea how your father feels about this pattern of spending to the point where he has to bail you out?"

Knowing when as well as how to bring up a pattern does require some practice. A good general rule is to stay close to what the patient is saying and follow the core algorithm. The most effective interpretations usually appear as carefully chosen reflections of the patient's own words. The therapist should also consider timing, avoid bringing up difficult issues when there is no time to follow through, and emphasize strength toward the end of a session. Otherwise, the therapist should let the process flow as intensely as the patient is willing to allow.

SUMMARY

In IRT, insight is said to have been achieved if the patient understands and acknowledges the accuracy and completeness of the case formulation. That is, the patient can identify (1) a problem pattern in terms of input, response, and impact on the self; (2) copy process links between a problem pattern and one or more IPIRs; and (3) wishes in relation to the IPIRs that support the problem pattern. When full insight is achieved, these three forms of pattern recognition (description, links, wishes) are accurate and are expressed in the three domains of affect, behavior, and cognition. The principal purpose of insight in IRT is motivational. It sets the stage for enabling the will to change.

Development of insight can be relatively rapid in IRT, but implementation of insight depends on developing a secure base, which for non-responders takes a long time. Security can be facilitated both within the therapy relationship itself and as the therapy encourages better relationships with contemporary important figures. Once acquired, security helps the patient muster the courage to apply insight—to let go of old fantasies and become free to engage in self-definition on his or her own terms. The chapter has discussed several activities that facilitate insight, as well as common errors.

NOTES

1. The CCRT method is reviewed in Luborsky, Popp, Luborsky, and Mark (1994). Other interpersonal assessment methods for use in research on insight include Cyclical Maladaptive Pattern analysis (compared to the CCRT method by Johnson et al., 1989) and Role Relationship Models (Horowitz et al., 1991).

2. Either a tailor-made system (ad hoc categories based on material at hand) or the QUAINT (Quantitative Analysis of Interpersonal Themes) coding system, which includes universal categories based on the Structural Analysis of Social Behavior (SASB) plus selected categories of affect.

3. Defined in terms of convergence between prior descriptions of the CCRT and assessment of CCRT in the therapy narratives.

4. Again, it is assumed that therapist discussion of the CCRT is correlated with patient awareness of it.

5. In particular, patient awareness of patterns involved in conflict. Objective methods of defining patterns, and of determining whether they are conflicted, can begin to test the psychoanalytic assumption that conflict underlies psychopathology.

6. The SASB model can also enhance the clinician's ability to see patterns and their links.

7. This intervention combines rules 1, 2, and 3 from the core algorithm. There are an infinite number of possibilities, and the clinician is encouraged to invoke more than one rule at a time whenever possible.

8. "Adherence" is observed if an intervention implements one or more rules from the core algorithm and does not violate any of them.

9. Most forms of supervision or consultation require patient consent. Clinicians should use good judgment as to when a generic consent-to-treatment form (such as the one provided in Appendix 3.1) is exceeded, and permission specific to a given consultation is required. For example, students in a practicum obtain signed permission from each case to discuss it in the group supervisory situation. The patient knows the supervisor's name and qualifications, as well as the identity of the class/group that will be hearing details of the case.

10. See "Summary and Conclusions" at the end of Chapter 5 (p. 188).

11. This problem has been introduced in Chapter 5 in the section "Does Attachment to the Therapist Facilitate Destructive Dependency?"

12. This has been described by Bowlby (1969, 1977) and discussed in Chapter 2.

13. The therapy relationship (Chapter 5) and insight (this chapter) are necessary but still not sufficient conditions for reconstructive change. Consistent implementation of the flow charts in Chapters 3 and 7 is also required to encourage the necessary experiential learning.

14. Because I did not independently check the security of Martha's attachment, and because attachment is so central to IRT theory, this interpretation is circular. However, it would be possible to do so, for example, by giving her the Adult Attachment Interview (reviewed in Hesse, 1999).

15. This term usually refers to a patient who is able to cooperate with and benefit from therapy interventions. It probably originally meant "person with a higher level of ego strength."

16. Martha learned in therapy how to DISCLOSE rather than BLAME when engaged in a dispute with her mother.

17. In IRT, the formal definition of an adequate level of detail is that the episode is SASB-codable. This means that there is enough detail to identify two interactive persons or forces, a focus, a judgment on the love–hate continuum, and a judgment on the CONTROL/SUBMIT to EMANCIPATE/SEPARATE continuum.

18. Now the episode sounds more as if the mother were SEPARATE in relation to the patient as she PROTECTed the sister.

19. Here, the code for the mother would be (among other things) IGNORE.

20. This would suggest ATTACK as an appropriate initial descriptor.

21. This sounds like ACTIVE LOVE.

22. Discussed in Chapter 2.

23. Complementarity is defined and illustrated in Chapter 4.

24. Usually through the principle of complementarity.

25. His demanding dependency (TRUST plus CONTROL) had elicited from the therapist a complementary position of coerced caregiving (PROTECT plus SUBMIT).

26. Referral to an outpatient therapist who could and would follow recommendations in the IRT discharge summary would have been ideal.

27. Some readers might object that this remark is too suggestive. Its purpose is to facilitate collaboration by explaining why there is interest in the past. If one simply introduces a question out of the blue, this does not indicate mutual respect in the relationship. Note that the statement is very general and does not suggest specific connections. There is room for there to be none, as illustrated by the examples in this paragraph.

28. The full-model SASB codes for the father's part of this scenario would be as follows: For the father, **136. Put down, act superior**; for the patient, *235. Appease, scurry* and *337. Restrain, hold back self*. The rule was this: "Suppress yourself [*337. Restrain, hold back self*], or you will wound [**121. Angry dismiss, reject**] your father who will then leave you [*221. Flee, escape, withdraw*]." In other words, the unusual rule here was that Bryan had to degrade and suppress himself in order to avoid rejecting and losing father. The link between his self-negation and the father IPIR constituted key insight.

29. This technique has been mentioned previously in Chapter 2. It is particularly helpful to use SASB coding to classify patterns in terms of attachment, control, separation, or hostility (which serves control, distance, or both).

30. SASB dimensions.
31. SASB coding can objectify the intuitive. The spider in the dream was menacing and generally included focus on other (the dreamer) that was hostile and had influence. A relevant point on the full model would be **131. Approach menacingly**. The complement, of course, would be <u>231.Wary, fearful</u>. The creature grew larger and went away (<u>228. Go own separate way</u>). Somebody invited it into a swimming pool (**142. Provide for, nurture**), where it became clear that the creature was playful and nice (<u>212. Relax, flow, enjoy</u>). These codes move from the hostile to the loving axis—and, indeed, summarize the fundamental therapy task that Mandy eventually mastered. She separated from old menace, gave up her self-hate, and came to appreciate all that she was and could be.
32. An approach explained by Theodor Reik (1949).
33. SASB coding makes the links very clear. The hymn was about PROTECT, and <u>TRUST</u> was its complement. The patient was quite sure that she could not trust her husband, and she wondered about the therapy. The dimensionality of the dream and the song were the same.
34. As usual, SASB codes of the narrative can help the clinician tag the quintessential issues in the narrative
35. DLL theory prescribes that the presenting problem is the derivative of an important attachment. The question explores the internalization of a key figure in relation to this problem of despair and emptiness.
36. The codes of this narrative would fall almost exclusively on "track 2" of the SASB full model, which plots variations on the theme of nurturance. The codes would be that the patient manifested *322. Ignore own basic needs*, which was an internalization of **123. Abandon, leave in lurch** or **122. Starve, cut out**. She yearned for the opposite—**142. Provide for, nurture**. Beth realized that she might not be able to accept it if it came her way (<u>242. Refuse assistance, care</u>), although she was able to provide well for others. She also felt amazement when seeing the result of nurturance in a colleague (*342. Nurture, restore self*), and outrage when seeing neglectful parents.
37. So that it can be SASB-coded.
38. Recorded with permission of all participants, and following disclosure of the reasons for making the tape.
39. Loftus et al. (1994) did not provide these citations to make the point that repression is clinically important. Nonetheless, the findings speak well to that point.
40. The ideal study would compare forgetting of salient welcome events to traumatic or otherwise unwelcome events. One obvious methodological challenge here would be to define salience. Trauma can be assumed to be salient. Perhaps the control condition should be memory for salient expectably positive events, such as going to the circus the first time, the day of graduation from high school, or the day of marriage. Defining expectable salience is important. Surely the control comparison should not involve memory of what was for dinner on July 1, 1990.
41. Classical psychoanalysts see conflict in terms of ego versus id or superego. The central purpose of defenses is viewed as blocking awareness (cf. Greenberg & Mitchell, 1983).

42. Patients with BPD are famous for lacking identity because they often suddenly change plans and trash the immanent realization of an identity they have been working toward. The underlying identity is to need the services of an important one, and this easily supports the lifestyle of being a nonfunctional, perpetually challenging patient.

43. For example, perhaps such a man had training to the effect that he had inordinate destructive power within the family. One way or another, he learned that passing thoughts, trivial gestures, crimes of omission, or maybe even his very existence could "cause" catastrophic reaction, even death. (See such a case in Benjamin, 2000c.)

44. However, it is no guarantee.

45. Within some cultures, there is a strong preference for family or friends to come in to a session separately, to give information out of the patient's hearing. I suggest instead that an informant attend the first session and share the perspective with the patient and relevant others. I am reluctant to hold sessions that exclude the patient (and, as a result, have lost a number of referrals). Therapist preferences on this will differ, but I believe that in the long run, it is best to have whatever is going on "put on the table." When informants have accepted the invitation to share their views with the patient, the result has almost always been constructive.

46. SASB codes of BLAME for the brother and wife, SULK for the patient.

47. If the clinician did not use the SASB model to explain complementarity, it would still be possible to speak of it in general terms: "It is often true that hostility begets hostility. If somebody breaks the cycle and there is underlying good well, better patterns can follow."

48. That is, therapy goal behaviors as defined by the SASB model.

49. In consultative interviews, there has to be "telling" if the patient is to know what goes in the consultative report. Cautions and considerations about whether and when to do this are discussed in Chapter 2.

7

Step 3:
Blocking Maladaptive Patterns

OVERVIEW OF METHODS OF
BLOCKING PROBLEM BEHAVIORS

It is difficult for nonresponders to stop doing what makes things worse for themselves and others. Suicidality, homicidality, and child abuse are among the more dramatic and alarming versions of their maladaptive patterns. Blocking these, as well as unblocking therapy stalemates, has a high priority in Interpersonal Reconstructive Therapy (IRT). According to Developmental Learning and Loving (DLL) principles of case formulation (Chapter 2), problem patterns continue because there are good internal reasons for them. Despite how nonsensical they appear to the rational observer, maladaptive patterns serve the purpose of offering hope that there will be, that there can be reconciliation with Important Persons and their Internalized Representations (IPIRs). It follows that the therapy must address and transform these internal reasons if the maladaptive behaviors are to cease and be replaced by better alternatives.

Self-Discovery as a Means of Reorganizing Motivation

Important components of the recommendations for step 3 of IRT, maladaptive patterns, appear in the third row of Figure 3.1. Self-discovery activities, shown in the center of the figure, address the problem motivation (Red) and help set new motivation (Green). Self-management activities, shown at the right, help get the job done. After self-discovery has led to credible challenge of the underlying sustaining motivation, then customary self-management activities can become quite effective, even if they previously have failed.

Seeing It Differently and Reacting Differently

Self-discovery helps people see situations differently and react differently. For example, Martha (see Chapter 6), who was dangerously suicidal in order to "escape" her mother's relentless control, gave it up when she fully understood the costs relative to the gains. Her motivation changed when she achieved insight. Given that she had adequate security to risk change, Martha was able to stop the suicidal behaviors, as she also began to develop better-differentiated responses to her mother.

Befriending and Valuing the Self

Befriending the self can also enhance the motive to block the problem behaviors. Many nonresponders have internalized hatred and do not easily think about what might be best for them. It is important that they be helped to find compassion for themselves when they were abused, ignored, shamed, and the like. Such appreciation can help them give themselves permission not to engage in problem actions. Discussions in Chapters 5 and 6 have made it clear that the therapy relationship can facilitate self-care, which includes blocking problem behaviors. Other benevolent relationships do the same.

Changes in Self-Management Following Initial Changes in Motivation

Insight does not complete the task of motivational reorganization, nor does the conscious decision to try to befriend the self. More often, the techniques discussed in Chapter 8 in connection with step 4 (enabling the will to change) are required before the patient can fully and effectively reorganize the underlying motivation. Nonetheless, awareness of a credible case formulation and a decision to treat the self better can start the underlying change process. It is important that patients learn early in therapy to relate dangerously maladaptive patterns to their case formulation. Understanding that their extreme behaviors are gifts of love often helps people to restrain themselves in the short term.

Changing Self-Talk and Behavior

One of the ways patients can block problem patterns is to change their self-talk. For example, a man whose rages are copies of his violent father's may decide to say, " I do not want to be like him any more. I am determined to learn to handle this differently. " Usually he will need some coaching in how to develop alternative responses to the situations that are likely to set off his rages. Simple assertiveness training may, for example, be very helpful to him, once he has decided that he no longer will provide violent testimony to his father IPIR. Mood-altering medications may also help him resist the old way of responding.

Invoking New Internal Models

Newly motivated patients may become better able to take advantage of role plays, during which the therapist models more adaptive self-talk and alternative ways to respond to a recurrent crisis situation. Patients can pick other models as well. The point is that they need a new image for themselves, a new interpersonal goal to work toward.

CRISIS MANAGEMENT

Standard Considerations for Crisis Management

Every clinician needs to know how to assess and appropriately address emergencies, regardless of theoretical orientation.

Commitment to a Hospital during a Crisis

If the health care provider perceives that there is a psychiatric emergency, such as threatened suicide or homicide, he or she should engage standard interventions designed to make it less likely that the violent event will take place. The intervention of last resort is to call the police and have the patient transported for safekeeping to a psychiatric hospital, or to whatever facility is appropriate to the situation. If for some reason the patient cannot be detained, there may be a duty to warn any known specific victims or close relatives who might help avert suicide.

Although calling the police is relatively easy for the clinician, it is not so simple to decide whether or not such coercive measures are necessary. Negative impacts of commitment can include the involuntary expense to the patient and possible demoralization over having a commitment on his or her record. Another problem stems from the fact that in psychodynamic therapy, the therapy relationship is central to therapy process (Chapter 5). Commitment carries a significant possibility of damaging the therapy relationship, because it can create feelings of resentment and betrayal.

Clinicians frequently confront situations where there are no really clear guidelines regarding how to weigh the pros and cons of using legal force to protect the patient or others on the one hand, and trusting the patient to control him- or herself on the other. Whereas trusting the patient usually seems the desired alternative, failure to implement hospitalization when the patient's Regressive Loyalist is dominant may result in serious injury to self or others. That, of course, is a result to be avoided above all.

Voluntary Hospitalization for Safekeeping

While forced hospitalization involves a high risk of introducing unwanted complications to the therapy relationship, voluntary (collaboratively chosen) hospitalization can be very helpful in the treatment of severely disordered persons. A freely chosen hospitalization should not be regarded as a failure. For example, by accepting safekeeping in the hospital, the patient preserves the option of growing later on. Other potential benefits include a cooling-off period in relation to significant other figures; desired delivery of a strong message to key figures; an opportunity to control medications and diet; the potential for consultation and helpful reassessment of what has been going on; and opportunities for new learning (e.g., groups that teach assertiveness, communication skills).

Literature on Suicidal Management

Assessing Suicidal Threats

Standard psychiatric texts, such as Janicak, Davis, Preskorn, and Ayd (1997, pp. 236–241), typically offer lists of risk factors for suicide—such as diagnosis, hopelessness, negative life events (e.g., death of a loved one, humiliation associated with financial ruin), a history of prior attempts, and time since previous hospitalization. Some of the other variables mentioned by these authors as relevant to suicide risk include gender, age, race, family history of suicide, social contagion, impulsivity, drug and alcohol abuse or dependence, number of alcoholic relatives, medical illnesses (e.g., respiratory disease; cancer), socioeconomic status, and certain biochemical features (e.g., lower concentrations of 5-hydroxyindoleacetic acid in cerebrospinal fluid).

Many practicing clinicians agree that the risk is heightened if the patient has specific, credible plans and the means to implement them. Situational factors perceived as overwhelming, deep psychological pain, and a very poor self-concept are among the traditional markers of potential for suicide. Use of alcohol and drugs when one is feeling suicidal is also widely regarded as very dangerous. Psychosis is another factor that increases the likelihood of destructive action. Agitation or impulsivity are especially ominous features because they suggest a propensity to act. Social isolation is not a good prognostic sign, because social support, if available, can serve as a vital antidote. Peruzzi and Bongar (1999) note that it can be important to explore attraction to death by asking about fantasies about life after death. Beck, Brown, and Steer (1989) have developed a scale to assess the degree of hopelessness, which they believe is a particularly potent warning sign.

Recent suggestions for how to weigh risk factors are offered by Joiner, Walker, Rudd, and Jones (1999), by Rudd, Joiner, Jobes, and King (1999), and by Peruzzi and Bongar (1999). In addition to considering the problem of interactions among predictors, there are questions about generalizing across populations. The idea that prediction should probably take ethnic differences into account is supported by a report from Morrison and Downey (2000). Their study suggested that African American college students, unlike their Caucasian peers, were unlikely to describe suicidal ideation unless asked directly. The authors reported that African American and Caucasian students responded differently to the Reasons for Living scale. Risk factors for predicting suicide in adolescents are not exactly the same as for adults (Garland & Zigler, 1993; Lewinsohn, Rohde, & Seeley, 1994).

Research studies that mark such actuarial factors and their interactions can be helpful, but the clinician still can feel overwhelmed with the task of reaching a valid judgment of risk for a given patient on a given day. The nonresponder population presents greater challenges in this regard, because they tend to exhibit high levels of many risk factors much of the time. Despite the ongoing, clearly discernible risk for some such patients, it is rare that anyone can be treated on a long-term inpatient basis. It is not possible to hospitalize everybody who presents with suicidal ideation along with risk factors like those listed here and elsewhere. The judgment as to how, when, and how long to hospitalize for suicidality or homicidality typically comes down to a best estimate of how acutely suicidal or homicidal the person is.

Managing Suicidal Threats

Methods for managing suicidal threats include medication to treat the related depression, panic, anxiety, and psychotic thoughts (Janicak et al., 1997). Clinicians often use behavioral interventions, such as no-harm contracts (Kroll, 2000), to try to contain dangerous behavior. As mentioned before, it is a good idea to assess and enhance the support network (e.g., friends, family) when a patient is dealing with a current stress (Kleespies, Deleppo, Gallagher, & Niles, 1999). Rosenberg (1999) has reviewed a cognitive-behavioral focus on dysfunctional suicidal thinking, including examination of ambivalence (which includes a life-enhancing part of the self; exploration of the possibilities that suicide represents rage directed inward, that it stems from retaliatory wishes, and/or that the person feels unable to convey how deeply he or she has been hurt; and clarification that the person really wishes to eradicate the hurt, not the self. This list of current suggestions from the literature that are specific to the management of immediate suicidal threat is only illustrative of current examples. It should not be considered exhaustive.

Impact of Suicide

In addition to ending all options in life for the deceased, suicide has a devastating impact on the individual's family and friends. Suicide of a parent is particularly likely to be destructive to children. To a much lesser degree, suicide also harms the clinician (Peruzzi & Bongar, 1999). In addition to the obvious sense of loss of a person with whom there has been an important relationship, the clinician may face malpractice action initiated by grieving family members or friends. Consequently, quite a bit has been written about how to cope with the stress added by the legal perspective. Jobes and Berman (1993) recommend that clinicians be familiar with relevant laws and ethics, maintain a written policy-and-procedures statement with respect to handling of suicidal behavior, assure clinical competency, and provide adequate documentation of assessments and procedures.

Literature on Homicidality and Its Management

Assessing Homicidal Threats

Other than quite a few papers on the ethical considerations involved in the duty to initiate hospitalization or other action by the police, as well as duty to warn potential victims, the literature on homicidal risk and management of such risk is sparse. Nor does the average psychotherapist have much training in how to recognize homicidal risk or how to manage it (other than, again, to notify proper authorities and potential identified victims). Yet every practicing therapist is likely to confront this problem sooner or later. It might be in the form of a patient who is disgruntled with his or her employer, coworkers, or even the therapist; a battering spouse/partner; a child-abusing parent or a parent contemplating infanticide; or an individual considering homicidal sexual assault.

It is likely that the risk of generic homicidality is increased if the male patient has homicidal thoughts, has a personality disorder or schizophrenia, and uses alcohol (Tiihonen & Hakola, 1994). Similar findings in a female population were reported by Eronen (1995). Rosenbaum and Bennett (1986) suggested that homicide can be associated with depression and suicide, as well as with a history of physical abuse as a child. These authors felt that real or fantasized sexual infidelity was a particularly lethal incentive for homicide. Homicidality toward current or former partners is a distressingly frequent outcome of domestic violence. Simon (1995) has provided a well-documented review suggested that the legal system could do much better at preventing fatal outcomes of domestic violence. Other fatal consequences of spouse/partner abuse can be seen in its association with enhanced suicidality in victims (Kaslow et al., 1998).

Parental violence toward children has been shown to be affected by financial stress, negative life events, and lack of social support, as well as by maternal depression and domestic violence (Levendosky & Graham-Bermann, 2000). There are new programs designed to enhance awareness of and to prevent child abuse (Golden, 2000). In the United States, rates of child abuse decreased from 1997 to 1998, Still, in 1998, over 903,000 cases of child maltreatment were substantiated after being reported and investigated. Forty-nine states reported a total of 1,087 child maltreatment fatalities (Golden, 2000). Distinguished professionals (Finkelhor & Dziuba-Leatherman, 1994) and politicians (DeLay, 2000) have argued that the victimization of children deserves far more attention that it presently receives. These pleas to curb and contain family violence have strong long-term preventive implications at the societal level. Individual clinicians can know that anything they can do to help patients avoid violence toward their spouses/partners and children could be extremely helpful in the lives of all family members and in society in general.

Finally, eroticized homicide deserves mention. Advocates of violent pornography argue that symbolic expression of an association between sexuality and violence reduces the likelihood of violent sexual behavior. The idea is that vicarious expression satisfies the need. On the other hand, advocates of learning theory suggest that the likelihood of sexual violence, including homicide, is very much increased by pornography. A noted sexual serial killer, Ted Bundy, provided compelling testimony in support of that hypothesis. He maintained that such pornography started and encouraged his violent sexual patterns, which resulted in the deaths of a very large and still undetermined number of young women (Michaud & Aynesworth, 1989). It is not reasonable to dismiss Bundy's observations simply as self-serving efforts at blame avoidance. A sample of 25 serial sexual murderers (with three or more known victims each) was compared with a sample of 17 single sexual murderers (with only one known victim each). The serial killers, like Bundy, had more paraphilias, more documented or self-reported violent fantasies, and highly organized crime scenes (Prentky et al., 1989). Hazelwood and Warren (2000, p. 267) also reported "a pervasive and defining fantasy life" in violent sexual serial offenders. A highly relevant review of research on sexual fantasy has been offered by Leitenberg and Henning (1995).

The implication of this perspective is that sexually based homicide could be reduced if the association between eroticism and violence were not so widely encouraged in literature and in the mass media generally. An attempt to disconnect eroticism and violence was implemented by Gidycz et al. (2001), who used a psychoeducational intervention intended to prevent acquaintance rape among college students. They provided subjects arguments in favor of rejecting rape myths, sexual aggression, and more. The intervention resulted only in less acceptance of rape myths—a change that was maintained at a 2-month follow-up. Such research studies with normal college students are not necessarily of compelling immediate use to the clinician working with severely disordered patients. However, studies like these can provide an entrée to discuss social (peer group) attitudes with patients who struggle to contain such violent behaviors as murder, rape, or physical abuse.[1] Discussion alone obviously will not suffice, but to the extent that the therapy relationship is meaningful, therapist mention of alternative perspectives may at least challenge fantasies of glory that the violent client may anticipate at some level.[2]

Managing Homicidal Threats

As mentioned above, not many discussions in the literature have clear implications and compelling usefulness for the clinician who encounters homicidal persons in his or her caseload. A brief but useful publication on this subject is a book chapter by Reid (1989). Some of the markers Reid discusses include intolerance of affect, humiliation, narcissistic injury, the belief that violence is the best choice of behavior, and a limited capacity for nonviolent alternatives. Reid cautions against simplistic views of the causes of violence, and reviews many treatment approaches. Reid (1989, pp. 552–553) first lists "organic/biological" treatments as a way to approach homicidality. Calmatives and sedatives (barbiturates, benzodiazepine) are frequently helpful. If the diagnosis suggests psychosis, then antipsychotics may also be indicated. Electroconvulsive therapy can help contain catatonic excitement. Janicak et al. (1997, pp. 157–159) make related and updated recommendations for handling episodes of acute violence with medications.

Longer-term prevention of violence is more difficult since "there is no 'antiviolence' drug that is specific for severe aggression" (Reid, 1989, p. 553).[3] Reid makes some suggestions for managing aggression, which include trials of maintenance neuroleptics for associated thought disorder, or lithium carbonate if there is an associated bipolar disorder. Propranolol can help inhibit violence associated with central nervous system trauma. Hormonal approaches are mentioned in association with sexual violence. Reid also marks for consideration temporal lobe epilepsy, hypoglycemia, and more. Reid advocates behavioral management of violence and suggests that the clinician conduct a functional analysis of the violence, based on a behavioral log. This procedure helps the patient see the process and consequences of his or her behavior. Work with the family can help the patient develop better alternatives to violence. Psychotherapy is sometimes recommended too, according to Reid. Finally, he suggests that there be attention be given to management of the social environment. Probabilities of violence can be reduced if the violent patient can learn to avoid certain kinds of family conflict and to take seriously the danger of using disinhibitive substances (e.g., alcohol or drugs).

CRISIS MANAGEMENT FROM THE PERSPECTIVE OF IRT

The General Approach

The IRT therapist will take coercive steps against the Red only as a last resort. He or she first tries to engage collaboration with the patient's Green

by discussing the dangerous (Red) behaviors in the light of the case formulation. For example, suicidal patients often feel overwhelmed, defeated,
and full of self-loathing. They report unbearable pain. Their prototypic
fantasy is that death will bring "escape" from all the pain. However, suicidal episodes do not represent escape from conflict, according to DLL theory. Instead, the case formulation is more likely to suggest that suicide represents acceptance of the destructive branch of the conflict between Red
and Green, and is yet another example of hurt and loss. If the patient can
begin to see the suicidal wish is a residual of relationships with IPIRs, the
destructive plan can become less attractive. Later—under conditions of
safekeeping, or after the patient is stabilized—there will be time and conditions that permit developing full emotional appreciation of copy process
links and underlying wishes. With full realization that suicidality is driven
more by residuals of outdated conflicts than by current stress, the desire to
die typically diminishes greatly.

An Illustration of How to Use the Case Formulation
to Block Dangerous Behaviors with a Reluctant Patient

A discussion with Jessica, the psychotic woman introduced in Chapter 1,
illustrates how a clinician needs to become very active in reviewing copy
process links during crisis. At these times "telling" may be necessary.[4] Recall that Jessica was convinced she had been a disruption to the lives of her
parents and siblings. She had lived all of her life with the perception that
they wished she did not exist. Jessica came to a session saying that she was
ready for discharge, and the therapist asked about suicidality. Jessica was
evasive, saying she was satisfied that she had gotten all she needed from
this hospitalization. The therapist was uneasy about the ambiguity in this
declaration.

THERAPIST: What does it mean when you say you have gotten all that you
     need from this hospitalization?

JESSICA: It means what it says.

THERAPIST: Are you saying you have decided to kill yourself, and that is
     okay with you?

JESSICA: Could be.

THERAPIST: Well, that is not OK with me. May we talk about this more?

JESSICA: No.

THERAPIST: That is unfortunate. If we can go no further today, I can only
     recommend that you are not ready for discharge yet.

JESSICA: But I am.

THERAPIST: Not if you are content with a suicidal decision. Are you sure you won't talk about this?

JESSICA: Well, OK. What about it?

THERAPIST: I hear that you see no other options, and believe that there is no other way to understand this. I remind you that what I offer is a chance to learn about your patterns, where they are from, and what they are for. Once you see all that clearly, you would be in a position to decide if you want to change or not. If you decide you don't want to leave things as they are, you may then be in a position to learn different patterns. Now it seems to me that your plan to kill yourself is an intense version of your habit of trying to please your brothers and sisters by serving them, and by staying out of the way as much as possible. So now, after this big blow-up at the family reunion, your plan to kill yourself looks like an effort to please them once and for all!.

JESSICA: Yes, it would.

THERAPIST: And that seems like such a shame. Here you have spent all of your life getting the inappropriate message that you are "in the way." It makes me very sad to think of that little girl shrinking in front of the TV, wishing she did not exist so her brothers and sisters could go play. The fact that you have spent your whole life trying to please them, rarely succeeding, and believing that you were their big problem is really tragic.

JESSICA: (*Quiet*)

THERAPIST: And now you go to the limit and do away with yourself as the ultimate gift.

JESSICA: (*Quiet*)

THERAPIST: Am I on the right track here?

JESSICA: Yes. (*Looks sad*)

THERAPIST: And I wouldn't be surprised if even going *that* far still wouldn't do it. I bet they would even bad-mouth your suicide.

JESSICA: (*Sobs*)

THERAPIST: (*After long silence*) So could we talk more about another way for you to cope with all the pain that has come from a lifetime of trying and failing to please them?

JESSICA: I guess so.

After the discussion of a goals in a longer-term therapy, the session ended as follows:

THERAPIST: How do you feel now?

JESSICA: Exhausted. Sad. Tired.

THERAPIST: Are you feeling like taking better care of Jessica, after all she has been through?

JESSICA: I think so.

THERAPIST: Good. Let's work on this again tomorrow. Once you clearly decide you are going to make up for all the bad years by being nicer to yourself, we can talk about discharge and about how we or your outpatient therapist can continue to work on raising Jessica with love.[5]

Exploring Reluctance to Apply the Case Formulation

As is often the case with people so entrenched in devotion to self-destruction, Jessica arrived at the next session suicidal again, as if no progress had been made in the preceding session. Figure 3.3 suggests possible ways of mobilizing therapy progress after it has stalled in this way. There, it can be seen that exploration of the therapy relationship is a good avenue to try. Again, Jessica's case provides an example:

THERAPIST: So we have developed the theory that you got the message you shouldn't exist because you were such a bother to everyone. So now you will give them what they want.

JESSICA: Right. If that is what they want, I'll do it.

THERAPIST: OK. We need to go back to discuss your willingness to give them so much power over you. But first let's talk about what we are doing. How do you feel about our relationship?

JESSICA: All right. But it makes me nervous.

THERAPIST: Nervous?

JESSICA: Yes. I don't think my family would like this very much.

THERAPIST: Can you say more about that?

JESSICA: Sure. They would tell me that I am just making up all this stuff about my being in the way. And my brother would be furious over what I said about him. I am the sick one. They would say you are putting ideas in my head.

THERAPIST: So they would be critical of this process.

JESSICA: Yes.

THERAPIST: Any idea why they would feel that way?

JESSICA: Well, like I said, I am supposed to be the sick one.

THERAPIST: Sounds like that means you are not supposed to get better. If therapy helps you feel strong, then therapy is bad. If you get ideas they do not like, they will try to discount you and attribute them to me. Then, of course, I will be criticized too.

JESSICA: Exactly.

THERAPIST: Do you think I have put ideas in your head?

JESSICA: Well, you make things very clear. But I don't think you put the ideas in my head. And I see that they make sense.

THERAPIST: You see that I am a friend of your strong part, your Growth Collaborator, and that makes me and therapy the enemy of those who seem to want you to stay the way you are.

JESSICA: I guess.

THERAPIST: So how can we get you to be on your own side? How can we get you to come on over to the side of the Green and work on your own side?

JESSICA: I can try.

THERAPIST: Great. I need you to do that, because, as I said before, I cannot do this alone. Therapy is a learning process, and you have to be active in your own learning.

JESSICA: OK. But I can't imagine being any different.

THERAPIST: I guess that is not surprising, since you have little experience being any other way. You have always tried so hard to stay out of the way and at the same time, to serve. Now we are talking about self-care and speaking up for yourself and all kinds of defiant things! Even choosing to live is defiant and altogether different.

JESSICA: You aren't kidding!

THERAPIST: Nope, I am not. And on top of the threat from defying old rules, there is fear of change. Everyone fears change of this sort. People often say, "If I am not depressed and suicidal, I have no idea what I would be like." It is so familiar that they cannot imagine anything different. We will have to spend quite a lot time working on what you would choose to be if you are able to get free of this old pain. But looking ahead can come later. For now, please understand that it is really natural to feel afraid about this kind of change, but it is possible to get over that fear—with time and support.

At this point, the process had touched on two common blockers shown in Figure 3.3—negative view of therapy, and fear of change—as well as on lingering loyalty to IPIRs mentioned in Figure 3.1, step 4.[6] Follow-up to a crisis session such as this one should review these themes, taking more time to fully develop the patient's ABCs.

A Flow Chart for Dealing with Threats of Dangerous Behavior

Figure 7.1 offers a sharply focused series of recommendations for managing a crisis, except when specific alternative procedures are required by local law.[7] The steps suggested in Figure 7.1 are followed while also adhering to the core algorithm.

Message Received; Checking Willingness to Explore Copy Process Links

According to Figure 7.1, the first step in crisis management is to let the patient know that his or her frightening message has been received. It is unwise to try to ignore cues about suicidality, homicidality, or other forms of dangerous behavior. Under most circumstances, it is appropriate to ask directly about hostile behavior when the clinician senses the possibility that the patient is contemplating such actions. Any affirmation of thoughts along those lines is pursued until it is clear that there may be specific danger. Once it is clear that dangerous behavior is the topic, the IRT therapist asks whether the patient is interested in exploring what might be inspiring the harmful thoughts and what might be done with or about them. If the answer is no, Figure 7.1 suggests that the therapist go over the case formulation and learning contract once again. This review should connect the current dangerous impulses to relationships with IPIRs. This process of moving from a cryptic hostile remark to clarity about definite suicidal planning, followed by treatment, has just been illustrated in the discussion about Jessica's suicidality in relation to her internalization of her siblings.

Consolidating the Decision to Challenge the Copy Process Links

After the review, the therapist again asks whether the patient wants to try to understand his or her current state better. If the patient does not agree to collaborate to control the crisis by examining copy process links and following the steps described in the next section, then the process must shift to symptom management, outlined in Figure 3.4 and discussed in Chapter 3. If the patient says yes, the process shifts to a more detailed exploration of the copy process links. The goal of this conversation is to consolidate the long-term decision to separate from the destructive patterns that presumably provide testimony to the related IPIRs. As indicated above, there probably will not be time to develop this theme fully during a crisis. It will take many subsequent sessions of reexperiencing the pain and despair associated with the relationship with the IPIRs eventually to complete all the steps required for coming to terms (described in Figure 3.2 and discussed in Chapter 3).

Successful crisis work does not require the patient's full acceptance of

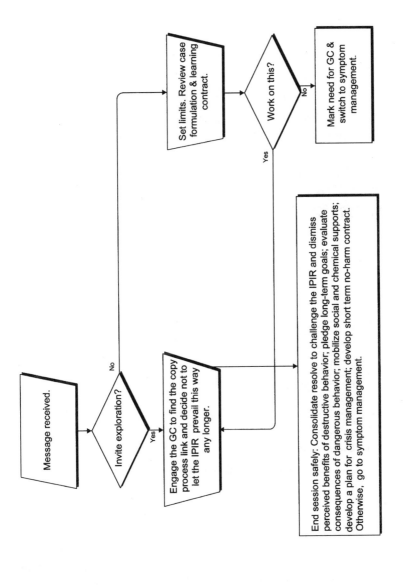

FIGURE 7.1. Dealing with threats of dangerous behavior: "There is no choice but to kill myself [him or her]."

the hypothesis that the destructiveness is based on a gift of love. The patient's primary need is to understand the copy process connections well enough to see that the dangerous behaviors are linked to important relationships in ways his or her Green does not wish to endorse. The patient also needs to have a specific understanding that there are better ways to handle the violent feelings and wishes (discussed below). Finally, the patient needs to be assured that he or she will have an opportunity to work on developing these skills, preferably in longer-term therapy. With this specific form of hope, the patient no longer is without recourse. Understanding, combined with a plausible plan for how to change things in the long term, usually makes it easier for him or her to engage in behavioral control for the short term. From that point on, several steps listed in the lower left-hand box in Figure 7.1 may be very helpful in ending a crisis session safely.

Defining and Challenging the Perceived "Benefits" of Destructive Behavior

Perceived benefits of suicide sometimes reside in fantasies about what the patient expects to happen if he or she were to succeed in self-murder. For example, it might be informative to invite Jessica to anticipate her siblings' reactions to her funeral. She would probably say that they would celebrate and be relieved. But pressed beyond that, she might stall. The dialogue could continue:

THERAPIST: How would it change their lives?

JESSICA: Not at all, except that they wouldn't have me to help out any more.

THERAPIST: How do you feel about that?

JESSICA: Sad for them.

THERAPIST: How about for Jessica?

JESSICA: It doesn't matter as long as they are happy.

THERAPIST: But if they need you to blame and use, how can they be happy if you are gone? To please them, maybe you should stay alive and suffer.[8]

Eventually, such a "crazy" conversation could edge toward recognizing and giving voice to Jessica's long-suppressed rage. More importantly, she would need to rouse compassion for herself. At the beginning, the therapist would be alone with the belief that Jessica should and could be treated better. As that view was shared, Jessica could be invited to fantasize about better, more effective ways to express her anger in service of distance from the internalizations. At the same time, she would be helped to start taking care of herself.

Setting Goals for Long-Term Learning

As mentioned in the section on consolidating the wish to challenge the copy process links, the patient needs to understand in concrete terms how therapy can help him or her find more satisfactory ways of relating to self and others. Generic hopeful remarks or promises that do not specifically address patient needs as defined by the case formulation are not likely to be so effective.

Consider, for example, such statements as "Things will feel better in a while," or "You have to learn to stop letting others bother you so much." Jessica, like so many nonresponders, would not be impressed by iterations of these general truths. However, their core meanings might be tailored in case-relevant ways that could reach her:

> "I know you have been in acute pain ever since the family reunion, and you feel you cannot stand it any longer. We need to understand how your intense pain reflects the years you spent trying to please your siblings, now culminating in what you see as an 'ultimate' failure. Your self-condemnation makes sense if you believe they have access to cosmic truth. On the other hand, it makes more sense to realize that you have let your siblings dominate your view of yourself quite long enough. Does all your service—all those times you have worked so hard to make things better for them—really count for nothing? Although it probably will take us some time to fully understand and appreciate what this all means, it surely is possible to do that. Your siblings just do not hold your passport to existence. You can take it back and reclaim your birthright, if we can help you find a way to focus your remarkable energy more directly on your own best interests. Somehow we have to help you see that your brothers and sisters are not in charge of the universe, as it once seemed."

This way of talking about Jessica's dilemmas would have many important features. It would be highly specific and case-relevant. It would address external stressors, but emphasize personal responsibility and choice. It would be empathic. It would invoke an interpersonal version of evidence-based therapy as it challenged her dysfunctional belief about herself with her own stories. It would redirect an obvious strength—her willingness to work hard—toward her own interests. It would clearly take the eminently reasonable position that she has a birthright to exist but has given it to others. The hope offered would be based on a specific formulation and treatment plan. The time frame would be realistic. Finally, the speech would be so "out there" that Jessica would have plenty of substance to consider as she decided whether to enter into a viable long-term contract to work on making things better.

Reviewing the Disadvantages of Taking Hostile Action against Self or Others

In general, patients need to see that by giving up through suicide, they lose the chance to learn how to change their behavior patterns and the responses of others to them.[9] It may also help to encourage a self-destructive patient to spell out the specific losses he or she would suffer if the suicidal or homicidal plan is implemented. In this process, the clinician needs to be careful to understand the suicidal wish from the perspective of the Red. For example, an ordinary observation about how sad it would be if the patient were to die now might embolden the Red if the case formulation has suggested that sadness is a way to achieve intimacy with an IPIR.

A likely Green loss for suicidal persons is the chance to help and see their children grow. Too many patients listen to a Red message to the effect that their children would be better off without them. This is unlikely to be true. Implementing a specific plan to help cope with whatever is bothering them about the children can serve as a powerful antidote to the idea that the children would be better off without them.[10]

A negative (or positive) perceived consequence of suicide that is easy to overlook relates the patient's spirituality and belief in the afterlife. As mentioned before, it can be very important to explore details of the patient's expectations of what might happen in the afterlife following suicide. Of course, a secular therapist should not discuss theological details of a religious belief system. However, if the patient has a destructive interpretation of his or her religion, referral to an appropriate spiritual counselor may help build Green. Therapist awareness of and support for positive spirituality can be a strong adjunct to therapy (Barlow & Bergin, 2001).

Exploration of the consequences of homicidal behavior is similar to the exploration process for suicidal behavior. However, severe social sanctions are added to the list of consequences for homicidal behavior. Sometimes patients need to be informed about state laws on this matter. Some inappropriately imagine that there are no consequences if their crime is judged to be due to mental illness. One deterrent for these folks may be to learn that in some states, a person who murders while mentally disordered is indeed treated; however, when recovered, he or she then has to stand trial.

Mobilizing Social and Chemical Supports

A collaborative discussion of the patient's current social situation may help him or her find alternative ways to deal with the current stress. Referral to likely community resources is often helpful. These may include lawyers, local agencies and facilities, a wise coworker, appropriately supportive and resourceful friends, and so on. The IRT therapist freely uses such resources chosen in relation to the case formulation. Such support almost always represents appropriate self-affirmation and self-protection.[11]

Use of medications for crisis management is likewise helpful. Of course, antidepressants take a while to become effective, so interim hospitalization may be required if other supports are not adequate. Antipsychotics can have a more rapid impact and help in implementing short-term behavioral management. One viciously self-destructive man was greatly reassured to know that he could quiet his voices with Haldol if they started telling him to stab himself again. In the meanwhile, we studied the impact of his developmental learning on those voices. On the basis of his case formulation, we constructed a self-management plan for quieting the voices if and when they started bothering him. When subsequent crises did come, he was able to banish the voices and keep control of his mind. He did not have to use the medicine, but the availability of the powerful pills gave him the audacity to prevail over his old internal programming. This man saw antipsychotic medication as the safety net under his tightrope. Such a collaborative attitude greatly enhances the effect of treatment, whether chemical or psychosocial.

Social skills training is another form of support. A minor version of skills training can be initiated if the therapist role-plays a particular situation that has been difficult for the patient.[12] Interpersonal skills training in general is especially likely to be useful to people who have learned absolutistic, all-or-nothing, black-or-white ways of thinking. Examples of these beliefs include Life is a jungle ("Everyone for him- or herself, regardless of the impact on others") or Life is a courtroom ("Right and wrong are the only choices. If you are right, I am wrong. If I am right, you are wrong. If I hate you, I am right. If I love you, I am wrong"). Softening of these beliefs can help defuse a crisis. For example, if the patient wants to die because of a recent mistake, a more modulated way of thinking (one with shades of gray) can dilute the suicidal impulse. This is, of course, an application of cognitive-behavioral therapy (CBT). In IRT, this use of CBT techniques is modified by adding the observation that a specific IPIR modeled this style. Hence the motive for all-or-nothing thinking is targeted, as well as the practice itself.

Developing a Structured Plan for Crisis Management

People who have a long history of responding to crisis with suicidal thoughts can be calmed down if the therapist is willing to hear out all the problems and help sort through them one at a time. Problem solving can require a form of advice giving about the problem-solving process. The recommendation to give specific help in problem solving defies a tradition that therapists do not give advice. Nonetheless, with clients whose Red is very active, structuring a process for successful immediate problem solving can be critical in negotiating a crisis safely. Let it be clear that IRT advice giving never takes the form of advising about any particular life choice, such as "Divorce him," "Buy the car," "Quit your job," or "Kick that kid out of the house." Although very active in directing the therapy process, IRT therapists do not advise patients about important life choices, even in crisis.

For example, consider Laura, a patient with an abusive history who was repeating her pain in an unusually exploitative divorce process. She was also trying to manage a rebellious and hateful adolescent son, to whom she always had deferred. Finally, she was hearing a voice that interfered severely with her work. Laura knew that if this continued, she would lose her job.

The therapist systematically discussed approaches to the divorce, the adolescent, and the voice. The husband resembled an abusive older brother and was repeating his attacking patterns in the divorce process. The therapist helped Laura seek the counsel of a reliable lawyer and follow instructions to protect herself materially. The adolescent son was responding to her deference with tyranny. He was beginning to resemble the brother and husband.[13] A plan for parent training was suggested, along with the promise of further exploration of links among the son, brother, and husband. The voice was marked as the most immediate problem, because without her job, Laura would have very few resources with which she could take care of herself. She did not wish to use antipsychotics, but they were listed as a requirement if she could not manage the voice on her own. The voice echoed the voices of her older brother and husband. There was a discussion of mental strategies that could help her resist the voice's destructive messages. For example, she was mobilized positively by the thought that to fall apart would make her estranged husband happy. She was in touch with enough anger at him to become determined not to listen to his "voice." These specific steps to address the three problems (divorce, adolescent, voice), combined with plenty of empathic support, helped Laura stabilize quickly and continue long-term therapy work on her gifts of love.

Obtaining the Patient's Agreement to a Short-Term No-Harm Contract

Before a session can be considered to have ended safely, the patient must agree to a short-term contract not to act on his or her homicidal or suicidal urges for a specific time period, depending on current circumstances. For example, the time might be until a week after an upcoming critical event. A more general version of a no-harm contract is that there will be no harm of self or others until the current crisis has been discussed for three successive therapy sessions. If necessary, at the end of the third session, there will be a discussion of whether a new short-term contract is needed. Ordinarily, three sessions is enough to help Green take over again. Then it is all right to revert to the basic long-term contract discussed below. If any session cannot be ended safely, then Figure 7.1 shows that the clinician moves to all-out symptom management (Figure 3.4).

Long-Term No-Harm Contracts

A therapist had followed the conventional procedure of asking a chronically angry patient at the end of each session whether he was suicidal or homicidal. He always said no, and that fact had been duly recorded for many sessions over a long period of time. One day the patient came to therapy with a gun, and murdered the therapist and himself. Clearly, his word that he was not homicidal or suicidal was not valid. This incident makes it very clear that simply asking an assessment question or securing a promise may not be enough. In IRT, such assessments and contracts depend on clear collaboration between patient and therapist. Collaboration can be assessed in the light of the case formulation and analysis of the therapy process.[14]

In addition to the short-term no-harm contract just discussed, IRT includes a long-term no-harm contract that applies to all outpatients except for those who clearly state that they are not suicidal (or homicidal or otherwise dangerous) and never will be. The matter is ended for these people who are unlikely to engage in harm to self or others with a comment such as this: "Please let me know if that ever changes." For people who have a history of suicide attempts or violence toward others, and/or who are presently struggling with dangerous urges, the long-term contract goes well beyond asking about suicidality and homicidality. Here it is:

> Will you agree to discuss your thoughts of harming self or others whenever they come up in therapy? If you are tempted to act on your destructive wishes, will you agree not to act on them—but instead to call me, reach me, discuss it briefly on the phone, and agree to meet me in an emergency meeting if necessary? Simply leaving a voice mail message will not fulfill the terms of this contract. When we talk on the phone, it will be very brief, because I do not do emergency therapy on the phone. I will only attempt to try to get in touch with your stronger (Green) parts, so that you will be able to make it until the next therapy session, when we can go over it all in detail. If that does not succeed, we may decide to have an emergency session. If that does not seem reasonable, we may have to turn to the hospital for help.

Some of the less common features of this long-term contract are as follows: (1) It is specific about procedures for how to keep the contract; (2) it does not ask for a blanket, open-ended agreement to contain harmful behaviors; and (3) the therapist, rather than a crisis line or emergency room, is identified as the person to call. Here are the reasons for constructing the long-term contract this way:

1. Specific procedures are described, because the Red parts of patients are wily and are sure to find a way around any generic agreement. The most likely violation of a broad agreement to call the therapist when a patient is feeling suicidal would be to leave a message such as the following on the therapist's phone: "You said to call if I felt like harming myself. I do. Goodbye," or "I called and you didn't answer, so now I am going to do it. Goodbye."

2. The contract does not take away the choice of harmful acts for all time; it only asks for specific preventive behaviors to be implemented. This is the case because it is not realistic to ask potentially dangerous patients to give an unlimited no-harm contract. Either they will refuse the contract, or they will have to lie. It is destructive to collaboration to put people in a position where they have to lie. The short-term no-harm contract, which does ask for absolutely no harm to self or others, is for a specific, short interval. People often can and will agree to meaningful absolute no-harm contracts for a brief period.[15] The time then "bought" can be used to build collaboration and mobilize the will to contain the Red plan and build Green strength instead.

3. Having the therapist be the first point of contact reflects the IRT goal of supporting Green, which typically (but not always) includes avoiding hospitalization. In IRT, the therapy relationship is central to the treatment, and the therapist is necessarily the only one who can use the therapy relationship to help during crisis. The IRT therapist knows the case formulation and can probably understand a patient's harmful urges in light of recent events. As is clear throughout this chapter, the case formulation can be used to block the harmful action. Moreover, the attachment to the therapist and the therapy process can provide a sense of future, along with the possibility of alternative solutions. The immediacy of contact with the therapist during the crisis makes it harder to forget the potential that therapy offers to the Green. This advantage is wholly contingent on collaboration.

IRT therapists can have many legitimate personal reasons not to be available after hours. These therapists can instead ask patients to call crisis lines or emergency rooms if they need contact outside of therapy sessions. As long as crises are viewed and discussed in terms of the case formulation, and as long as therapist interventions conform to the core algorithm, the therapy is IRT-adherent.

Standard Tools: Hospitalization, Commitment, Duty to Warn or Notify

If the IRT therapist is not sure that there is good collaboration and that a no-harm contract is valid, he or she should consider hospitalization, commitment, and duty to warn potential victims of homicide or concerned relatives of a suicidal patient. These actions, as well as referral to a crisis service that is not IRT-adherent, constitute a switch to symptom management (see Figure 3.4). The discussion of the related literatures at the beginning of this chapter has shown that there are many usual and customary ways to assess and deal with suicidality or homicidality. There is no attempt to review or prioritize them here. Once the flow of events shown in Figure 7.1 has switched to symptom management, IRT is interrupted or even terminated. Usual and customary rules take over.

Hospitalization itself will not include the IRT approach unless a service has people specifically trained in IRT. It is relatively rare that a patient needs to be hospitalized while in IRT, but the option and willingness to hospitalize for symptom management is a vital adjunct to IRT.

"Outpatient Hospitalizations"

If the patient wants a port in a storm, or a period of rest and rehabilitation (R&R), a "prescribed vacation" can be a good idea. The plan is implemented so that there are adequate promises for safekeeping and nonstressful companionship. It would be unwise, for example, to send a suicidal person on a vacation with someone with whom there is mortal psychological combat. Similarly, a desperate wife enmeshed in an abusive marriage should not be sent to a remote place essentially to do full-time battle. Rather, she might do well on such a vacation with a wise and kind aunt, or friend from work, or an old college buddy. There needs to be reasonable access to health care if necessary. The idea is that a benign vacation will directly address the need for R&R, can be a lot cheaper than hospitalization, and will probably be more fun. Naturally, this plan demands a solid collaboration between therapist and patient. Without trust and good collaboration, the plan will not be safe.

The therapist and client can create other versions of an "outpatient hospitalization." These plans provide a break in routine, and some way to optimize safekeeping. Staying with an attentive friend while taking sick leave is one example.

Handling a Crisis by Telephone

Sometimes, especially early in IRT, the clinician may receive a desperate call at an unscheduled time. Handling a crisis by telephone presents special challenges, because the threat can be real, but the clinician is not physically present to see nonverbal cues. Communication is necessarily compromised. In addition, the call may come at a time when the clinician is otherwise engaged and not ready or able to focus intensely on the caller. Furthermore, the steps in Figure 7.1 cannot be implemented properly during an unexpected, brief phone call. All of these factors indicate that a clinician should attempt only brief and minimal interventions by telephone.

Basic Steps

Here is a short list of basic steps that need to be included in handling a phone crisis. Good first questions are "What's going on?", followed by "Where are you?" If the patient hangs up, or won't agree to safety by the end of the conversation, the therapist then has a choice of whether to ask a family member or even the police to go check on the patient. Asking whether the patient has been taking prescribed medications and whether he or she is hearing voices (including what they are saying) is part of assessing the patient's state and the immediacy of the danger, as is asking whether the patient has been using alcohol or illicit drugs. If the patient is dangerous and in a chemically altered state (i.e., medication overdose or use of illicit drugs/alcohol), the IRT therapist immediately defers to external controls (family members or police officers take custody).

If the patient is sober, the conversation can continue. If there is a threat of suicide or homicide, it is wise to ask whether the patient has the means (razor, gun, rope, etc.) available. If so, then before the conversation ends, it is good to ask that he or she get rid of the means immediately. Examples of ways to do this include asking the patient to flush the blades or pills, and asking the patient to direct a responsible family member to remove all guns from the house right now. If collaboration seems weak, it may be necessary to ask to have a responsible family member speak on the phone, so the therapist can hear that the support person will assist in follow-through.

The optimal outcome of such an episode is to end the conversation with a trustworthy short-term no-harm contract, including an agreement to meet soon and discuss the threat of dangerous behavior in ways described in Figure 7.1. Usually this emergency appointment will take place the next day. The therapist is well advised to anticipate that there may be a need to transport the patient to the hospital at the end of the emergency session. Asking a family member to bring the patient to the session and to be available after the session is one way to approach that logistical problem.

If a safekeeping agreement cannot be reached by the end of the phone conversation, then the therapist can ask the patient to go to the hospital immediately, to be taken to the hospital by a family member or friend who is present, or to go by whatever means makes sense under the conditions. It is helpful if the therapist agrees to be available by telephone to talk to the intake officer, with the patient's permission. If the patient will not agree to go to the hospital, then the therapist may need to call the police or other appropriate authorities to assess and commit him or her if needed. If possible, it is a good idea to give the police a specific idea of what to expect when they arrive on the scene.

In all of IRT practice, including after a crisis telephone conversation and/or an extra session, it is important to document the event according to the rules of the covering agency. For IRT private practitioners, entry into the IRT data base in the Between-session contact? and Emergency? sections suffices (see Figure 3.5). The record should include the usual components of the SOAP algorithm discussed in Chapter 3 (i.e., subjective patient report, objective data, analysis, and plans).

Pitfalls to Avoid in Handling Crisis Calls

It is not unusual for patients, especially new ones, to believe that they can get free extra sessions if they call on the telephone with a crisis. Another common patient belief is that the crisis call will provide a test of the therapist's caring. Willingness to spend a long time giving encouraging messages will establish that the therapist is "there." This, of course, is very Red and does not need to be enabled. Crisis calls in IRT are brief, and there may be a charge for them if they abuse the therapist's good will or if they are too frequent.

Automatically "pulling out all stops" in response to crisis calls can set a pattern of crisis-based hospitalization that may not be necessary. Turning to the hospital as the first alternative can convey the idea that the patient cannot mobilize the strength to manage him- or herself, when that may not be the case. It can cause needless expense to the patient and to the health care system. Clinicians need to hospitalize when necessary, but also to remember the story of the boy who cried wolf.[16] However, every crisis is potentially serious, and so its handling deserves the clinician's most careful attention, reflection and action.

Handling a Crisis That Emerges at the End of a Session

Sometimes patients will "drop a bomb" at the end of a session by announcing that they are suicidal or contemplating some other dangerous or precipitous behavior. The clinician has to take a few minutes to assess the situation, but is far less patient and interested than if the topic had been brought up earlier in the session. One way of dealing with this is to say, "Oh, that's terrible. How come you didn't bring this up earlier today, so we could have had some time to talk about it?" After the patient explains that he or she was afraid to discuss it (or says something comparable), the therapist says, "Clearly, we need to discuss this carefully. Can you wait safely until next session?" If the answer is no, the clinician may offer an extra session later in the day or early the next day. Again, the clinician asks whether it is safe to wait. If not, then something like this is said: "I need to know that you will keep our safety contract until the next session, or I am going to ask you to go to the hospital now." The clinician tries to get the name of a person who can accompany the patient to the hospital, and either calls that person directly or trusts the patient to do so. Ordinarily, the patient must either give a credible short-term no-harm contract or be escorted for safekeeping. If the patient refuses a safety contract, refuses an extra appointment, and refuses to go to the hospital, the clinician must commit the patient if he or she meets legal standards for commitment. After an exchange like this, most patients learn to bring up important issues regarding dangerousness early in the session. If they do not, by definition IRT cannot continue, because such patients require too many of the symptom management activities described in Figure 3.4.

FOLLOW-UP AFTER CRISIS

Rudd, Joiner, and Rajab (1995) studied 188 subjects in suicidal crisis and reported that those who refused further help showed avoidant, negativistic, and passive–aggressive personality traits. Their prediction was that those personality traits would lead to recurrent crisis. Clearly, it is important to try to help such people remain in treatment and work on their problem patterns. As mentioned above, an inpatient experience that helps the patient develop a well-focused case formulation and an associated long-term treatment plan can motivate serious participation in follow-up outpatient work.

After resolution of a suicidal crisis, patients in IRT need to explore their feelings about it, even if they have managed to avoid hospitalization. Some declare that the crisis proves they have made no progress and never can recover. The basic approach to this discouraged condition is to listen well to the concerns in a collaborative way. Before corrective action is taken, regressive talk must have a full hearing. During this debriefing, the strategy is to help the patient understand that the episode is a repetition of an old scenario and can be understood in terms of ordinary learning processes. Therapy progress can be plotted as the motion of a pendulum suspended from a moving chain on a track. There is a lot of back-and-forth movement, but there is also gradual progress in the chosen direction. Learning is never absolute. There are better days and worse days, just as in any other kind of learning. This way of normalizing regression or "backsliding" can help the patient maintain morale.

REDUCING INTENSITY AND FREQUENCY OF CRISIS

Crisis is less likely if both the therapist and patient clearly understand that crisis management interferes with therapy work. IRT is in full gear only when the patient and therapist are engaged in the activities described in Figure 3.2 as coming to terms. Dealing with crisis does not involve much therapy, other than marking the underlying motivators and focusing on how to block them. It is primarily a series to steps needed to preserve life and the later option to return to therapy work. Unfortunately, nonresponders too often think that the excitement of dealing with crisis is therapy. In reality, efforts to deal with crisis can enable patterns that make long-term disability more rather than less likely.

Anticipating Crisis via the Case Formulation

The Growth Collaborator is enhanced if crisis can be anticipated and avoided. Many patients will feel pleased if they realize that they are no longer plagued by constant crisis. Many techniques appropriate to IRT crisis management can also be used to avert crisis. For example, both situations call for use of the case formulation to defuse a potentially dangerous scenario.

Suppose the patient has a jealous IPIR that attacks whenever the patient is successful or happy. In such a case, progress in therapy is likely to precipitate a crisis. The clinician who anticipates this can help the patient to learn to do the same. For example, the therapist may say toward the end of a session when successes have been noted, "Given your past responses to success, I am getting nervous about what your Red might do about this." If the patient recognizes the threat, he or she can consider corrective self-talk and alternative constructive activities if needed after the session. There can be rehearsal of a plan to tell the IPIR that he or she "has had control too long and has done too much damage." The self-sabotaging person can decide to inform the Red internalization, "The Green is in charge now. The Green knows it is [the present year], not 20 years ago, when [name of the IPIR] could directly affect my daily life." Concretely separating "then" from "now" is often very helpful to patients trying to resist instructions from the past.

In anticipatory interventions, more time can be devoted to work on the underlying motivators then in crisis, when there is an immediate need to manage dangerous behaviors. In addition, anticipation helps the patient begin to break destructive patterns of responding to particular stresses. He or she learns to practice habits that serve a newer and Greener concept of self.

Developing a List of Distracting or Constructive Activities

Crisis can be averted or managed by having the patient construct a list of attractive constructive or distracting activities to choose from when thoughts of dangerous behavior become intrusive. Common examples of such activities include watching a "junk" movie (but not one related to the problem thoughts), taking a walk, calling a specific friend, or engaging in a hobby.

It can help to suggest that the crisis-prone patient not dwell on stress between sessions. Instead, he or she should to try to use the list of agreed-upon distracting or constructive activities. However, such patients also need to agree that they will focus directly on core issues related to the problem thoughts at the next therapy session. In those sessions, the therapist provides the initiative and structure needed to examine and give up (Figures 7.1 and 3.3) destructive behaviors.

Monitoring the Therapy Relationship

The IRT therapist constantly monitors the "temperature" of the therapy relationship, especially for crisis-prone cases. Many therapists can intuit when something is wrong.[17] The therapist tries to identify any subtle hostility in its various forms, such as indirect attack, resentful compliance, withdrawal, or the like. When those behaviors are felt or noted, it is probably time to ask, "How are you feeling about our work now?" The question may uncover anger at the therapist. It may well be based on an actual error or interpersonal offense by the therapist; if so, the therapist's misstep must be acknowledged and trust rebuilt. On the other hand, if the patient has distorted a therapy event, the therapist needs to clarify what really happened and work toward understanding in light of the case formulation. Whatever the cause or context, the reader is reminded that ruptures in the therapeutic alliance always need to be repaired before therapy can go forward (Safran & Muran, 1996). This is unusually important whenever there is a threat of dangerous behavior. For example, suppose that a patient, Mike, has reported increased suicidal wishes and that the therapist has just asked how he feels about therapy today:

MIKE: Not great. Last time it seemed like you didn't want me to be here, and I felt just terrible afterwards. It's been that way all week. I didn't even want to come today.

THERAPIST: Yes, I was feeling tired and distracted last time, and I did ask you to repeat something you had already discussed. It's really bad that my lapse reminded you of an old injury. It is natural that it hurts a lot when anybody acts like your dad, and especially hard if I do. But, I think that I don't do that very often, and in many ways am different from your father. Does that seem right to you?

MIKE: Yes, but last time I really was uncomfortable.

THERAPIST: Thank you for bringing this up. I ask that you keep doing it whenever you feel something is not right in our relationship. I will try to acknowledge my part in any problems and hope that you too will be willing to learn from talking about our work together. Today maybe we can explore this to see what we can learn from it.

If the patient is narcissistic,[18] the discussion might emphasize the fact that other people have their worlds too, and that it is not catastrophic if they don't center on the patient. If the patient is passive–aggressive, the learning might center on yet another reconsideration of likely consequences of the "solution" of revenge. If the patient is dependent, the learning might center on building personal strength, or on how the patient did not fall apart even though the therapist was not focused on the problem. And so on.

Eliciting and Discussing Fantasies about the Therapist

Destructive fantasies about the therapist can relate directly to crisis behaviors. Naturally, fantasies will differ according to the case formulation. This section provides brief illustrative descriptions of some of the more frequent fantasies that can contribute to suicidal behavior. A common theme of such fantasies is that when the therapist is finally mobilized to attend properly, the patient's internal balance will be set right, and there will be peace and reconciliation with the IPIRs.

Here is a therapist reflection of a common fantasy of this type: "I hear that you feel I could help, if only I would. It sounds like you feel your problem is that I don't really understand how completely desperate you are. If I did, then I surely would do something more helpful." The belief that escalating self-harm will bring effective understanding by an omnipotent figure, followed by relief from pain, can be inspired by earlier modeling of others' nonresponsiveness that finally was mobilized under conditions of extreme need. For example, a patient may have had a chronically demanding and relentlessly punitive parent, who for just one time was compassionate when the child had an experience of physical or psychological trauma. Templates like this can lead to the idea that intensified self-flagellation, unbearable need, intolerable pain, or abject humiliation will somehow rouse the therapist to bring relief.

Some patients believe that their death will deliver deserved punishment to the therapist. From their perspective, the therapist should know how much harm rather than help has been delivered. Once that is understood, the therapist will shape up and deliver something worthwhile. Never mind if a patient has to die to achieve this goal.

Other patients are devoted to besmirching the therapist's reputation by this dramatic demonstration of treatment failure. Again, the ultimate unconscious plan is that once the therapist is "brought down," he or she will begin to do his or her job properly. Some confuse the therapist so completely with parental figures that they will escalate their suicidality even as they do not pay their therapy bills,[19] all as a desperate test of love.

This illustrative list of involves distortions of the therapy relationship that are illogical and profoundly unrealistic. But that does not matter.

What drives behavior is perception, not reality. The therapist needs to be ready and able to hear such statements, and to talk about them so that perception and reality can be squared in a compassionate and understanding manner. In IRT, the distortions are ultimately resolved through coming to terms as shown in Figure 3.2. The reader is cautioned that merely running through this or other lists of possible destructive fantasies about the therapist would be inappropriate. In every case, the clinician tries to match the exploration of fantasy about the therapist to actual data about the current state of the therapy relationship and the specific case formulation.[20]

Trying to Confine Distress and Symptoms to the Therapy Sessions

It is not unusual for patients, especially those who have been in many different treatments, to believe they are really doing important work when they are so upset by sessions that they are hardly able to function afterward. This is taken as evidence that they have "gone deep" and are really "heading toward uncovering basic issues." There is a kernel of truth to this perspective. Remembering and discussing problem experiences will naturally be upsetting. Moreover, one cannot come to terms with problem IPIRs without encountering the painful memories associated with the problem patterns.

Nonetheless, one of the earliest instructions to new IRT patients is to try to learn to confine distress as much as possible to the therapy sessions. Therapy is a learning process devoted to enhancing Green. Efforts to keep the Growth Collaborator strong include efforts to enhance, not interfere with, daily function. In addition to setting the expectation that upset will be confined to the therapy as much as possible, patients are given 15-, 10-, or 5-minute warnings (depending on the situation) before the end of the session. This compares to a "cool-down" after a workout. When the warning is given, the conversation switches to here-and-now topics and to adaptive techniques if necessary.

Another helpful way to contain upset due to therapy is the defense of isolation. Patients can be taught how to store and how to retrieve material that has been isolated. For example, suppose the therapy dialogue has involved remembering beatings when the patient was a child. The patient has been reexperiencing a range of feelings about it, including terror and rage. The therapist can invoke isolation in the last 10 minutes of the session by saying,

> "This is really important work. Our goal is to view that stuff from the perspective of a healthy adult, so you can see it for what it was and understand how inappropriate and unjustified it is to treat a child that way. Once you truly understand that you did not deserve that treat-

ment and that the issue could have been handled better, you may feel less vulnerable to it. We probably will need to discuss this several times and to view it from several angles. But for now, let's leave that work to therapy sessions. Therapy is the place to think about those times and to reexperience and reconsider them. They have done enough damage already, so let's agree to let it all that stay right here."

In subsequent sessions, this whole speech can be telescoped in various ways—for example, "10 minutes. Are you OK with this now?" or "Time shift! Then is then. Now is now." These are but two of many ways of concretizing the principle of working with state-dependent memory without inspiring contagion.

This version of isolation invokes an intellectual understanding of the issue and seeks to contain it in an assigned place and time. Pathological isolation would, of course, permanently cut off all access to the ABCs of the experience. This version of isolation merely specifies when and where the experience can be accessed. In subsequent sessions, with a few well-chosen words from the original narrative, the therapist can trigger all the affect and memories from the previous sessions. Sometimes patients enjoy picking their own trigger words for regressing—and, more importantly, trigger words for returning to the here and now. They and their loved ones appreciate their increased functionality, even while they are in therapy.

This use of isolation with regard to painful memories does not mean that there is no work to be done outside of therapy. To the contrary, very important and well-focused homework assignments are discussed in Chapter 9, in connection with learning new patterns. There it becomes clearer that IRT learning about self and others takes place both within and outside of therapy sessions.

The Expectation of Rapid Stabilization

IRT places a high priority on, and usually succeeds at, stabilization early in treatment. However, if IRT were stopped as soon as there was symptom remission, rapid recurrence of symptoms would be expected. The typically dramatic effectiveness of IRT in the short term is dependent on patient comprehension of the validity of the case formulation and the long-term commitment to get help in coming to terms with it. The case formulation and the therapy contract help enable the will to resist the inner destructive forces.

Here is an example of how that works. When one is starting therapy with an individual with Borderline Personality Disorder, the parasuicidal behaviors and constant threat of need for hospitalization are usually contained within just a few weeks except for isolated later flare-ups. If not, the patient in IRT is invited to consider the possibility that the therapy "may not be working." Maybe he or she should consider another approach. With the possibility that the therapy may have to be discontinued for lack of acceptable progress, the patient usually manages to contain or at least greatly reduce the intensity and frequency of the crises. In such an emergency, the patient is reminded, "This is not therapy. This is work we have to do so we can get back to therapy. I hope we can do that soon." Since the patient usually knows that the IRT process is authentic and valuable, he or she appropriately fears the threat of losing the opportunity to work in IRT.

It should be noted that if patients are using drugs or alcohol in ways that lead to crisis, they may not be able to mobilize enough Green to be able to meet this standard. In that case, treatments focused on control of their alcohol and drug use will need priority, as discussed in Chapter 3. IRT will have to wait until the Green is no longer so compromised by chemistry.

THERAPY-BLOCKING BEHAVIORS NOT USUALLY INVOLVING LIFE-AND-DEATH ISSUES

Nonresponders often get stuck in therapy because of habits that interfere with treatment. In addition to the crisis behaviors discussed above, therapy-interfering behaviors include poor attendance in therapy; failure to actively engage enough Green in therapy; relentless self-sabotage, even if not necessarily involving life crises (e.g., self-cutting, increased use of drugs or alcohol, gambling, reckless driving, failure to pay bills); and violations of therapy boundaries, such as intrusions into the therapist's personal life (Yeomans, Selzer, & Clarkin, 1992). Various contingencies have been suggested for violations of therapy rules and protocol (Neale & Rosenheck, 2000). For example, it is not unusual for therapists to ask personality-disordered individuals to agree that if they miss a certain number (say, three) of therapy sessions within a prescribed treatment, therapy is automatically terminated (Piper, Rosie, Joyce, & Azim, 1996). If they engage in too many therapy-interfering behaviors, therapy ends (Linehan, 1993). Though such issues are familiar to every clinician, there is relatively little research on specific forms of limit setting and their relation to outcome (Pam, 1994).

The IRT administrative approach to many of these problems has been presented in Chapter 3 under the heading "Administrative Issues." Whenever possible, such issues are approached on an individual basis in terms of the case formulation. All interventions are delivered according to the core algorithm. The discussion of Figure 3.3 in Chapter 3 has illustrated the method. This section presents additional specific techniques that may be helpful when one is using the procedures described in Figure 3.3 to deal with behaviors that are blocking the therapy process.

Limit Setting

Soft Limit Setting in IRT

As usual, a problem event is to be understood in terms of the case formulation (Chapter 2). Interventions are to be delivered according to the core algorithm (Chapter 3). As noted in Chapter 3, if a patient has good reason to miss sessions, and this behavior is not a manifestation of the Regressive loyalist, there is no problem with missing sessions. Therapy resumes when the patient is able and willing. This policy accommodates people who may have unpredictable and unusual work or travel schedules. It can also be reassuring for people who are terrorized by coercion of any sort. However, if three sessions are missed in a way that suggests the Regressive Loyalist is running the "schedule," this has to be addressed in the context of the case formulation. In this situation, contingencies for the missed sessions may have to be put in place. For example, the patient is given time slots that are maximally convenient for the therapist if there is a history of many cancellations. Individuals with Passive–Aggressive Personality Disorder are most likely to present this particular challenge. Fighting with them is a mistake, because it only repeats very old patterns. From the perspective of the IRT therapist, a missed session is seen as a loss that patients may choose, and it is rare that limit setting on attendance is needed once that is understood.

Verbally expressed anger at the therapist needs to be identified, acknowledged, and eventually subjected to soft limits. As always, the behavior is related to the case formulation—for example, "You are as angry with me as you have been with your mother, and I can see why we seem the same to you." From there, the steps in Figure 3.3 are explored. Hostile words are allowed for as long as required for the patient to see the connections to the IPIR. However, the IRT therapist does not sit for endless sessions as the target of furious shouting or gratuitous meanness. Such Red behaviors have a chance to be heard, but they are not allowed to dominate the therapy. IRT theory does not prescribe that "getting it out" comprises cure. A therapist is not required to take ongoing emotional abuse. Once the anger is understood in terms of the case formulation, it, like any other repetitive maladaptive pattern, is blocked until it has been replaced by more constructive patterns.[21]

In curbing fury at the therapist or others, it can be helpful to invite the patient to name his or her furious state in terms that connect it in some clear way to the relevant IPIR. For example, if a woman is having a tantrum like those she used with her father, then she provides a name for herself in that state. After eliciting agreement that having tantrums is no longer adaptive, the therapist may then explain that he or she will call the patient by that name to help her learn to block the raging. In subsequent sessions, the therapist might say, "OK, [name], that's enough now. I'd like to talk to [patient's Green name]." Together, patient and therapist then review the therapy episode as described in Figure 3.2, coming to terms.

Strict Limit Setting in IRT

Soft limits are set on therapy behaviors that are characteristic of the Regressive Loyalist but not physically harmful to self or others. Strict limits are set on behaviors that provide material threat. Nonresponders and other severely disordered individuals can present intolerable challenges to the therapist him- or herself. Examples include trashing the therapist's office, threatening to burn down his or her home, stalking the therapist, and making threats to the therapist's person or family.

These and all other material threats are immediately greeted with strict limit setting by the IRT therapist. Aggressive behaviors targeted at the therapist quickly lead to methods of symptom management (Figure 3.4) if they do not yield rapidly to discussion of the case formulation and steps outlined in Figure 7.1 for dealing with threatening behavior. Threats to the therapist are handled like threats to anyone else, except that the therapy relationship—a vital antidote to aggressive behavior—is also its target. A model for handling such a threat is illustrated in the following situation, which involves romantic interest in the therapist that may be accompanied by murderous wishes. Indeed, sexual and murderous wishes are often closely related, and the method for dealing with them is essentially the same.

Suppose a psychotic male patient falls in love with his female therapist and begins to sit in his car outside her home in the evenings. Stalking is always serious, since it can be followed by physical violence, whether sexual or not. The IRT therapist would mention this in the first session after she noticed it, and follow the steps in Figure 7.1. Responses to the patient's declarations of love (or murderousness) can be affirming, gracious, and informative without demeaning the patient, as in this example:

> "I appreciate that you are so pleased with [or enraged about] me and our work together. I think there really is a potential here for you to learn to feel much better about yourself, and to relate to others in ways that will be a whole lot more satisfying for you. But, as I have said before, therapy is an opportunity to learn about your patterns and to grow. It is not a place where your needs can be met directly by me. I enjoy working with you and would like to continue. But I cannot do that if you are going to focus on me so intensely and exclu-

sively. The therapy has to be about you working on you. These behaviors directed toward me [list them] have to stop completely and immediately. If they don't, we are going to have to [list reasonable symptom management possibilities shown in Figure 3.4]."

Considering the *Klute* Syndrome

The *Klute* syndrome (Benjamin, 1996a, Ch. 6), mentioned in Chapter 3 and included in Figure 3.3, is present if patients have eroticized the interpersonal patterns inherent in their chief complaints. If present, this problem can doom therapy to stalemate. The *Klute* syndrome is discussed in more depth in Chapter 8.

BLOCKING MALADAPTIVE PATTERNS OUTSIDE THE THERAPY RELATIONSHIP

This chapter is restricted to a discussion of crisis behaviors and other behaviors that directly block the therapy process. Examples of how to apply Figure 3.3 and 3.4 to other problem behaviors appear throughout this book.

SUMMARY

When there is a need to block problem patterns, the IRT therapist addresses underlying motivation that has been marked by the case formulation. Self-discovery facilitates motivational change. Once the process of changing underlying goals is underway, self-management activities offer a mechanism for seeing, feeling, and acting differently in problem situations. The chapter applies these principles to two problem areas: (1) crisis management, and (2) therapy stalemates that do not necessarily involve life-and-death matters.

Several specific steps are recommended for any session that involves a threat of dangerous behavior (Figure 7.1). If use of the recommended procedures fails to yield adequate self-management that resolves the crisis, IRT switches to symptom management (Figure 3.4). IRT therapists and patients work hard to reduce the number and seriousness of such crises—both because they are dangerous, and because they seriously interfere with the central therapy work of coming to terms (shown in Figure 3.2). Reduction in the frequency and intensity of crises can be achieved rapidly in IRT. This effect usually depends on understanding the case formulation and the promise of a long-term working relationship with the therapist. The strength of that relationship (Chapter 5), and the insight (Chapter 6) about case formulation (Chapter 2), are what help people learn rapidly to minimize their crisis and other problem behaviors.

NOTES

1. IRT takes a definite position on what is normal (the rationale appears in Chapters 2 and 4). Homicide, spouse/partner or child abuse, rape, and the like are defined as pathological and are not arbitrary value choices. Sexual practices that support these behaviors are therefore seen as problems to be addressed with collaboration from the patient's Green.
2. Not long after Charles Whitman gunned down people on a Texas campus, I had a patient tell me that he was thinking about doing the same thing. He seemed surprised as I looked alarmed. He hurried to "reassure" me that I might therefore have my picture on the cover of *Time* magazine.
3. Lee and Coccaro (2001) have recently reviewed research on the neurochemistry specific to aggression, and report that decreased serotonergic responsiveness is associated with impulsive aggression. They propose that the prefrontal cortex and other regions of the brain are involved in the expression of aggression. Work is proceeding on the relevance of serotonin, other neurotransmitters, and neuropeptides to aggressive behavior.
4. Another time for "telling" is during a consultative interview, discussed in Chapter 2.
5. If Jessica were an outpatient threatening suicide for these same reasons, the decision might be that if she stayed Green, she wouldn't have to go to the hospital. The session could end safely if she agreed that she could maintain that attitude until the next appointment, and that she would go directly to the hospital (or do whatever the contract called for) if necessary for safekeeping. Of course, the relationship would have to be strong enough that the therapist knew Jessica would keep her word and was not just lying to get out of the office and on with a suicidal plan.
6. This clinical example again shows that the clinician draws upon all steps, flow charts, tables at any time. The diagrams and tables are guides for the clinician. They are not exhaustive, and they are not computer programs.
7. For example, in many states reporting incidents of child abuse is mandatory. In some circumstances, such reporting could interfere with the therapy relationship and collaboration in ways that increase rather than decrease the probability of abuse. Nonetheless, the law and professional norms take precedence.
8. In terms of the Structural Analysis of Social Behavior (SASB) cluster codes, this paradoxical instruction would command (CONTROL) Jessica to comply (SUBMIT) with her own rule that she must please them (SULK) and suffer (*SELF-BLAME*). However, it would also reframe the charge in a way that eliminated suicide (*SELF-ATTACK*). Her Red part would be, in effect, hoist on its own petard. The reader should be cautious in using paradoxical communications, however, because they can misfire unless they clearly block Red and enable Green.
9. I have sometimes shown the SASB model to people during crisis to demon-

strate concretely how their patterns have contributed to their current problems, and to show specific alternatives. Here is an example: "You have been amplifying BLAME, because that is the language of your family. That draws for SULK, counterBLAME and *SELF-BLAME*. No wonder things never get better! But look at the opposites, AFFIRM and DISCLOSE and *SELF-AFFIRM*. These are what happen when you learn to switch from hostile control to friendly affirmation." This educational intervention has been very successful at remoralizing despairing people to the point where they can agree to work hard to try to learn this new way of relating.

10. Referral to parent training is one way to do this. Patients who have previously not responded to parent training can be referred again after they understand links between their present parenting behaviors and IPIRs.

11. Agency AFFIRM is internalized as *SELF-AFFIRM*; agency PROTECT is internalized as SELF-PROTECT.

12. In such role plays, the therapist can be guided by the SASB model, which specifies antidotes that are content-free. For example, if the patient is in a blaming fury (BLAME) or feeling defeated and helpless (SUBMIT, SULK), the therapist can model appropriate assertiveness (AFFIRM, DISCLOSE) in ways that will have a much better probability of succeeding. It is important to remember that the therapist should not role-play a Red person, because that is likely to weaken the therapy relationship.

13. Through the principle of complementarity. For example, hostile compliance (Figure 4.2) draws for hostile control.

14. SASB codes of the therapy process can be compared to SASB codes of the case formulation.

15. The reader is reminded that sometimes no-harm contracts are not enough. Other people may have to be notified, or commitment proceedings may have to be initiated.

16. As readers may recall, this is an old tale about a shepherd boy who delighted in the village response whenever he cried, "Wolf!" After a while, the villagers tired of false alarms; then, of course, the wolf *did* show up, but nobody responded to the call.

17. A more precise way to assess the condition of the therapy process is to SASB-code it.

18. Discussion in this paragraph is based on my "case formulations" for each of the DSM-IV personality disorders (Benjamin, 1996a).

19. Therapists contribute to this fantasy when they imagine that their love will heal and that the therapy fee is just an inconvenient, somewhat incidental "necessity." In IRT, the therapist knows that treatment is hard work and the fee meets the therapist's needs in a fair exchange. The therapist "owes" the patient nothing other than to do good work. However, IRT theory does not preclude loving one's work and the people one works with.

20. SASB coding can be an effective aid in this process, because it accurately characterizes the therapy process and provides well-operationalized links to the case formulation.

21. Examples include DISCLOSE, TRUST, *SELF-AFFIRM*, *SELF-PROTECT*, and *SELF-CONTROL*.

8

Step 4: Enabling the Will to Change

The Interpersonal Reconstructive Therapy (IRT) therapist consistently targets the underlying motivation that maintains the problem patterns. The purpose is to help the patient come to terms (Figure 3.2) with the Important Persons and their Internalized Representations (IPIRs) that have been linked to problem patterns through copy processes. Giving up those wishes clears the path to change. During therapy, the Red part of the patient pursues old wishes, while the Green part supports constructive growth. Nonresponders typically begin therapy with significantly more Red than Green (Figure 1.1). The domination of Red might be called resistance in generic psychodynamic therapies. Letting go of old hopes that support resistance is perhaps the most difficult part of IRT. This chapter, on enabling the will to change, is primarily about how to encourage the patient to do that and to grieve for the losses.

LITERATURE ON MOTIVATIONAL CHANGE

Motivational Change by Abreaction

A popular view of the change mechanism in therapy centers on catharsis and abreaction. Many clients believe that if only they can remember key childhood traumatic incidents and get it out, all will be well. They believe they will feel better following catharsis, and will easily fall into more normal patterns of relating to self and others. However, experienced therapists are aware that recall does not automatically bring relief. Instead, a rather long period of "working through" must usually follow the recall.[1]

In their summary of beliefs about catharsis, Kosmicki and Glickauf-Hughes (1997) note that since the time of the ancient Greeks, there has been debate over whether remembering childhood trauma "provokes" or "purges" passions. In the domain of modern psychotherapy, catharsis was invoked first by Breuer and Freud. Freud later decided that affect associated with remembering is only a by-product of the uncovering that leads to insight. Subsequent psychoanalysts disagreed and argued that abreaction, the result of successful catharsis, is itself central to cure. That view remains prevalent in practice. However, Kosmicki and Glickauf-Hughes provide plenty of evidence that controversy on this matter is not resolved.

Meanwhile, within the domains of health and social psychology, additional interesting and informative studies have appeared. For example, Greenberg, Wortman, and Stone (1996) review the literature establishing that disclosure of experienced trauma does improve physical health. However, their own perplexing findings, if replicated, would suggest that simply reporting trauma—whether real or not—can have a beneficial effect on health.

Models of Change from the Addictions Literature

Helpful empirical studies focusing specifically on changes in motivation to give up drugs and alcohol began to emerge in the 1980s. These interventions have centered on efforts to help patients focus on consequences rather than causes of the problem behaviors. The studies are "bottom-line-oriented" and are not based upon any particular theory of psychopathology. In 1985, W. R. Miller provided an important review of interventions that had been shown to promote motivation for change in alcohol use. Helpful techniques included advice giving, providing feedback (including videotapes of the self when drunk), setting clear goals, role playing and modeling, maintaining contact between the client and treatment provider, and setting contingencies. Unsympathetic to the widely practiced confrontative approaches, Miller added that therapist hostility was not helpful, whereas empathy and positive expectancy did enhance outcome (W. R. Miller, Benefield, & Tonigan, 1993). In a recent review of subsequent studies, Yahne and Miller (1999) confirm earlier results establishing that the nature and intensity of treatment do affect outcome.

Prochaska's transtheoretical model of change (Prochaska, DiClemente, & Norcross, 1992; Prochaska et al., 1994) has been shown to describe stages of change in a wide number of empirical studies. According to this model, there are five stages of motivation that can reliably be identified as predictors of change: precontemplation, contemplation, preparation,[2] action, and maintenance. Although the work was initially applied to alcohol/drug use and smoking, it subsequently generalized to other behaviors to be diminished, such as over- or undereating and domestic abuse (Murphy & Baxter, 1997). In addition to these applications, the transtheoretical model has been used to assess stages of change in encouraging desirable behaviors (e.g., using of condoms, using sunscreen lotions, seeking mammography). Many of the change studies establish that people in the earlier stages of change are more resistant to treatment. Although the transtheoretical model is not typically invoked in studies of psychotherapy, Hoglend (1996) reported that motivation for change and realistic expectations of therapy were significant predictors of good outcome and long-term follow-up in brief dynamic psychotherapy.

A major implication of the work with the transtheoretical change model is that treatment approaches should vary with stage of change. For precontemplators, the emphasis needs to be on developing understanding of the need for change. Contemplators need to be helped to decide to make the change. People in the action stage need structure on and support for actually making change. And people in the maintenance stage need help in resisting the temptation to regress. Having firmly establishing the prognostic significance of stages, the research literature has more recently turned to what motivates people to move from one stage to another. For example, when treating eating disorders, Woodsie, Blake, Kaplan, Olmsted, and Carter (2001) described a pretreatment intervention called motivational enhancement therapy. Dench and Bennett (2000) explored motivational procedures that enhanced problem recognition and reduced ambivalence about giving up alcohol. As expected, these methods improved treatment response. Continued work on how to move people from one stage to another should prove to be useful.

Motivation to "Get Attention"

There is a popular belief that patients do what they do "to get attention." An extreme example of this perspective was provided by a psychiatry resident, who explained that a woman who had severely gouged her abdomen and both thighs had done so simply "to get attention." Such acts of self-mutilation must be driven by more than a need for attention. He agreed that it was unreasonable for the woman to mutilate herself just to get attention, but observed that she had a thought disorder. An alternative interpretation involving her IPIRs made more sense to the patient and to her outpatient therapist. On the other hand, seeking attention is not irrelevant to Developmental Learning and Loving (DLL) theory, because seeking attention can be a derivative of attachment. For example, individuals with Histrionic Personality Disorder (HPD; Benjamin, 1996a, Ch. 7) define themselves in terms of their ability to entertain and charm important figures. In this very specific way, people with HPD do need to seek attention. However, attention-seeking behavior in these people is specifically linked to an IPIR and is a manifestation of pathology, not an explanation for it.

Motivation via Manipulation of Secondary Reinforcers

Manipulation of secondary reinforcers has sometimes been used to motivate change. A very sensible perspective of this sort has been offered by Lecomte, Liberman, and Wallace (2000, p. 1312), who suggest that clinicians use "interviews or questionnaires that list numerous objects, persons, activities, and settings, and then assess the client's perception of the value of each item. Such surveys help identify the type of reward that might be useful for motivating the client. If properly assessed and delivered, reinforcers can increase the clients' skill acquisition, attainment of goals, and feelings of self-efficacy." In other words, preferred items are used as positive incentives. If manipulation of secondary reinforcers suffices for desired change, there is no need to invoke the more complex procedures of IRT.

Moral Choice

Moral choice, which enjoyed some success in institutional milieu therapy at the end of the 1800s, has more recently been applied within Glaser's Reality Therapy. A recent review of this technique in motivating change, which has yet to be tested empirically, is offered by Linneberg (1999).

Summary and Implications for IRT

Among the reviewed approaches to the problem of motivating change, the transtheoretical model enjoys the greatest empirical support. Targeted treatments based on this model appropriately emphasize external controls and incentives specific to the target behaviors. By contrast, IRT focuses on the will to change interpersonal patterns and wishes in relation to IPIRs. This task is inherently more difficult to pinpoint than is the assessment of behavioral outcome variables, such as number of cigarettes, ounces of alcohol, or calories that are consumed. However, assessments based on the Structural Analysis of Social Behavior (SASB; see Chapter 4) do provide well-operationalized evaluations of problem patterns, IPIRs, copy processes, and outcome. With these clear definitions of patterns and representations, the concepts in DLL theory and IRT are specific enough to assess changes in IRT in terms of stages proposed by the transtheoretical model.[3]

Collected notes from IRT sessions that seemed to enhance the will to change fell easily into groups that did compare well to four of the stages of change described by Prochaska et al. (1992, 1994). (1) The IRT version of the precontemplation stage can be called confronting the gift of love. (2) The stage of contemplation becomes enhancing motivation to give up the wishes. (3) The stage of action can be termed actually giving up the wishes. (4) Finally, the maintenance stage can be called resisting the wish to go back.

The balance of this chapter sketches some ways to mobilize the will to change in IRT, wherein the targets are attachments to IPIRs that support the problem behaviors. The major section headings mark IRT equivalents of the transtheoretical stages of change. Each stage is discussed in terms of the two classes of activities listed in Figure 3.1: self-discovery and self-management. The activities for step 4 mentioned in Figure 3.1 are included, along with a number of additional ways to enhance the will to change.

PRECONTEMPLATION: CONFRONTING THE GIFT OF LOVE

The first stage in enabling the will to change is to recognize and acknowledge the need to give up the wishes in relation to the IPIRs. People who have not yet become aware of copy processes and their gifts of love can be compared to "precontemplators" in the transtheoretical model of change. Since motivation is based on early attachments, it follows that well-focused, accurate discussions of the past are likely to be necessary but unlikely to be sufficient to motivate change in IRT. Greenberg, Rice, and Elliott (1993) have shown that effectiveness is increased if therapy sessions are structured to focus on current events and their historical roots. Once the patient sees clearly that his or her problem patterns are related to feelings and thoughts about early relationships, he or she may become more willing to consider new ways of being. After understanding the case formulation, the patient is ready to move from precontemplation to contemplation of change. Here are some ways to facilitate that change.

Self-Discovery

Becoming Willing to Explore Links to the Past

Patients vary greatly in their willingness to consider links between their current problems and past patterns. Whereas some are eager to review alleged past "crimes" of family members, others are quite insistent that their childhoods were happy and there is no point in reviewing them. This latter group may believe that to talk about family members in any but the most glowing terms would be unspeakably disloyal. A third group is too terrified or disgusted to give the past another millisecond of their time. A collaborative therapist rarely presses a patient to explore past connections when he or she is unwilling to do so. For example, patients who have suffered overt physical and violent sexual abuse may find talking about the past to be as appealing to them as is revisiting deadly jungle battles to a veteran. That perspective is reflected in the following example, along with the therapist's attempts to explain the need to revisit the past in order truly to leave it behind. The patient, Julia, was describing how it felt to try to survive chronic and severe physical and sexual abuse:

> "You put a lot of energy into not feeling whatever you are feeling. You don't know if you can get to the end, if there is an end. You have to put yourself in some kind of a trance. If you are in any normal state of mind, you could not get through it. But you have to remember, too, to stay on guard. The balance between remembering and forgetting is important."

Then, reflecting on what it would be like to remember, she told the therapist:

JULIA: If the plan is to put me back there and open up my eyes and see what is going on, I can't. You can't be there with eyes open. (*Crying*) I can't do it.

THERAPIST: This time it is safe. This time you are not alone. This time it won't last.

JULIA: I understand. But I can't really go back there.

THERAPIST: Those times need to be reexperienced in the present light, so they do not affect your dreams, your mood any more. You need to experience the fact that those people [named] are not there any more. They are not here.

JULIA: There are moments when I have this dazed feeling. It is involuntary time travel. You cannot be both places at once. You cannot be here and know what it was like. If you are there, you are there. You can't even think about this.

THERAPIST: The point here is to bring them together.

JULIA: I think I can understand what you are saying. I am not there yet.

In people so severely traumatized, it is important to back off after the goals and methods of exploring the connection in terms of the ABCs have been made clear. Julia needed many subsequent sessions within which to begin to trust the therapist and others in her current adult world. After she had time to enhance her sense of security and strength, she was able to discuss the past with enough distance to be able to reconsider it from a current perspective.

Seeing the Copy Process Links

After the patient has agreed to collaborate to explore the past in relation to present problems, developing skills at recognizing the gifts in action can begin. At this stage, it becomes especially important not to commit a "telling error" (see Chapter 2). Beginning IRT therapists are likely to be so excited when they see the connections and the gifts of love that they want to jump in to tell their patients the whole story right away. However, unless this is done in a profoundly empathic context and in an obviously collaborative way, the predictable response to "telling" is for the patient either to deny the validity of the formulation or to leave therapy abruptly.[4] If someone has lived with a given idea about him- or herself for decades, discrepant information is very difficult to take in all at once. For example, imagine you have spent your whole life believing you are stupid, and the Army tells you that its assessments suggest you are a genius. Even though the test scores may be "objective," and even though the news may be "desirable," it is difficult or even impossible to believe. Any radically new information about the self is unlikely to be absorbed until it is encountered in a context in which the patient is an active participant and essentially "puts it together" for him- or herself. The IRT therapist may have the map, but the patient has to travel the road. The great educator John Dewey taught long ago that we "learn by doing." This is as true in psychotherapy as it is anywhere else. Once again, it is apparent that the therapist is a teacher and guide, not a hands-on "fixer."

Identifying the Gift of Love: Unmasking Old Loyalties, Rules, Fantasies

Like any good guide, the therapist maximizes the learner's independence. At the same time, he or she constantly tries to keep the patient focused on problem patterns, copy processes, and related IPIRs. This optimal process is illustrated by the following exchange. Bonnie had an alcoholic boyfriend who was unpredictably loving and critical, as was her alcoholic father. Everyone in her family wanted her to kick him out of her apartment, but she could not. She was wondering why it was so hard for her to deal with the problem of her cruel boyfriend.

THERAPIST: Who does he remind you of?

BONNIE: Dad, of course. I tried to fix Dad, and now I am trying to fix my boyfriend. I don't understand this. I thought that I always did the opposite of what Dad thought or wanted.

THERAPIST: But here it is. Same old, same old.

BONNIE: Well, why would I do that?

THERAPIST: Why would you try to fix Dad?

BONNIE: Oh. I see. So he could be nicer to me.

In this brief exchange, the IRT therapist was clearly "pushing" Bonnie to recognize a copy process and its purpose. Bonnie was actively involved and collaborating. The therapist knew that Bonnie was recapitulating patterns learned with her father with partners, but needed to elicit the details from Bonnie herself. Again, the optimal "interpretation" was essentially given by means of intensely focused reflection that led the patient to make the actual connection.

Identification and consideration of the gift of love constitute an excellent ending for every discussion of a current problem incident during the precontemplation stage. Consider a patient who despairs over a long history of painful situations and consequences. After acknowledging the ongoing suffering, and developing agreement about the gift of love, the therapist may take an approach to breaking up the pattern that goes something like this:

> "You are right. You have wasted your talent, and many years have flown by in horrible misery. How many more years do you think it will take before you can convince your parents to apologize for the consequences of their actions and make it all up to you?"

Or:

> "It is truly painful to realize it never can again be as it was. It was wonderful, but it did not prepare you to make it on your own. So now you either have to begin to make the best of adjusting to your present condition, or begin the lengthy and boring process of developing the skills you need to become the person you could have been, the person you want to be."

Statements like these are, of course, tailored specifically to the actual case history and the current therapy dialogue. They occur in a collaborative context and flow naturally from and with clear relevance to any immediately preceding material provided by the patient.

After many such episodes, the therapist may hear something like this from the patient:

> "You have been hammering on that for so long. I really see it now. They are not ever going to apologize or give me what I need. They had a really rough time themselves. I have got to do this myself."

At that point, the patient has engaged the will to change.

Self-Management

Collaboration as a Necessary Condition for Change

Chapter 5 has suggested that good collaboration[5] helps provide a secure base, which is needed to make major changes at step 4. Motivation for change usually cannot be forced by confrontation, aggressive interpretation, or attempts to take control of the process. On the other hand, examples throughout this book show that though the IRT therapist is not invasive[6] or rude, he or she nonetheless is not passive. As indicated in the preceding discussion, he or she constantly invites the patient to reflect on current patterns, copy process links, and gifts of love.

Collaboration can be blocked by patients' conscious belief that if they learn too much about themselves, they will have to make changes they are not ready or willing to make. An appropriate approach to this problem is to suggest that recognition does not necessarily mandate action. For example, one patient was afraid that if she looked closely, she would discover her husband was too much like her hated father, and she would no longer want to be married. The IRT therapist responded by commenting that if she discovered she had married for the wrong reasons, or that she was really unhappy in her marriage, she still could choose to stay married. In this example, the fact there is no necessary link between understanding and action can be used to short-term advantage.

Most often, collaboration is compromised by feelings and thoughts that are not so conscious. The patient comes to therapy intending to change, but is unlikely to be aware that change will require giving up cherished wishes.

Agreeing on a Therapy Model

IRT offers a learning model of development and of therapy change. This can clash with other models of therapy. Common examples of models with very different treatment implications are the cathartic model, the "remember it" model, the "auto mechanic" model, and the "courtroom" or "justice" model. Although expression of affect and remembering critical experiences are surely important parts of IRT, they are not stand-alone paths to change. As indicated earlier in the review of the literature, simply "remembering" is not reliably helpful. Similarly, "blaming the family" can be iatrogenic if it merely repeats a problem pattern, which it usually does. Another less than optimal approach is to try to fix problems for patients by, say, giving good advice to enhance self-management. Experience shows that with nonresponder patients, good advice is likely to fall on deaf ears.

The cathartic model is so widely used that it seems important to explore the potential for its misuse in more detail. If a patient rages to try to force the internalizations to change, the battle will be lost. The IPIRs will "win." Consider Ann, who was a gifted writer but had been essentially nonfunctional for years. Her highly judgmental mother had criticized her relentlessly and predicted she would have a lonely and useless life. Ann was fulfilling that prophecy. She had no problem expressing anger, and raging made things much worse in her daily life. There had been quite a number of sessions discussing memories of interactions with her parents and siblings, and these inspired great fury. After each new adult experience with rejection and apparent failure, the IRT therapist had consistently encouraged Ann to free-associate to her thoughts and feelings. If she tagged anger, the therapist asked her what she wished this anger could accomplish. A wish for a more loving, affirming mother usually became apparent. The anger was to force her mother to change her behavior toward Ann. Then the therapist would give some version of the learning speech and explore one or more relevant versions of how the present situation surely sounded like what the mother expected. Ann's consistent reliving of her mother's prophecy suggested that Ann at some level was agreeing with her mother. Finally, after a trip home, Ann said, " It is starting to sink in—the part about me living up to her expectations in an effort to prove her right. I really ought to find a better way of loving her." Then Ann sobbed for a long time. This recognition of the need to contemplate giving up the wish marked the beginning of the major behavioral changes that ultimately characterized her reconstruction.

The "justice" or "courtroom" model of therapy is also common and problematic. Other than noting patterns, links, and gifts of love, the IRT therapist does not judge the patient or people in his or her world. Good versus bad, and right versus wrong, are defined in IRT in terms of the therapy goals of baseline friendliness, moderate enmeshment, moderate differentiation, and balance of focus. These values inherent in the goals of IRT do not include the parts of interpersonal space that would define "winners" and "losers."[7] The IRT goal is not achieved by dispensing justice.[8] Instead, healing in IRT comes with letting go of old wishes.

Confusing description with judgment, many patients (and some clinicians) believe that drawing connections between problem patterns and family interactions is equivalent to blaming the family—usually the mother. If IRT patients believe that description means judgment, then a simple discussion of copy process links can seem like parent blaming. This in turn can agitate the Red and generate problem behaviors, such as self-punishment. If the therapist and patient take the justice model to the point of confronting family members, great rage and suffering within the family may follow.

Showing empathy as the patient describes links may be seen as therapist agreement that injustices have been committed. With that belief, adherents of the justice model will go home and rage at family members. They may even declare, as they dispense judgment, that the therapist "said so." Whether or not they are confronted, families that adhere to the justice model may be very threatened by therapy. Some family members may therefore refuse to support therapy, and actively vilify the therapist and any other family members who participate in therapy. The courtroom or justice model costs these families dearly.

Joseph, a college professor, was a loyal and devoted family member who could not let go of the justice model. The following exchange illustrates a therapist attempt to release him from this assignment. He had come the therapy after viciously slashing his arm, and in this session he was engaged in a spate of verbal self-shredding. He had slowly come to realize that the severe beatings he had received from his mother were highly inappropriate. The therapist asked what he thought about what he was doing as he escalated his self-vilification. He explained:

JOSEPH: I tend to blame myself.

THERAPIST: It sounds like it is important to know whom to blame.

JOSEPH: Of course.

THERAPIST: Well, this is not a courtroom.

JOSEPH: I am pretty big on blaming myself. That might translate to having to blame somebody. The only thing I have really come to terms with so far in therapy is that even though I had misbehaved, it was not anything that bad. The consequences were excessive. But I have not stopped blaming myself.

THERAPIST: So thinking about how you were beaten severely for small "crimes" helps you be less harsh on yourself. But you still blame yourself?

JOSEPH: I guess.

THERAPIST: Well, I hope that we can find a way to get out of the courtroom and just try to learn about patterns, where they are from, and what they are for. If you can see that clearly, perhaps you can make more of your own choices on your own terms.

Joseph had a very difficult time giving up his devotion to the courtroom model. He had been punished inordinately, and so he punished himself to excess. It seemed just. When he realized that his punishments had far exceeded the magnitude of his "crimes," his own self-punishments became milder. They did not disappear entirely, and he still gave ultimate value to the justice model. Many repetitions of conversations about differences between the justice model and the IRT goals of a normative position of basic friendliness, with moderate degrees of enmeshment and moderate degrees of differentiation (described in Chapters 2, 4, and 5), are necessary with people like Joseph.

In sum, people come to therapy with a wide variety of assumptions about what therapy is and how it works. The IRT therapist tries to be explicit about the IRT model of therapy during the first session. This is accomplished by giving a version of the learning speech (Table 2.5). But since understanding takes place in degrees, it is often necessary to remind the patient of the implications of the IRT model. Nowhere is this more important than when the therapist is trying to set up the willingness to give up devotion to gifts of love that sustain problem behavior patterns.

CONTEMPLATION: ENHANCING MOTIVATION TO GIVE UP THE WISHES

Contemplation is the next stage in enabling the will to change. The core change in IRT is to give up wishes and fantasies in relation to key IPIRs. Greenberg and colleagues (e.g., Greenberg & Foerster, 1996) have provided rare and important data on the problem of transforming internalizations. By analyzing 11 successful and 11 unsuccessful episodes of attempts to resolve "unfinished business," these investigators found that constructive change in the relationship with a key internalization was enhanced by intense expression of feeling, expression of need, shift in representation of other, and self-validation or understanding of the other.

In IRT, this process of giving up destructive residual effects of the attachment to the IPIR compares to the process of letting go of a maladaptive love affair—another form of addiction.[9] Usually the addiction to a "bad" lover is not forgone until and if the issue is forced by (1) painful awareness of how costly the relationship has been, and (2) finding a more adaptive alternative. Condition (1) is facilitated by full understanding of the case formulation. Condition (2) becomes more likely when the patient realizes that living in the present can be more satisfying than living in the past. These changes are facilitated by the following self-discovery and self-management activities.

Self-Discovery

Realizing How Much the Fantasy Has Cost

Some of the most wonderful moments in IRT come when patients actively consider the costs of what they have been doing, and then declare, "Enough is enough. This has got to change." Of course, because learning is gradual, such moments of revelation usually need to be repeated more than once.

Virginia had spent her life fulfilling her father's prediction that she would "screw up" anything she tried to do. Her success at failing both in work and in love was remarkable. She had made multiple suicide attempts and could stay drunk for months on end. With the help of Alcoholics Anonymous, she built a fragile sobriety and began IRT, where she quickly grasped the "total picture." Her case formulation suggested that she was supposed to mess up and then suffer greatly. When things got bad enough, her father would step in and rescue her. In the first year of IRT, she took many good steps toward rebuilding her life. However, she continued to have difficulty separating herself from a boyfriend who specialized in both loving and trashing her. Gathering up her will to deal with him, as well as to get a better job, she observed, "I need to give up this suffering agenda. This is ridiculous. I have decided to try being happy and see if it works. I have felt like I am the gate knocked by a ball in a pinball machine. Some event comes along and knocks you flat. I am sick of this." Her subsequent progress demonstrated that she had mastered her ambivalence and was ready to be Green.

Sometimes the therapist needs to be more active in helping the patient realize how much the repetition of old patterns costs. For example, a teacher became extremely upset every time a student came to her with a patently absurd story of why he or she had done badly on a test. This type of student would claim that everything was the fault of someone or something else. The student's explanation rarely included the fact that he or she had not done the homework. Every time this scenario appeared, the teacher diagnosed it as "complete crap." She may have been accurate in her description, but our therapy problem was her internal rage and her consequent dysphoria that would last through the day and on into the night. Her anguished response to students who presented in this way was excessive.

The therapist had to be fairly active to shift the focus from ruminations about the students to situations that they reminded her of. The root of her feelings of rage and helplessness was in her family, whose members rationalized and denied the extent of their problems as they presented an innocent front to the community. As an adult, any pretension to innocence in a context of likely guilt reminded the teacher of years of familial abuse and hypocrisy, and of all the related feelings she had as a child.

"*Sunset Boulevard* syndrome" (SBS) may be one of the more difficult fantasies to leave behind. It follows a pattern described in the classic 1950 movie directed by Billy Wilder, and starring William Holden and Gloria Swanson. *Sunset Boulevard* is about an aged Hollywood star who cannot face the fact that her time of glory has come and gone. Nonresponders with SBS, like the elderly actress, were also once adored and served. To cope, they needed to do little more than "show up," and occasionally to have a temper tantrum to get others to hurry to fix any problems.

The parent of a person with SBS, working with his or her own injuries, may have believed in the "empty tank" theory of development. This perspective suggests that if all of a child's needs can be met, all will be well. Frustration of needs, failure to fill the tank, must be avoided at all costs. Well-meaning though it may be, such a model deprives the child of a chance to learn to cope with life's challenges. A most sinister version of SBS emerges if the parent adds to this indulgent focus a highly inappropriate but nonetheless erotic (nonviolent) sexuality. If the erotic liaison includes the perception that the parent could not function without proximity to the child ("You are my only, my 'real' love; I cannot live without you"), the prospects for change approach zero.

Helping people with SBS see the costs of their adjustment is particularly difficult, because everything has seemed so fine.[10] The problem is the world, which won't shape up. Whatever the details of their history and version of the pattern, the point at which people with SBS have the most trouble is when their life situation calls for self-restraint and sustained effort. For them, impulse control and hard work belong in another universe. Nobody has modeled it for or demanded it of them. It is not unusual for people with SBS to resolve their dilemma by becoming professional patients. In therapy, needs are expected, and warm concern is provided most of the time.

The IRT therapist needs to help the patient with SBS get a glimpse of how exciting good functioning can be, even if it is terrifying and boring to work on developing the requisite skills. The person with SBS needs to find the idea of taking responsibility attractive rather than fatal. He or she needs to see clear ways to achieve a more functional lifestyle. The latter vision can sometimes be facilitated by a rehabilitation counselor who can outline a program for skills building, one level at a time. However, the patient will only be able to make use of the training—whether it is entry-level vocational rehabilitation, social skills training, a return to college, or something else—after the decision to give up the addiction to the providing IPIR. Letting go of the gift of love is a lot easier if people with SBS have present-day associates who appreciate them for their strengths rather than their weaknesses, and for health rather than disorder.

Changing the View of the IPIR

Differentiation from a problem IPIR is often facilitated by the patient's coming to understand that the IPIR was severely limited in his or her ability to deliver the parenting behaviors that typically have been the focus of all the yearning. Even a person with SBS who has had a "lover" parent needs help in seeing how impaired the parent must have been to need to center so much on one particular child. If sexual abuse was included, the identification of parental impairment and limitation is made easier because the behavior is so obviously out of line, but talking about it is much harder.[11]

The quest for "perfection" in family image is still another major blocker to developing a realistic perspective on an IPIR. This is illustrated by a lethally suicidal inpatient who had a prolonged struggle with accepting the case formulation, which she nonetheless acknowledged made sense. Emotionally, she was convinced it would be better for her to die than to think her parents had not been perfect. The breakthrough came when the student IRT therapist asked her whether she thought her parents might have Red and Green parts, just as she did. This simple concept released her to acknowledge that there were some Red behaviors in her mother and father, and then to think about the impact of these behaviors on her. The Red–Green model allowed her to at least discuss the effects of her parents' Red parts on her, while reassuring herself that they still had Green parts.

Another example of changing the view of the IPIR comes from Jack, who had trouble controlling his temper, especially with loved ones. He had repeatedly noticed that he was behaving like his father, and that recognition did help him manage his anger much better. However, the template persisted, and it continued to be a struggle for Jack to keep from blowing up. Just before he turned a corner, the following conversation took place. The night before, he had briefly lost his temper again with his wife.

JACK: I love them. I get angry with the people I love the most.

THERAPIST: You have to care to get angry.

JACK: (*Sobs*)

THERAPIST: Sound like this is something you experienced yourself?

JACK: Yeah.

THERAPIST: Who in your life would hit you and love you at the same time?

JACK: My dad. I knew he loved me dearly. I always knew. But his ways were so filled with anger and control. I so did not want to be like him.

The therapist began to enhance Green by underscoring Jack's current loving and thoughtful behaviors. Very soon thereafter, during a trip home, he saw his parents as frail and as struggling with their own injuries and limitations. That experience seemed finally to settle his determination to stop copying his father. After mastering a period of panic from loss of identity, he became increasingly comfortable relating in more accepting ways with himself and others. Jack became "another person."

Engaging Anger in the Service of Differentiation

In IRT, anger is viewed in terms of its interpersonal purposes, whether it is directed toward an actual figure or toward an internalization. After anger is vented, the IRT therapist usually asks what the patient wishes the target of his or her anger would do. The answer should imply that the raging will yield control, distance, or both.[12] Since the goal in IRT is to differentiate from destructive IPIRs, it follows that constructive anger would serve the purpose of distance from IPIRs, whereas destructive anger would serve the purpose of enmeshment.

If a patient is enraged about abuse that prevailed in childhood, any therapist would naturally be inclined to facilitate expression of anger. The abuse was wrong, and outrage is appropriate and just. Clearly, there is much relief in telling a story of abuse to an understanding person. Another possible result of telling the story is enhanced attachment to the listener. If the listener is a therapist, whatever healing forces are present in the therapy will probably be intensified.

Nonetheless, even as the clinician needs to hear that anger, he or she must take care not to fuel or prolong it. Seeking justice by confrontation or other means is rarely indicated in IRT. Subsequent personality change will depend more on what else the therapist can do to facilitate letting go of the gift of love to the abusive IPIR. Consider the prototypic patient who becomes furious with parents after reflecting about some form of abuse. To be sure, it feels better to be indignant than to be helpless. An angry shift out of helplessness is a vital first step on the way to healing. But when the indignation goes on for session after session, it is likely to become a form of continuing the suffering. Instead of facilitating the ongoing psychic hostile enmeshment, the clinician does well to focus more on the wish that supports the indignation. When the wish is gone, the anger will disappear. Then the patient will be freer to learn new ways of relating to others.

If anger in therapy is about relations with current figures, then the recommendation not to dwell on anger about past injustices is modified. Although letting go and distancing from expectations associated with internalizations from the past are recommended, the therapist does not urge separation from current loved ones.[13] Current rage is facilitated and then discussed in terms of whether it serves the purpose of control or distance or both. Those current goals and wishes for control or distance, rather than the anger, are the ultimate foci of the therapy discussion. As indicated before, neither extreme of control or distance is consistent with the goals of IRT. For ongoing relationships, the ideal is to have neither total enmeshment (total control or submission) nor total differentiation (total emancipation or separation). The goal is to love each other without power struggles and without resorting to living parallel, nonintersecting lives. This goal of warm, balanced mutuality has been sketched in Figure 4.4.

Whether current or past, the interpersonal translation of angry wishes into control or distance is often assisted by asking questions like these: "If your mother [parent, spouse/partner, child] could hear you now, what would you hope she [he] would do or say?" or "What is the best possible response your [parent, spouse/partner, child] could make to help you now?" The answers will vary tremendously in form. They may touch on apology, compliance, humiliation, suffering, restitution, rescue, love, or something else. But most variations can be translated into control or distance.[14] Once the goal is clear, the dialogue can turn to deal more directly with that purpose. For example, "Are there other ways you could get away from her [him]? If you had total control of her [him] every minute, what would you do? Are there other ways to meet that need?"

To help the clinician begin to listen for anger in interpersonal context, here are some examples of the two basic types. An example of constructive anger that would lead to freedom from a problem internalization would be the following: "It makes me livid to think that he did that to me all through my childhood. I can't stand the thought that he still has any effect on me at all." By contrast, the kind of anger that would not contribute to letting go of the fantasy would be this: "She never did love me. That b**** makes me furious. I would like to wring her neck and teach her a lesson. She absolutely ruined my life." This rage would bear the tell-tale signs of a desire to control by changing history, if not the future. As expressed, it would be unlikely to lead to letting go. Nonetheless, a constructive follow-up of this statement might be possible if the clinician were to ask how she ruined the patient's life, and the details eventually led the patient to conclude:

> "She really is totally limited in her ability to focus on anybody but herself. I know that can never change. I guess when I wanted her to show some concern about me too, I really expected more from her than she could give. I need to find somebody who is more balanced."

To review, if anger seems to be trying to change, resurrect, or otherwise influence an IPIR, it is not consistent with the goals of IRT. It should be "aired" but not encouraged. If, by contrast, the anger can lead to a perspective that enhances the wish to distance from a destructive IPIR, it is consistent with the IRT therapy goals. If the anger applies to a current desired relationship and not just to an IPIR, then the relationship needs to be reviewed with a goal of developing more warmth and more balance on the enmeshment–differentiation continuum. If there is ambivalence about the relationship, the possibility of total separation may be the patient's choice, after efforts to improve it to the satisfaction of participants have been made.

Reconsidering Perceived Family Wishes

It can be helpful to consider family norms in a broader social context. For example, Merideth was discussing her extreme anxiety when things were out of order:

> "I grew up in a family where there were Absolute Rights. One of those was having things be neat. Mother says there is a God-given way to set the table. The rest of the ways are wrong. Dishes have to be in the

dishwasher exactly the right way. You can only use two pieces of toilet paper."

Showing her emergent perspective and humor, Merideth added, "I don't have that one!" Her realization that such rules are neither universal nor particularly reasonable was one of her many steps toward freedom from her severely constrained and self-punitive lifestyle.

Sometimes there is a critical realignment when patients realize that their families are most loving when they themselves are "down." For example, Jan, a talented gardener, noted that her extended family members were devoted to staying together and protecting themselves from the evil world. She could not understand this, because their lives were so completely miserable. She knew, however, that the family disapproved of her leaving the hometown.

JAN: I understand they are very much afraid of anything outside the family. In fact, I was amazed when they welcomed me back last visit.

THERAPIST: That was when you were broken and despairing.

JAN: Well, yes.

THERAPIST: So that brings us again to the question of whether your ongoing despair means you still want to follow their rules.

Jan continued to struggle for a while with her apparent determination not to be happy. She would embrace everything dreadful in her life and ignore all the bright spots. Eventually she did accept that the "rules" for belonging were to be dependent and broken, and that she could choose the opposite—to be strong and whole.

Self-Management

Allowing Compassion for and Tolerance of Self

According to copy process theory, people who are treated like trash think of themselves as trash. One way to encourage more benign attitudes toward the self is to (1) facilitate reexperiencing of the perceptions and feelings the patient had as a child when interacting with relevant IPIRs, while simultaneously (2) asking the patient to comment from an adult perspective on this child's situation. In this exercise, the patient both reexperiences early trauma and evaluates it from the distance of adulthood. The nearly universal response to this strategy is to feel vulnerable as a child and, at the same time, to be outraged and grief-stricken as an adult. After eliciting the reexperiencing of the childhood position, the therapist asks the patient,

"What would you do if you saw this happening to another child?" Reliably, patients will suggest something that would protect the child—such as: calling child protective services, trying to get the child out of there, telling the parents to go to parent training class, and so on. These observations represent having compassion for the self.

Sometimes this exercise centers on self-concept. For example, Larry reflected on the impact of his having to identify and address the needs of others in order to avert disaster.

> "You lose your self-identity when your world centers on somebody else. And I had that growing up. At the time I was learning self-worth, there was little opportunity to be me—to be a significant individual. Some of that has served me well. I have learned to be hypersensitive to others' needs, and I use that in work. But some of it has not. I remain a sucker for needy people who give nothing back."

Seeing these patterns helped Larry begin to look after himself more. He needed further sessions to reexperience how it felt to be so self-negating for so long. He needed help in feeling compassion for the little boy whom nobody looked after. The discussions that evoked wishes and feelings when he was a child, along with his evaluation of the situation as an adult, were important components of his ability to begin to reach a point of better self-care.

Sometimes movies will trigger compassion for the self. When their situation is replayed in the theater, people can have compassion for the protagonist. This compassion can then be transferred to themselves in their own world. An example of a movie likely to do this for some is the 1996 film *Shine*, starring Geoffrey Rush, Lynn Redgrave, and Noah Taylor—the story of a schizophrenic man with an ambitious, abusive father who is determined to have a famous son. One patient identified with the sister who watches the beatings of her brother and can do nothing about it. Explaining her extreme upset at the movie, this patient said,

> "It reminded me you are not safe anywhere. Everything looked fine. Then all of a sudden, any second, anything can happen, and there is nothing you can do about it. I never could understand how the next day people could act like nothing happened."

In the movie, she could see that there truly is nothing the girl can do to save her brother from these attacks. This helped her to be less harsh on herself for failing to save other family members from her father's rages. Having the pattern validated in "the outside world" helped her give more credibility to her view on the family situation.

Empowerment via Children

Taking the perspective of children helps inspire Green behaviors. Patients' sensitivity to and caring for their children typically emerges sooner than the ability to care about themselves. Given clear understanding of the copy process links, this inherent love for offspring can rather quickly override the pressure to carry on family tradition and attack self or others. Sometimes suicidal impulses can be blocked by asking patients to imagine their children's reaction to such an event. The perspective can mobilize the patients' will to see that their children "have it better" than they did themselves, and to continue the fight to break the generational cycle of suffering by finding better solutions to current stresses.

Being Willing to Be Starkly Honest with Oneself

A patient realized that she was very uncomfortable when people would praise her work. She said,

> "Part of what is keeping me uncomfortable with these notions of success is being deeply distrustful of the viability of the world out there. I have lived expecting the world to fall apart around me. I feel more at home in situations that are not working. They are a more familiar world. I know what it is about to live on the edge of disaster. I worry that maybe I am capable of keeping myself in that kind of situation when it is not necessary."

Such complete openness and candor about the present situation can provide a huge boost to the will to change.

ACTION: ACTUALLY GIVING UP THE WISHES

Self-Discovery

Grieving for the Losses

One of the saddest parts of IRT comes when a patient realizes how many years, opportunities, and other irreplaceable things have been lost out of devotion to old rules and values. Sometimes the pain of visualizing the full extent of the waste is simply unbearable. Patients can wish to scream, pound the wall, or otherwise "go crazy" when they fully let in the meaning of what has happened—of what they have chosen. Again, this affect is usually driven by a wish to change things, to reverse time, to take control of what is long past. Until the physicists come up with technology for going backward in time, however, the only resolution of this dilemma is eventually to accept things as they have been and are. This is akin to confronting a death. Something very important is gone and will never return. It is over. It was what it was. It is what it is. As is the case with the death of a loved one, there is nothing to be done but accept it, to feel the full force of the sadness and loss, to be with it for a while—ideally, with the support and understanding of trusted other people. The wish to make happen what could not and cannot be is over. This is Green grief. Sometimes patients concretize this stage by holding a "memorial service," or even a "funeral," to help grieve for their losses. In time, acceptance will be achieved; the person can then move on into the future, determined to make the most of whatever time remains.

Therapists can facilitate the Green grieving process by listening well and being empathic. They also can provide appropriate optimism about "where to go from here." In the case of grief in therapy, unlike grief for a death, optimism is usually justified. Now that the weight of the past is lifted, there can be new opportunities and options. In this particular sense, the grieving stage of therapy may be more like being let out of prison. Here is a fragment from a grief-based session for Lou:

LOU: It is clear I was not cared about. (*Sobs*)

THERAPIST: They just did not care about you as you.

LOU: (*Continues sobbing*) If I had been what they accused me of, it would have been just fine. If only I really had not cared about anybody and was only concerned about myself. It is still incomprehensible—their ability to hurt me.

THERAPIST: Sometimes parents misperceive a child as somebody from their own past.

LOU: Well, they did always say I looked like Dad's father. (*Long silence*) But now the war is over. Nobody won. It is time to move on. It definitely makes sense to realize that if I didn't care about what they did to me, than nobody would care at all. I was thinking the other day about how I always did things in opposition to them. But now I can just do things right.

Letting Go

Letting go of the fantasy is the end point of the action stage. A woman who had "had tons of different kinds of therapy" began nearly every IRT session for 2 years with detail about what a very hard time she was having just surviving. This typically was followed by fury at her mother for giving her such a bad start in life. Her childhood had, in fact, included severe abuse (mixed in with adoration). Ignoring justice, the IRT therapist was stubborn in trying to find the purpose of the ongoing focus on injury and anger. It always came down to wishing that her parents had been and would now be different. The mother should apologize and, more importantly, should now do what she could to make things better. The father should listen to and respect her. After many repetitions of this scenario, the pattern began to change. One time, after a visit home, the patient described her experience as follows:

> "You would be really proud of me. I did good. I feel really good about it. I did a lot of observing. It was very interesting. It was hard. I was careful not to meddle. I saw my parents as little kids themselves. I am feeling a sadness come over me now. (*Tears*) I am wondering if I have replaced a lot of things with anger. Like sadness. I realized if you accept it, it will dissipate."

After years of unending and intense pain, this wise woman found peace and acceptance in the idea that her rage could not bring the love she needed and wanted. When she gave up the impossible wish, she was ready to let go.

Forgiveness

Forgiveness is closely related to, but not the same as letting go. According to the *American Heritage Talking Dictionary* (1997), forgive means "to excuse for a fault or offense. To pardon, to renounce anger or resentment against. . . . To refrain from imposing punishment on an offender or demanding satisfaction for an offense." Since IRT does not support the justice model, forgiveness is not required. For people who must have justice, however, forgiveness may be the only route to letting go. Forgiveness therapy has reportedly helped heal victims of sexual abuse (Freedman & Enright, 1996; Worthington & Rachal, 1997). However, it is not difficult to find individuals within the population of nonresponders who do not improve with forgiveness therapy. Marie, introduced in Chapter 1 and discussed again in subsequent chapters, was one such patient.

Internalizing New Figures

In Chapters 3 and 5, I have suggested that the internalization of the therapist, along with other currently important figures, is an important part of the therapy change process. The most desirable version of internalization of the therapist is simple generalization of the therapy learning. Patients frequently report that they thought about what the therapist would say as they encountered an old problem and gave a new response.

There are also toxic versions of internalization of the therapist. If a therapist's behaviors support an unrealistic fantasy, the process of internalization will enhance old problems. For example, a patient who has been dependent on a powerful and sexually abusive but supportive IPIR is likely to yearn to be specially connected to the therapist. In this case, unless the therapist is palpably different from the IPIR,[15] the therapy connection is at risk of intensifying problem patterns. Fantasy feelings about the therapist need to be acknowledged, linked to the IPIR, and discussed as ideas whose time has expired. The more the therapist can convey genuine warmth and appreciation for strength, and not for dependency, the better. If health-inducing therapist attitudes can be internalized, the reconstruction is facilitated. Of course, this is not easy. One such patient explained with candor how it felt when she faced the destructiveness of her attachment to the therapist: "It is easier to think of being close to you than to understand what this is about and face the intense sadness about what happened and what still is between me and my father. Right now, I feel intensely overwhelmed and suicidal." Clearly, the Red part of this patient preferred to realize the ancient wish by having the therapist become an iatrogenic replacement for the father. She admitted that it would be easier to let the therapist "replace" her father than to develop an altogether new pattern. Once again, it is vital in such a case that the clinician think about therapy process in the light of the case formulation.

Yet another form of evidence for the role of internalization of the therapist arises after serious old habits have been blocked, new ones have been developed, and then there is a break for some reason in the therapy connection. Perhaps the patient or the therapist goes out of town for several weeks, or maybe insurance payment problems cause an interruption in treatment. Under these conditions, it is not unusual to see a regression to old habits. When that happens, it takes an indeterminate number of sessions to restore the newer patterns. It seems that internalization at first is fragile and requires some time to consolidate. The therapy "dose" needs to be maintained until the old proclivities are well extinguished and new patterns are well established. Perhaps this compares to treatment of a highly resistant infection with long-term doses of antibiotics. If the treatment is stopped too soon after symptoms disappear, the problem returns. It will be very important eventually to learn how to tell when internalization is stable enough that therapy sessions are no longer needed to support it.

Another helpful internalization for many people is their version of a spiritual guide. Chapter 7 has included a discussion of supporting this resource when it is Green, and seeking help from the clergy when it is Red.

Compassion for IPIRs

These examples show that a visit to the family of origin during the later stages of therapy can crystallize the therapy learning and consolidate the new identity. Instead of being seen as judgmental, withholding, cruel, incompetent, critical, and the like, parents can be seen as vulnerable, possibly well-meaning, but very much limited by their own injuries and experiences. With the clear perception that the well is dry, it becomes much easier just to "give up" the old expectations. Necessarily, patients then begin to relate to their parents in more dignified ways. One man summarized his new, more benign behavior with his parents: "It felt good to behave like this with them. For years I did not know if I was right or wrong. Now I know that I am good enough, I can trust myself."

Self-Management

Constructing New Goals and Ways That Feel Right

Change both follows from and leads to self-discovery. Sheer "willpower" is an important part of change, too. For example, one woman had been defined in her family as the "crazy." Her history was dominated by overwhelming love and control. Every detail of her existence was hand-picked and closely monitored by her very concerned mother. One of her most reassuring traits as an adult was to have the badge of being a terrible housekeeper. When the case formulation made it clear that she had to be messy to exist, she said,

> "I am scared to think of myself as having my house in order and functioning well. Then I would not be able to make a statement. This mess in my house is my voice. The mess is my being. But I think I am sort of getting it now. I could exist in other ways."

Another way to set goals at this stage is to (1) imagine the outcome of ongoing behaviors according to the gift-of-love wish; (2) compare the wish to the actually expectable result; and (3) replace the wished-for goal with the normative one (described in Chapters 4 and 5). For example, suppose a mother describes a pattern of unreasonably demanding behaviors in her teenage daughter. The daughter nags and demands, and eventually the mother relents and spends an inordinate amount of money on whatever items the daughter feels she must have. Both the therapist and the patient agree that a pattern of such indulgent spending may cause the daughter to develop inappropriate expectations and to fail to acquire skills at living comfortably within her means. Still, the mother is unable to resist. She continues to be an "easy hit," and the daughter's demands escalate.

The exercise of imagining what happens if this practice stops might yield the belief that the daughter will love her if the mother buys whatever is wanted, but hate her if she does not. It might also reveal that the patient is determined to spare the daughter the humiliation she herself endured as

a teen, with only hand-me-down clothes to wear and with none of the ame-
nities that the other kids had. This conversation makes it clear that the
patient is trying to love and be loved by her daughter. But instead of love,
their exchanges lead to a demanding and blaming daughter and a helpless,
exploited, and resentful mother. This situation can be improved if there is a
clear therapy discussion of how the mother is trying to correct for her own
injury, and how that solution is actually not working.

The primary job of a parent is not to elicit love from the child. Demanding that a child to love a parent is an inappropriate and inauthentic
burden for the child. Nor is the primary job of a parent to keep a child
from having any pain in life; that is impossible. With some help from the
therapist, the mother may consciously decide she wants to let the daughter
know she is loved, and also to help her learn to choose wisely so she can
live within the family means. This new goal will be based on the more general idea that parents should strive to provide a safe home base from which
the child can go out into the world with realistic confidence, grow strong,
and thrive. Clinicians may find this general developmental learning model
to be helpful in discussing goal setting with parents.

Accepting or Rejecting Responsibility Appropriately

A healthy person (see Chapters 2, 4, and 5) accepts neither too little nor
too much responsibility. By contrast, externalizing patients come to therapy convinced that all difficulties are due to someone or something else.
Internalizing patients come to therapy convinced that everything that goes
wrong is surely their fault. Either extreme is a problem. The goal of achieving a balance in responsibility taking should be clear.

Ellen, an internalizing patient, was excessively self-critical and wore
herself out trying to address everybody's needs but her own. She believed
she had no right to expect anything for herself. One therapy conversation
went like this:

THERAPIST: Every baby needs to be hugged and loved.

ELLEN: Love is not an entitlement.

THERAPIST: It is not? Evolution helps us arrive ready to hug and be
    hugged. It is a part of a chain of reflexes needed for survival [see
    Chapter 2].

ELLEN: So I blew it. I had my chance.

Here Ellen took responsibility for her failure to develop a good attachment. She believed she was responsible for her own development even as
an infant! She needed 2 more years of therapy work to come to believe that
affection is more important than control in human relationships. If an

internalizer like Ellen had participated in a treatment that emphasized "responsibility taking" independently of case formulation, she would probably have increased rather than decreased her self-blaming. Within IRT, she eventually developed better balance and self-care, as well as less exploitative friendships.

Patients with SBS, discussed earlier, are externalizing individuals. One explained her perspective on the matter of taking responsibility:

> "I am angry I have to choose. I don't want to make a choice. I don't want to be responsible for this. I want to scream, 'I hate you. You brought me to this. You worked to strip away all the defenses and walls and things I protected myself with. Part of me despises you for that. Let me die. Let me have ended it rather than continue to struggle and deal with it.' "

Fortunately, this woman also had enough Green to realize that raging was an old and inappropriate way to try to cope. She knew she would need to accept the pain of having to make choices that were her own. Her failures would be hers—but so would her successes. Once she understood and accepted the reality that competence was not a crime, and that responsibility taking was an appropriate form of assuming control of her own affairs, she became interested in working toward some long-term goals. If she had been in a treatment program that indiscriminately encouraged people to "accept help," she might never have become able to take charge of her own ship.

Dealing with Fear of Feelings

For many patients, fear of feelings creates a large barrier to enabling the will to change. The task of reexperiencing early pain and then viewing it from an adult perspective is daunting. It can help to remind the patient that although feelings are painful, they will no longer be punished if expressed in therapy. And nobody will be destroyed if the buried feelings are heard in therapy sessions. After the patient lets the memories and feelings flow in sessions, therapist acceptance and empathy can help the patient experience those old intense feelings and remain sane.

Enduring the Pain of Giving Up the Fantasy

Giving up the fantasy that an IPIR will finally relent and become more loving is at the core of reconstruction. It has been mentioned in several contexts and is not reviewed further here, other than to note that patients do need to engage their willpower to "hang in there" even as the grief hurts so much. Pat, who had expected she would end therapy in a state of clear happiness, explained:

"I always thought I would have intense positive feelings at the end of therapy, not just balance. I have said that perhaps one of my problems was an addiction to the intensity of feeling that hurting and being hurt provides. You have said that happiness is not as intense, but more comfortable. I think I needed time and space and some protection to allow me to understand whether I have had balance and happiness. I think I don't recognize what others consider to be happiness or love or peace. The thing I have had to bury or distance from is that promise of intense happiness. I let myself believe it. It had to be true to keep doing what I was doing. (*Sobs*) I am not sure I should believe it any more."

Pat did manage to cope with this disappointment and maintained her gains very well.

Changing Klute Syndrome Practices

"I have a good imagination and I like pleasing. . . . Don't be afraid. I am not, as long as you don't hurt me more than I like to be hurt. I will do anything you ask. You should never be ashamed of things like that. You mustn't be. . . . There is nothing wrong. Nothing is wrong. I think the only way any of us can ever be happy is to let it all hang out and, you know, fuck it."

So goes the voice-over at the beginning and at selected other points in the 1971 movie *Klute*, starring Jane Fonda and Donald Sutherland, and directed by Alan J. Pakula. Fonda plays a would-be actress named Bree, who earns her living on the side as a call girl. The voice-over is from one of her "tricks" early in the movie. A client wants her to let him act out some violent sexual fantasies, and she agrees—"as long as you don't hurt me more than I want to be hurt." Some time later, John Klute (played by Sutherland) is commissioned as a private detective to locate a missing corporate executive. It is believed that the executive may have been Bree's customer, and it develops that he may be the one who has been harassing her with obscene phone calls and letters. The viewer learns through cameos from her psychotherapy why Bree likes to do tricks: She knows what she is doing and feels in control. Much of the movie is about her evolving relationship with Klute, who is loving, protective, and loyal to her. She abuses him badly and is confused by his consistently kind and loving acceptance. She lets her self-destructive tendencies reign when she rejects Klute in favor of renewing her contract with a hated pimp. She even tries to stab Klute with scissors. This does not deter Klute. Eventually he does for her what her long and expensive psychotherapy failed to do: He breaks through her manipulative cynicism and creates a willingness to make a commitment to another person. The stakes are high in this conversion: Klute rescues Bree her from her murderous and terrifying stalker (with a surprising identity). Just before the rescue, Bree is forced to listen to a tape recording of her own invitation to combine sex and violence (quoted above) by the man who is now about to murder her. Then he plays a tape of his most recent fatal enactment of that fantasy with Bree's friend, a strung-out call girl colleague. The murderer explains: "There are little corners in everyone that are best left alone. Sicknesses and weaknesses, which never should be exposed. . . . I never was fully aware of mine, until you brought them out."

The scriptwriters may be saying that the murderous perversion lurks in the unconscious and can be unleashed by opportunity. Another perspective is that whatever is practiced in fantasy is likely to be unleashed in practice. A learning theorist would favor that interpretation. I have been repeatedly impressed over the years with the fact that when patients fail to respond to treatment despite apparent collaboration, a valid case formulation, and a modest interval of treatment, it is likely that they have, in effect, eroticized their chief complaint. I call this the *"Klute* syndrome" (Benjamin, 1996a, Ch. 6). Examples include being tormented by repeated scenes of degradation and humiliation, and having sexual fantasies with the same effect; being repeatedly rejected, and having sexual fantasies about unavailable people; feeling that others are always in control, and having sexual fantasies of being helpless; and so on.

The implication of this finding is that when cases seem to be "stuck," it may be time to explore the possibility of a connection between sexual gratification and a specific interpersonal pattern. Surely it is true that if present patterns are supported by ongoing sexual fantasies and satisfaction, the will to change will be minimized. If such a connection is found, the option of sexual reprogramming can be offered as a powerful way to enable the will to change.

Tamara, a hard-working lab technician who suffered from loneliness and a sense of missing out while others thrived, had the *Klute* syndrome. She had been extruded psychologically from her family, having been "diagnosed" from an early age as being too difficult to live with. In all likelihood, this assigned role was based on her physical resemblance to her father's overprivileged younger sister. It turned out that Tamara's gift of love—namely, a life of rejection and loneliness—was buttressed by a wholly compatible sexual fantasy.

TAMARA: I want to try to talk about the sexual fantasies. It is so hard to even think about. I told you that when I come, I cry. You asked what it was about. I couldn't answer before, but it feels like the same feeling I have when I feel somebody really cares about me. When people are good to me. I never expect someone to really be caring about me. Orgasm feels like I have been given something I am not supposed to have and can't expect to have again.

THERAPIST: It means you cannot have love, pleasure, dreams. That is not for you.

TAMARA: Yes. For me, it is more like a starving person is grateful when somebody hands them a loaf of bread.

So Tamara had eroticized her experience: Even having a loaf of bread was not for her. This is not an unusual defense, even if it has not been recognized in the psychological literature. People do get through difficult situations by trying to imagine them as pleasurable. I first encountered this general idea when I took an early (1960s) version of birthing classes. The instructor was totally enthusiastic about the approach, and announced that the next day she was to have a tooth pulled. She declared she would not have any anesthetic because she would use the birthing techniques. I dropped out of the class right away.

The strategy of imagining pain is pleasurable can be adaptive, particularly if there are no other alternatives (e.g., anesthetic). But if chronic pain is supported by sexuality, the pleasure link must be broken if the patient wants to get rid of the pain. This may require sexual reprogramming. The technique is simple, but nonetheless quite difficult to implement.

The patient is invited to choose a new fantasy, and the therapist makes sure that it has interpersonal dimensions of normality.[16] The patient is instructed to introduce the new fantasy at the moment of orgasm, and is warned that this may totally ruin the sexual experience. But the patient must decide to invoke it anyway and keep doing it until it no longer ruins the orgasm. After that, he or she should introduce the fantasy earlier and earlier in the sexual process, until it has totally replaced the old fantasies. This will be very difficult, but the choice is clear.

Patients need to be supported and encouraged to use their new rather than their old fantasies as often as possible. They will complain, regress, blame, ignore, and be quite creative at avoidance. Of course, the IRT therapist never engages in a power struggle over this. In fact, the method is so powerful that a patient is well advised not to make any sudden life decisions while using it. The patient must engage in it only as rapidly and so long as he or she is willing. All of the control belongs to the patient. The therapist only offers a rationale, a method, and support for better choices.

MAINTENANCE: RESISTING THE WISH TO GO BACK

A recent study on maintenance of sobriety from the addictions literature (Downey, Rosengren, & Donovan, 2000, p. 743) reported higher rates of abstinence for individuals who did not like to see themselves as substance abusers: "The perception of discrepancies between substance use and self-standards was an effective motivator of abstinence even among those who reported previous use of substances to dampen self-dissatisfaction." This study might suggest that maintenance of the decision to give up old patterns will be facilitated by consolidation of the sense of a new self. The new self no longer has to do things the old ways. It is free of the influence of old suffering; it is "free to be."

Self-Discovery

Dealing with Panic over "What Now?"

Successful IRT often comes to a point where the patient becomes anxious or even panicky about what comes next. Here are some direct quotes:

- "Who will be in my head after they are gone?"
- "I am afraid of leaving everything, of losing things. Part of me is dying."
- "I'd like to keep a part of the dream and not feel like everything has been wasted."
- "Who will I be if I am not what I have been?"
- "I think I might be a hologram. Without them to pull the switch, I won't exist."
- "The more I see myself doing this, the more horrified I am. How stupid and pointless and unnecessary. How incomprehensible it actually is."

Each person creates his or her own startling imagery that conveys the depth of the nothingness the person feels at this time. This, more than any other period in therapy, marks a clear turning point. From here, there is a huge temptation to go back to the beginning and not venture forward again. One patient explained,

> "This is what I want to do. In the past, trying these new good things would have bothered me a lot, and I would not be in this situation. I couldn't tolerate it. This is a time to see how comfortable I can be with doing what I feel like doing. It might be hard, but I need to try."

To counter the pull of the familiar, the therapist needs to provide strong support to give the patient the security to continue on the journey to the other side of disorder. An important first step is to reassure the patient that it is entirely normal to feel this way at this point. Almost all patients are disoriented and upset to learn that their underlying goals have been for naught, and that they must change in order to do and be better. As suggested before, full realization of the case formulation is akin to experiencing the death of a loved one. Moving on alone is frightening and, in addition, can feel like an unacceptable betrayal of an old relationship.

As the therapist provides empathic support for these difficulties, he or she can also help by pointing out how the patient's recent positive changes are consistent with the agreed-upon therapy goals. It is also important for the therapist not to hold out false promises. Personal disclosure can help keep expectations realistic. Occasional mention of a therapist's own minor personal challenge, or even defeat of some sort, can serve as a reminder that therapy does not eliminate life stress or pain.[17] All that therapy promises is to diminish self-defeating and destructive patterns and to enhance new coping skills. Life is sure to provide many opportunities to use those new coping skills!

Confronting the Wish to Stay Stuck

After the bridge to recovery has been crossed, wishes to go back to the old ways can be resurrected. Althea, a high school teacher, had been suicidal for many years prior to starting IRT. She had been relatively free of suicidality until she experienced a severe stress about 2 years into the treatment. Because of the recurrence of strong suicidal wishes, Althea needed an emergency session. That meeting averted hospitalization, but at her follow-up appointment the very next day, she continued to struggle with suicidality. Althea had resurrected an ancient litany of all the reasons she was bad, deserved to die, ought to be a different person, and so on. A discussion of the case formulation yielded her view of her perceived failure:

ALTHEA: I am angry I have so much insight, and yet I hurt so badly. It is not fair. I've been thinking this for some time. What is all of that insight good for? How much of this is some sort of biological/biochemical primary problem?

THERAPIST: I guess I'll pass on that question today. We can come back to it later if you wish. But for now, let's take a look again at how this episode started. The thing that was so hard for you this week was the public display of respect and affection you got at work. I wonder if you are frightened of change?

ALTHEA: Yeah. For sure.

THERAPIST: You don't know if you can trust what is happening?

ALTHEA: [Lengthy speech spelling out those fears]

THERAPIST: So the glass is half empty. Getting better is worse.

One could rightly conclude that Althea had a pessimistic cognitive set. There had been evidence for that in her many years of prior treatment. In IRT, the emphasis changed to the underlying motivation for that negative cognitive set. For Althea, getting better violated the definition of self that she developed in relation to a "Red" parent. Progress therefore created a sense of panic and despair. After she was reassured that progress could be understood as a threat to her old self, and that regression is also a normal part of learning processes, her mood and perspective stabilized. The suicidality disappeared once more, never to return.

Frequently, as in Althea's case, clear evidence of progress can threaten the stability of the reconstruction. Sometimes thought experiments can be helpful to explore why good news is so bad.

THERAPIST: Let's imagine that your family could be here to hear us talk about this success. What will they do?

PATIENT: My father would tune out, and my mother and brother would feel inadequate and threatened. My sister would be proud.

In this instance, going through each family member's anticipated reaction made it clear that the patient was most worried about threatening her brother, who was overtly hostile, and her mother, who would back him up. Working with the fear of their disapproval and resolving the wish to comply with their expectations allowed her to maintain her new gains.

Self-Management

Self-Discipline

At this last stage of step 4, the IRT patient is fully aware of his or her patterns, their copy process links to an IPIR, and the need never again to heed the old wishes. In a sense, this stage requires the same willpower that a person with an addiction to substances like alcohol or food has to use: He or she simply says "No" to the wish. This is entirely up to the Green. A few recommendations for how to support this decision follow.

Considering Rewards and Losses in Recovery

The distinction between activities that facilitate self-discovery and those that facilitate self-management is not necessarily sharp. One intervention that seems more closely related to overt patient choice is to decide to bring the patient's spouse or partner to therapy to discuss current issues and therapy goals. Relationships with significant others constitute an ever-present force in psychotherapy. It is helpful to assess whether the spouse/partner supports recovery, and to enlist his or her help whenever possible.

Most significant others want patients to change for the better, but the details envisioned may or may not be consistent with the treatment plan. If, for example, a patient is depressed and dependent, and the spouse/partner is interested primarily in improved obedience and service (e.g., better housecleaning, sex on demand), IRT goals will not be embraced by the significant other.

A session or two that makes each partner's wishes clear and relates those to therapy goals can enhance the collaboration and speed the therapy process along. For the spouse/partner who insists on more service, it is fair to acknowledge the expectation that each member of the relationship will fulfill his or her role. However, it may be good to reconsider and redefine understanding of desired outcomes in terms of the two-circle model in Figure 4.4. IRT for couples is a large topic that cannot be reviewed here, but the basic idea is that IRT will seek to develop strengths in a patient to enable friendly mutuality. This means that if the patient is depressed and dependent, he or she will, in the light of the case formulation, be invited to agree to try to become more assertive[18] and actively participate in creating a viable relationship. Most people really like this idea. If they do not seek friendliness, moderate enmeshment, and moderate differentiation, IRT is not a good choice for them.

For instance, Marcia's partner demonstrated an ability to help her Growth Collaborator. Marcia qualified for a diagnosis of HPD (Histrionic Personality Disorder, as defined interpersonally in Benjamin, 1996a). The label of BPD (Borderline Personality Disorder) had been given to her by others. Marcia was tiring of her life of crisis and pain, and found a new boyfriend whose strength she admired. Her first episode of "losing it" happened shortly after she began IRT. She brought her new boyfriend to therapy so he could understand how crazy she was. The IRT therapist, however, debriefed a recent crazy episode and related it to the case formulation and the therapy goal. The partners were shown the model of mutuality in relationship in the top part of Figure 4.4. Both enthusiastically endorsed that goal. From then on, Marcia worked consciously on not rerunning the gift-of-love scenario by being a dramatic nut case. Her boyfriend was truly constructive. He was attentive and supportive, but did not attempt to rescue or dissuade her from her next few crises. In turn, she began to take pride in acting in a balanced way, and he responded extremely well to this. The relationship was tremendously helpful to her rapid progress, which included no further suicidality or desperation dramas.

By contrast, another patient who also had collected the label of BPD from a long list of therapists qualified for a diagnosis of Passive–Aggressive Personality Disorder (Benjamin, 1996a). Her partner did not support her. In fact, he refused to have anything to do with therapy. The patient commented, "Maybe some things are already too late. He has apprehension about what I am doing in therapy. Something will change that will be hard.

I am losing a part of me. Some of what we shared is gone and trashed." A partner's opposition to change makes therapy harder, but not impossible. In that case, the patient continued to work hard and to change, and the relationship did survive after all.

Tolerating Variability in Progress

It is not unusual for people to feel impatient with their progress and themselves. Therapists need to remind discouraged patients that learning is a gradual process with ups and downs. Falling back is normal, and sometimes people need to realize that they can only tackle a complex task a piece at a time. In Chapter 7, the model of a pendulum moving on a track has been offered as a metaphor. Patients who make good progress and then lapse back into suicidality, despair, raging, and the like can often be remoralized by reminding them of that moving pendulum. The idea is similar to trend analysis in the stock market. There may be notable ups and downs on any given day, but the longer-term trend is more informative about where the process is headed.

In addition to realizing that ups and downs are expected, patients (and therapists) need to come to terms that there is no way to a quick, easy reconstruction of personality. Progress comes only with hard work and time, and with willingness to progress a piece at a time. If, for example, one wants to learn computer programming, one does not expect to do it overnight. Rather, the learner gets an overview of what lies ahead at first, and then the dreary process of practice begins, one step at a time. Here is an example of a patient's recognition of that truth in IRT. Miranda came to IRT with her life in shambles after many therapies and many suicide attempts. She had made considerable progress in IRT, in the sense that she was no longer overtly self-destructive and had begun to mobilize herself to the point of taking part-time work. One day, she had the urge not to keep her therapy appointment. However, she decided to make herself come, even though she felt frightened by the reappearance of a problem boyfriend and discouraged as to whether she ever could change. She explained, most insightfully:

> "A certain amount of me is fed up enough with this program I have had going all these years to do something about it. So I figured I could take this panic piece out and try to deal with it while it is happening. Now I have already got myself into the problem situation again. This time, I decided there wasn't any good to come out of feeling so panicked. I realized I was not stopping to take care of myself. I wasn't eating. I wasn't going to come to therapy. I wasn't doing things to try to make myself feel better. I was just losing time by getting upset. I decided I have to take a break one way or another—either by feeling bad, or by

doing things to make myself feel better. I see I am not going to solve the whole problem now. But I can at least consider: Is this panic really necessary?"

Making the Right Choices

Miranda's suggestion that she needed to decide not to panic was extraordinarily honest, and required a huge amount of trust in the therapist and therapy. More than once, I have seen inpatient staff become unsympathetic toward a chronic patient who, during an IRT interview, discovers that his or her symptoms can be understood in ways that might imply there is a choice to have them or not.[19] Therefore I would guess that some readers might dismiss Miranda's example as atypical, as not representative of "real" panic. But in truth, this woman's anxiety (as well as depression and more) was long-standing and well verified by all manner of conventional diagnostic procedures. She had been treated with a variety of medications and different therapies. At this time in IRT, she was beginning to implement genuine self-management. It was an act of will, but it most certainly did not mean that her symptoms had not been genuine. The learning speech includes the basic idea that treatment seeks to help patients become able to make such choices. Recognition of the role of choice should never encourage clinicians or family to "blame" patients for their disorders or for their resistance to treatment.

In short, making the right choice requires that the patient understand the case formulation, have a secure base in the therapy, and be remoralized to the point where he or she can make the decision to give up old loyalties and decide truly to work on recovery. For people who have a lifetime pattern of disability, this necessarily requires a very long, painful, effortful, frightening process of learning better ways of relating to self and others.[20]

NOTES

1. In Chapter 3, working through has been more rigorously defined as coming to terms, as shown in Figure 3.2.
2. The preparation stage was a later development in this change model (Prochaska et al., 1994), and is not always represented in studies using the model. It is not included in the IRT parallel descriptions of stages in enabling the will to change (see text headings).
3. The transtheoretical model evolved in the context of treatment for alcohol and drug misuse. By contrast, IRT is not proposed as a primary treatment for substance use disorders. Rather, it is assumed that substance use is under control before coming to terms can be attempted. The reason is that the internal strengths that are goals of IRT interventions are severely compromised by use of alcohol, cocaine, cannabis, prescription pain medications, or other chemi-

cals that distort affect, judgment, and the ability to learn. Situations where treatment of alcohol and drug misuse dependence preempts IRT are mentioned in Chapters 3 and 7.

4. I have recently learned that it is also possible to wait too long to give the case formulation. The case of the perceptive student therapist who had a clear case formulation by the end of the first session but said nothing about it—and whose patient terminated abruptly after four sessions—illustrates this (see Chapter 2, note 1).

5. Collaboration has been compared to "horse whispering" by W. R. Miller (2000). He explains that the popular movie *The Horse Whisperer* was based on the "join-up" method of Monty Roberts for training and rehabilitating horses. Miller notes that his "client centered directive therapeutic style and horse whispering each teach respect for others' autonomies and choices and move with rather than against resistance."

6. Except during crisis, and sometimes in a one-time inpatient consultation, as noted in earlier chapters.

7. Winning and losing typically involves BLAME/SULK, CONTROL/SUBMIT, and IGNORE/WALL OFF.

8. The distinguished feminist philosopher Claudia Card of the University of Wisconsin–Madison, notes: "According to Rawls [1963], the justice model can be based on fairness. Fairness is a distribution of the benefits and burdens of social cooperation that should be acceptable to everyone involved and justifiable to parties in every position" (personal communication, 2002). According to Rawls and Card, then, the IRT goal of friendly and balanced reciprocity does invoke the fairness or justice model. However, because patients so often define "justice" in terms of a perceived need to redistribute blame and extract restitution, I continue to use the term "justice" to describe the idea that punishment needs to be meted out and restitution is in order. I prefer to think of "fairness" as a different and broader term that is distinct from justice and clearly included as a goal in IRT.

9. In some patients, the gift of love may be considered to be an addiction.

10. Except for the virulent versions that involve sexual abuse.

11. Discussions of sexual abuse are unlikely to succeed in a healing perspective if they fail to include the fact that there were elements of pleasure and collusion from the patient. If this does not happen, the patient knows that the therapist doesn't know "the whole story," and hence any reassurances are empty. Once again, the blame model severely interferes with discussion and understanding.

12. According to the SASB-based interpretation of anger discussed at length in Benjamin (1989).

13. If a current loved one is a parental figure, the ideal is to let go of old expectations and to develop current friendly reciprocity. However, by definition, reciprocity requires participation from both parties. If that is not possible, then ordinary civility (if not genuine warmth) can emerge after the old expectations have expired.

14. With help from the SASB model. Note: If the wish is that the other will die, is this control or distance? This is not a simple question. Often the patient must then be asked, "So if she [he] dies, then what happens? Remorseful reunion in

heaven? Just suffering in hell? No possibility of further contact?" These subsequent answers can usually be coded in terms of domination or distance.

15. In addition to not having any sexual interest in the patient.

16. I have often been asked what a "good" fantasy is. My answer is a "normal" one as defined by the SASB model (see Chapter 4): friendly and moderately enmeshed or differentiated. But, ideally, this is not a fantasy; rather, it is a lived baseline. Hence the ideal is not to need a fantasy at all, but just for a person to love the person he or she is with, "as is."

17. Discussing a personal major life stress would carry a high risk of overwhelming or otherwise frightening the patient. If kept to the level of daily struggles (e.g., a normal-weight therapist mentioning efforts to control weight and exercise in a case-relevant context), there is less danger that boundaries will be violated. Please see Chapter 5 for a discussion of IRT-adherent personal disclosure.

18. With the understanding, based on the SASB model, that ASSERT is not at all the same as CONTROL.

19. The most dramatic and upsetting example of this occurred when a patient with Schizophrenia and dozens of hospitalizations in her record came out of "word salad" during an IRT interview. She told the poignant tale of how and why she went crazy. To me, of course, it all made sense. I still saw her as severely damaged and as needing years of skilled treatment, supplemented by medications to recover. But I noticed she was discharged with her diagnosis changed to Factitious Disorder.

20. Defined in Chapters 4 and 5.

9

Step 5: Learning New Patterns

After a patient's grieving over lost wishes and lost opportunity resolves, new hope can support realization of Interpersonal Reconstructive Therapy (IRT) goals. Figure 9.1 shows that at this final stage of IRT, the Green becomes large compared to the Red. That is, the Growth Collaborator (GC in Figure 9.1) now predominates. The Regressive Loyalist (RL in Figure 9.1) shrinks to a smaller size, but does not disappear completely. At times of extreme stress or fatigue, the Red may reemerge. Supported by full awareness and choice, the patient who completes IRT will consistently resist the Red habits and instead opt for the IRT goal behaviors, described below.

During this final step of IRT, the therapist provides helpful structure as the patient practices new interpersonal and intrapsychic patterns. The therapist also remains alert to the need to help the patient resist the pull to go back to the old Red ways. For both these purposes—learning new patterns, and resisting the pull to regress to old patterns—there must be continued self-discovery and self-management activities. These activities are described in this chapter, following a brief review of IRT goals.

THE GOALS OF RECONSTRUCTION

Interpersonal Goal Behaviors for IRT

The IRT "graduate" will function from a baseline of friendliness toward self and others that includes moderate degrees of enmeshment and moderate degrees of independence.[1] In addition, there will be a good balance between focus on self and focus on others. He or she will be fully self-defined and yet remain connected with others. In very specific situations,[2] ideally normal persons will have short-term access to extremes of enmeshment or separation and to hostile or sexual behaviors. Hostility will serve to

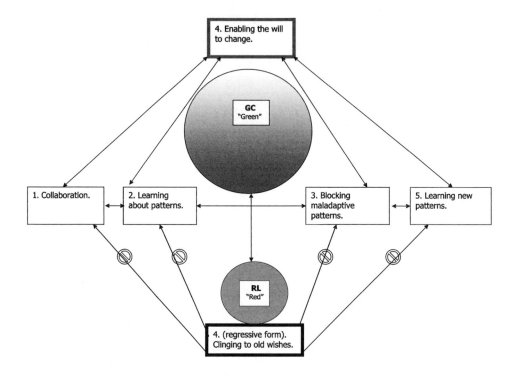

FIGURE 9.1. The five steps at the end of therapy, with emphasis on the conflict between the Growth Collaborator (GC) and the Regressive Loyalist (RL) at step 4. (Compare this with Figure 1.1.)

achieve control or distance, and sexuality will be associated with affection and attachment.

Goal Affects and Cognitions Accompanying Normal Interpersonal Behaviors

The affect and cognitive models paralleling the SASB interpersonal and intrapsychic model suggest that IRT behavioral goals are accompanied by specific desirable affects and modes of cognitive function. Affects (Figure 4A.2) that parallel the baseline behavioral goals include the following: Accept, love, and nurture; Be centered, delighted, and hopeful. According to the affect model, many other positive affects are composed of these six. For example, serenity is between centered and delighted. In specific, contextually appropriate situations, extremes of affect (e.g., murderous hate, passionate sexuality) are also accessible. In other words, the ideally normal person usually has comfortable and well-modulated baseline affect.

Parallel cognitive styles (Figure 4A.3) are as followed: Understand, Enhance, and Concentrate; Be expressive, optimistic, and well-directed. According to the cognitive model, many other effective modes of cognition are composed of these six. For example, creative would be between expressive and internally directed. Extreme variants of cognitive style (e.g., narrow focus; very broad scanning) can be exhibited appropriately in specific contexts. The ideally normal person has an effective, balanced, and positive cognitive style. All-or-nothing thinking[3]—described so well by Beck, Rush, Shaw, and Emery (1979), and frequently found in nonresponders—does not prevail.

Awareness and Choice Supported by Integrated Behavior, Affect, and Cognition

The person who achieves these ideal therapy goals will be fully aware of his or her interpersonal and intrapsychic motivations and patterns, as well as their associated feelings and ways of thinking. He or she will make benevolent, contextually appropriate choices with maximal degrees of freedom. As a person implements skills in awareness and choice, his or her behavior, affect, and cognition will function in an integrated manner appropriate to the interpersonal context.

ASSUMPTIONS AND VALUES INHERENT IN IRT GOALS

1. *IRT goals may be inappropriate for some individuals or cultures.* The IRT goals just described are based on the developmental assumptions presented in Chapters 2, 4, and 5, and stem from evolutionary data and reasoning. As discussed in Chapter 5, the IRT goals of friendliness, and of balance in focus as well as in enmeshment–differentiation, are not culture-specific. When the stated goals are not compatible with the declared norms of individuals or groups, IRT should not be utilized.

2. *IRT goals are not focused on justice.* As noted in Chapter 8, IRT therapists do not typically support wishes for confrontation, revenge, or justice. A victim of abuse, for example, may successfully conclude IRT without ever hearing an apology or receiving restitution. The IRT therapist tries to help the patient understand the wish for revenge or restitution in the light of the case formulation. If the patient continues to direct a blame pattern toward family members or other persons, it is treated as a repetition of any other problem pattern.

3. *The justice model prevails if there is threat of harm to self or others.* The legal system is required to maintain social order. In Chapter 7, it is made clear that when there is threat of harm to self or other, work with the

links to Important Persons' Internalized Representations (IPIRs) ceases. Symptom management, which includes the justice system, takes over. The IRT therapist uses clinical judgment to decide when the switch should occur.

Suppose, for example, that an IRT therapist were to find that a male patient contemplating murder had a violent, cruel, and punitive parent who was saturated with righteous indignation. Suppose too, that this potential murderer were to recognize that society forbids killing, and that he also has a clear sense of right and wrong. He would argue that the killing is right and just in this instance. In so doing, he would be copying and providing testimony to cruel parental rules and values. His social learning would have taught that life-threatening violence is the way things are done. This case formulation might explain the murder if the patient were to go ahead and commit it, despite all appropriate efforts in therapy to prevent it. But the patient would need to understand that he still has to be referred to the justice system to face the consequences dictated by society. Similarly, a retrospective IRT case formulation for a murderer would not exempt him or her from social justice.

AN EXAMPLE OF EMERGING RECONSTRUCTION

Here is an example of a patient who was beginning "the final approach" to reconstruction. Sasha had a long-standing pattern of having her partners center on her; otherwise, she would truly become terrified. She would react to separations with angry recriminations and reckless threats. She chose partners who tolerated her yelling, and who complied with her wishes if she punished them by withdrawing her affection. Her relationships were stormy. In a session during which she had actively been connecting her current patterns to those she had learned within her family, she said:

SASHA: I want to not have so much of my "damaged-ness" be there. But it is really hard to stop it when it is happening.

THERAPIST: You have noticed a lot about your patterns this week, and you are even more aware you want to be free of old habits.

SASHA: Yes. I am going through stuff a lot faster than I used to. I cry intensely, but only for a short time. I am interested in turning this around. Even as stuff happens, I have a voice that says, "Well, wait a minute." I try to think about what is happening and what I really want to do. Last night, my boyfriend stayed at work late and canceled our dinner plans. Instead of getting all unhinged, I just called a friend to make different plans. My evening really was quite pleasant.

Here are the SOAP notes from that session (see Chapter 3):

Subjective: Highly reflective. Making connections, and actively disrupting repetitions of old patterns (to be devastated and desperate in response to being left out).

Objective: Is in transition. No longer reflexively reacting to perceived abandonment with old patterns (panic, intense crying, threats). Has replaced chaos with constructive alternative (chose a pleasant evening with a friend).

Analysis: Realizes she is treating partners as if they were her father. Says she is tired of the damage from these patterns and is showing new responses.

Plan: Continue to support blocking of past patterns and emerging ability to show normative patterns in relationships.

THE NATURE OF LEARNING IN IRT

Measuring Progress in IRT

Most learning processes are gradual, including learning in IRT. Early in therapy there will be examples of new patterns, but they will not predominate until step 5, as termination approaches. IRT therapists and patients need to remember that learning is a gradual and variable process. In Chapter 7, therapy learning has been compared to a swinging pendulum moving along a track. There is overall movement in the desired direction, but there is also considerable movement back and forth.

When IRT Can Be Brief

IRT promises to help nonresponders move toward therapy goals, albeit slowly. There are instances when IRT can be accelerated. Some people can take more rather than less frequent focus on the case formulation and the gift of love. If the patient requests accelerated treatment, perhaps for administrative reasons,[4] it can be attempted. The clinician needs to watch carefully for signs that the process is going too fast. Cues that there is a problem might include frequent changes of subject, becoming silent, and disagreeing with a case formulation that has been previously affirmed. Even in sessions that show no indications of resistance to acceleration, it is good to say something like this: "I really have been leaning into you on this today, and I hope it has not been too much." Quite often, self-selected accelerated patients respond, "I like it. Thank you. I want to really get going, and what you are doing is very helpful." Or "I like this 'hypertherapy.' "

Uninterrupted collaboration is essential to accelerated IRT. It is very important to remember that many patients cannot respond to accelerated

IRT. Individuals with passive–aggressive traits (Benjamin, 1996a) or with *Sunset Boulevard* syndrome (described in Chapter 8) are examples. Evidence of collaboration[5] may be the best guideline as to whether the pace is acceptable. If collaboration prevails, acceleration can continue.

A Very Brief Review of the Four Steps Preceding Step 5

In Steps 1 and 2 of IRT, while developing collaboration and insight, the patient reviews specific current problem patterns in the light of recent input, response, and impact on self. Links to IPIRs are identified. In step 3, after recognizing these connections, the patient begins learning to anticipate and block repetition of the problem patterns. In step 4, as the patient makes the decision to stop repeating the old patterns, he or she needs to accept loss and determine to move ahead in new ways. Finally, as the old urges recede, new patterns can be learned in step 5 and can prevail. At step 5, as for the first four steps in therapy (see Figure 3.1), two classes of activity facilitate change: self-discovery and self-management.[6]

For example, the patient first learns to recognize an ancient urge: "I want so bad to cut myself now." Then he or she links it to the IPIR: "When cutting myself, I can both express my anger at him and, at the same time, agree with him that I should suffer. Maybe that will make him love me again." Next, the patient chooses not to implement the old pattern: "I am tired of all that. I know it does not work, and I really don't want things to be like they once were. I am going to 'kick the habit.' " Focus then shifts to the desired alternative: "Instead of acting like he is still the center of my life, I am going to assert myself in a friendly and well-defined way. It feels really good to be able to do that. It isn't easy, but I am going to keep doing things that can help me change my life for the better."

LEARNING NEW PATTERNS THROUGH SELF-DISCOVERY

According to Figure 3.1, self-discovery at step 5 involves (1) accepting what was and is, and moving forward; and (2) making mindful and benevolent choices. Self management at step 5 includes (1) identifying and practicing new, constructive patterns; and (2) resisting the wish to go back to old ways. These boundaries suggested by Figure 3.1 are permeable. For example, the decision to resist the wish to go back is based on self-discovery, but success in resisting that wish depends on self-management. The activities sketched in Figure 3.1 are frequently characteristic of the respective steps, but they are not exhaustive. In fact, "anything goes" at any time in IRT—so long as it is consistent with the case formulation and follows the core algorithm.

Accepting What Was and Is; Moving Forward

Figure 9.1 makes it clear that the Red does not disappear. This means that patients will continue to experience wishes to remain loyal to old rules and values. Self-discovery activities mostly focus on maintaining motivation to move on beyond the old rules and values.

Fear of Newness

As evidence of new learning cumulates, people in IRT often become uncomfortable with the loss of habitual ways they have practiced for so long. Changing from the old ways is disorienting for any learner. One patient, Lori, offered a clear description of this problem:

LORI: I feel uneasy doing things for myself that will help rather than hurt me. This is a bubble that will burst. It will all crash back down, and I will be in rubble and ruin again from the past. I don't trust good stuff to keep on happening.

THERAPIST: What have you learned in therapy about that feeling?

LORI: If things are going well, I sabotage them. I am a crisis management girl. I have to have several fires burning at once. But, really, I don't trust fate, and I feel guilty. I am doing better and don't deserve it.

THERAPIST: Who says that?

LORI: Dad, of course.

Lori was having another learning episode about her need to be in trouble in order to be psychically close to her father. This time, through recognizing her discomfort with progress, she could move a step ahead of the threat to regress to old ways.

Confronting Remorse and Regret

In addition to having to deal with fear of new patterns, recovering patients often look back on past behaviors with remorse and regret. They need considerable support in tolerating the pain of accepting what was, so that they can be freer to focus on what is and is yet to be.

Consider Jenny, who carried the bipolar label and had an old pattern of issuing ultimatums. One day, she reflected on her behavior at church, when she had insisted an event be run a specific way, while others on the committee failed to agree. Because they would not comply, she abruptly both quit the committee and left that church altogether. Two years later, as she reflected on the episode, she said:

JENNY: I have alienated people. I can see that I offended them. I left a bad taste. (*Tears*) There are so many things I have not dealt with gracefully. I think I just cannot deal with people.

THERAPIST: Stop! You are showing great courage to acknowledge your problem patterns. But to admit them does not mean that you will repeat them forever. Where did you learn to say, "my way or the highway," anyway?

JENNY: (*Laughs; cries*) I know it is tied to that Mom stuff. But I did lose good friends then.

THERAPIST: Yes, you did, and that is sad. But now you are more aware of what you don't want to do any more. If you had that situation again, how would you handle it?

JENNY: Well, if I could not bear what was happening and could not get the process to change, I could just resign a little later by saying, "I have too many responsibilities." I didn't have to tell them they were all wrong and I wanted nothing to do with them. I can see that I put them in a very awkward position. I really could have handled it better.

THERAPIST: Right. So now you see you just had some learning to do, and you have done it!

Making Mindful and Benevolent Choices

The Experience of Awareness and Choice

After the case formulation is fully appreciated and the decision to let go of old rules and values has been made, the IRT patient can choose to respond to a given challenge in either the old way or a new way. With therapist support, the new way will become the choice more often than not.

Paul was perplexed by why he seemed terrified to make a commitment in a relationship. He yearned to get married, but whenever a relationship started to move toward commitment, he abruptly lost interest and withdrew. He never could anticipate this reaction, and yet it happened over and again. As he puzzled over where he might have learned this pattern, the therapist asked:

THERAPIST: Did your parents model constancy?

PAUL: Yes, of course. They were together forever and ever. Very miserably. I don't know what I felt totally or precisely during those years—except a clear awareness of tension and hurt from my mother, and distance from my father. Their relationship must not have been a positive model for me, and it would be very logical that I would have concluded somewhere along the line that I would want nothing to do with such a binding, yet empty and tense, relationship.

THERAPIST: So commitment is not very attractive.

PAUL: Exactly. Why go there? My mother totally yearned for something more. She repeatedly said how unsatisfied she was at all levels. So why wouldn't I expect the same thing? If I commit to anyone, I will be deprived as she was. (*Long silence*) I like this "awareness and choice" idea. Awareness is potentially liberating. It says to me that my inadequacies in relationships don't mean I am worthless. They are understandable responses to some pretty unfriendly conditions.

Paul's fear of intimacy had other roots too, but this particular perspective seemed to help him resist the urge to flee, so that he could and did explore his next relationship in considerable depth.

A Family Conference: An Opportunity to Choose New Patterns

As mentioned in Chapter 6, a well-planned family conference that is tape-recorded for later review in individual therapy can allow the patient to learn about his or her patterns in the family context. Another possible function of a family conference in IRT is to give the patient an opportunity to choose to practice new patterns in a place where it may matter the most.

Mack, age 37, had had two severely self-destructive psychotic episodes, and frequently emphasized that he loved his parents dearly. They were in many ways very supportive, but his mother planned for his every moment. Through listening to a family conference tape, Mack realized that his mother would repeat her plans for him over and over, never acknowledging his protests or alternative suggestions. He compared it to the pattern of his voices, which also gave repetitive commands and accepted no discourse. Mack resolved to assert himself until his view was acknowledged. Not long afterwards, he reported on a conversation with his mother that had a new pattern:

"I have been rude to my mom a few times. Maybe therapy has caused it because it happened right after our last session. She said, 'You could be getting a new job over at the [name] bank.' I told her, 'It just is not happening.' She did not hear me, and so I shouted, '*It is not happening*! I am not going to keep hearing the same stuff over and over without my feelings on the issue being considered.' "

Mack was able to continue asserting, and his mother was responsive. She stopped giving him so many instructions for how to live his life, and was able to engage in more balanced exchanges with him. He had no further psychotic episodes.

LEARNING NEW PATTERNS
THROUGH SELF-MANAGEMENT

Seeking and Practicing New, Constructive Patterns

The Decision to "Just Do It" the New Way

Step 5 emphasizes teaching and learning desired new patterns. If the process of practicing new patterns falters, it can be helpful to remind the patient of interfering links to IPIRs. In the following example, the therapist did this while including other therapy steps as well. The exchange included therapist understanding (step 1), an invitation to look at the consequence of contemplated action (step 3), a connection to the case formulation (step 2), and affirmation of the patient's decision to behave differently (step 5).

Mabel, a financial advisor, had been taking antidepressants for many years. She was an expert in relation to customers, but crippled in relation to bosses. She was extraordinarily conscientious, always overwhelmed with too much to do, and severely depressed. Her willingness to be exploited was driven by the belief that she was responsible for whatever went wrong. After 2 years of IRT, she began to stand up for herself and resist unreasonable assignments at work. In the following example, she had just described an incident wherein she had been appropriately assertive on her own behalf.

THERAPIST: So this shows that you can assess a situation now and not automatically assume it is your job to take care of everything.

MABEL: Right. And I have to be careful to size up my own responsibilities properly, so I can discard those nagging beliefs that always make me feel so guilty and unfree. But I don't give those up well. [She describes another current overload assignment.]

THERAPIST: Who is responsible to see that gets taken care of?

MABEL: Harry, the branch supervisor.

THERAPIST: OK. Maybe if you simply refer those folks who are upset about this to him, he will have a chance to deal with it. If you take care of it, he won't even know there has been a problem. Then he will be unlikely to change the set-up that is creating this problem.

MABEL: Yes, I see that. But I feel so strongly I should do something myself.

THERAPIST: Can you connect that feeling to what we have been discussing?

MABEL: Oh yes. I have always wanted to fix an impossible, broken [family] system. It is really important I learn how to stop doing that now before I teach a new system to do the same thing all over again.[7]

THERAPIST: What a good idea!

It is clear that Mabel understood the case formulation, but still struggled to resist the old pulls. She resolved to work harder on this issue. In this episode, she demonstrated that she fully understood the role of complementarity (defined in Chapter 4) in creating and maintaining system patterns. At the time, her depression had remitted to the point of no longer needing medications. She needed only a small boost to stay on her new trajectory.

Another example of self-management via deliberate decision making during step 5 is provided by Alice, a very bright college dropout. Alice had been making remarkable progress out of her depression, as confirmed by friends and associates. Toward the end of her year-long therapy, Alice recognized a pull from her mother to stay nonfunctional. She said:

ALICE: I am trying to do great things. But Mother is critical. She plans to resign from her job, and says I should do the same. The way she feels about herself is the way she wants me to feel. She wants someone at her same level of disappointment, and tries to make me that person. It is so unhealthy. I don't want to do that.

THERAPIST: You don't want to join your mother in chronic misery and suffering.

ALICE: Definitely not. I think I am going to move to an apartment. I do not want to keep hearing these things from my mom. There is no way of knowing when it will come out if I live home. Well, I suppose I could learn how to take the blows. Just brush them off. Still, they hurt deeply.

Alice clearly saw the IPIR-based pull to nonfunctionality. She also understood differentiation. She contemplated achieving it through physical separation and at the same time, challenged herself to separate psychically.

Behavioral Techniques for Teaching and Learning New Patterns

Linehan's (1993) dialectical behavior therapy (DBT) for Borderline Personality Disorder provides useful training exercises that help patients enhance their skills at managing affect and relationships with themselves and others. The counseling literature also offers specific suggestions for how to enhance interpersonal skills. For example, Johnson (1972) described some useful experiential exercises for interpersonal learning, and Gordon (1970) taught empathic listening[8] to parents. Gordon's instructions for parents can also be helpful to fighting couples.

There are numerous behavioral skills-building presentations targeted at specific helper populations, such as school teachers (Braswell & Kendall, 1987), social workers (Nerdrum, 1997), executives (McEwen, 1997), nurses (Aschen, 1997), couple therapists (Jacobson & Christensen, 1996), and others. Such resources typically seek to enhance skills in assertiveness, communication, and stress management (e.g., Gelder, 1997); self-management (Braswell & Kendall, 1987); self-talk (Ellis, 1973); self-regulation (Cousens & Nunn, 1997); self-efficacy (Goldbeck, Myatt, & Aitchison, 1997); self-esteem and self-reinforcement (Overholzer, 1997); relaxation (Hamberger, 1997); and conflict resolution (Feeney & Davidson, 1996). Some of these publications (and others) also focus on the use of behavioral techniques to address specific symptomatic presentations, such as anger management (Hamberger, 1997), road rage (Lowenstein, 1997), anxiety (Aschen, 1997), couple difficulties (Jacobson & Christensen, 1996), battering (Hamberger, 1997), and perpetration of sexual abuse (Witt, Rambus, & Bosley, 1996).

In IRT, applications of such behavioral techniques are guided by the case formulation. Consider as an example, the behavioral technology of managing self talk. The IRT therapist embraces the idea of teaching new self-talk in terms that relate explicitly to the relevant IPIR. New self-talk, such as "I am not a vicious, mean, selfish person," in IRT becomes "That is just me talking to me like my father did. I know now that I simply want my views to be acknowledged and considered." In general, any behavioral technique becomes IRT-adherent if it is chosen in relation to the case formulation, and implemented according to the core algorithm.

Use of the Therapy Relationship to Model New Patterns

Use of behavioral technology and interpersonal skills training is not the only way to encourage new patterns in IRT. Another important method is to let the therapy relationship provide a model for new ways of interacting. An example of an approach that emphasizes the therapy relationship as an agent of change is time-limited dynamic therapy (Strupp & Binder, 1984). Examples of therapist behaviors that provide good models include empathy, respect, caring, and encouraging experiencing. Strupp and Binder wrote:

> Ideally, all aspects of the therapist's behavior should satisfy one fundamental criterion: it should provide the patient with a constructive experience in living. The therapist sets an example of caring, reasonableness, predictability, maturity—in short, presenting the best model of adult behavior of which he or she is capable. This is done as consistently as possible throughout the course of therapy. (1984, p. 137)

The idea that the patient may internalize therapist behaviors is important in IRT. However, in Chapters 4 and 5, there was discussion about why the therapy relationship is not a complete model for a love relationship. The problem is that the therapist focuses exclusively on the needs and concerns of the patient. His or her own needs are met by the therapy contract, and are not personal. By contrast, in a normal interpersonal relationship, focus on and consideration of personal needs are fully reciprocal. Although the therapy relationship models goal behaviors for focus on other, it does not include the full complement for focus on self.[9] If a patient expects his or her spouse/partner to act like a therapist, there will be an imbalance of focus in the marriage.

Use of the SASB Model to Teach Interpersonal Skills

Another effective way of enhancing new interpersonal and intrapsychic skills is to use the SASB model as a teaching tool. Feedback from the SASB Intrex questionnaire ratings of self and others helps develop and explain the case formulation to the patient. A summary of this approach appears in Benjamin (1996b, 2000b); extensive details are given in Pincus and Benjamin (in preparation). Several examples of how to facilitate interpersonal learning using the SASB model have been presented in Appendix 4.1 of this book. Here is an especially important example.

Assertiveness and dominance mean the same thing to many people. Oppressed and depressed patients will be reluctant to speak up on their own behalf, because they believe that would make them be like their dominant oppressors.[10] The SASB model makes it clear that "I will do it my own way" is the antithesis of "You must do it my way." They are not the same at all. "I will do it my way" is focused on self and is independent. "You must do it my way" is focused on other and is enmeshed. Most patients quickly see the difference between assertiveness and dominance when shown these two points in terms of the geometry of the SASB model.

For example, Adam reported that he'd had another fight with Alma, his wife, over how to handle their teenage daughter, Sheri. "I told Alma that she was not letting Sheri test her independence. I said she was approaching Sheri with too much control. If she did not stop, things would keep on blowing up." A skilled clinician and/or an SASB coder could see that although he was talking about independence,[11] and wanted to be helpful[12] to his daughter and his wife, he had in fact been critical[13] of his wife. SASB-based clear descriptions of his intention, in contrast to the actual process he used, helped Adam learn to communicate more effectively with Alma. He needed to learn how to disclose and inform without taking over or putting his wife down.

To help Adam learn another way of handling this problem, the therapist modeled a position of friendly differentiation from his wife:

THERAPIST: What if you were to say something like this to Alma another time: "It sounds like Sheri has thought through her plan fairly well, though I admit it makes me uncomfortable too. It may be one of those times that she needs to be allowed to find her own way. My impression is that she gets very angry when she feels you [Alma] are managing her too much, and so Sheri does what she wants anyway. Why don't we just tell her what we are worried about, and let her decide for herself? We can let her know we are available if she needs and wants our help."

ADAM: I see.

THERAPIST: The main idea here is that you keep the focus on your own views and feelings, and express them clearly as a separate person. You remain friendly, and don't try to force things by backing up your position with criticism of your wife. This way of relating shows respect for and trust in both your wife and your daughter. Of course, the outcome is not guaranteed, but you already are appropriately prepared to let your daughter do her own learning.[14]

Adam understood the difference between focus on self and on other. He could also make the distinction between enmeshment and differentiation as shown in the SASB model. This helped him replace control with disclosure. He began practicing friendly differentiation from his wife. Adam appreciated having a specific and clear understanding of how and why he needed to change his patterns of behavior in difficult situations like this.

Role Plays

In role plays, the patient assumes the roles of various key figures. In order to model constructive alternatives, the therapist plays the role of the patient, not of a difficult other person. As indicated before, if the therapist plays the oppressor rather than the patient, there is a significant risk of contaminating the therapy relationship and enabling the problem patterns. Instead, the therapist models the therapy goal behaviors of friendly balance of focus, with moderate degrees of enmeshment and of differentiation. These are shown in reaction to the challenges mounted by the patient, playing the roles of problem IPIRs.

Consider Elaine, who was scheduled to meet with one of her company's executive vice presidents (VPs) to discuss a pending request that she do something for another division. Elaine did not want to do this and saw it as possibly fatal to a different project she was currently working on. The therapist used role play to help Elaine practice saying, "No, thank you." To prepare for the role play, Elaine first reviewed all the reasons she should not be given the pending assignment, and described her alternative proposal for how the problem could be solved fairly. Her analysis was lucid and constructive. Informed with these details, the therapist was then ready to play her role, while she played the anticipated role of the demanding VP. Elaine took the VP's position with gusto and became quite intimidating. In the role of Elaine, the therapist disclosed her position without becoming attacking, sulky, defensive, or withdrawn. After a while, Elaine said, "I see. I'll try that." She did. Although the meeting was not a disaster, her unwanted assignment was still pending after the meeting. A few weeks later, the VP called, told her about new information that supported her position, and told her she had been right. He declared that he was going to try another approach to this problem, and Elaine could stay on her current project.

Of course, role plays by no means always lead to the hoped-for outcome, as in this instance. Even if they do not, the patient nonetheless gets a better sense of how he or she might behave in difficult situations. In the long run, friendly disclosure and effective listening with appropriate teaching and trusting behaviors represent optimal ways of handling problem situations. Their use will encourage everyone in the patient's system to function in the normative region of interpersonal space.

Self-Help Reading and Peer Groups

Self-help reading in behavioral therapy, as well as self-help peer groups (e.g., Alcoholics Anonymous) can be useful when the patient wants to practice self-management. Various books and other publications teach patients how to manage psychiatric symptoms. Examples include anxiety (White, 1995), binge-eating disorder (Carter & Fairburn, 1998), smoking (Sykes & Marks, 2001), and alcohol misuse (Humphreys & Moos, 2001). Another well-represented literature for self-help has to do with recovery from sexual abuse (e.g., Lynch, 2000). An overview of the entire self-help literature as of the early 1990s was prepared by Santrock, Minnett, and Campbell (1994). Increases since then in available self-help references and the implications for health care professionals have been noted by Norcross (2000, p. 370): "A massive, systemic, and yet largely silent revolution is occurring in mental health today and is gathering steam for tomorrow: self-help efforts without professional intervention. The self-help revolution traverses multiple disciplines and entails diverse activities." Norcross notes that self-help activities typically occur independently of professional treatment.

The self-help literature sometimes takes an adversarial position toward health care professionals, and vice versa (Lynch, 2000). An IRT therapist embraces self-help enthusiastically at step 5. The main caveat is to assure that the self-help activity is consistent with the case formulation. For example, suppose that the self-help book is about enhancing self-esteem, and the patient's maladaptive patterns stem from an addiction to receiving praise that originated with excessive adoration during childhood. In that case, it would be important for the therapist and patient to carefully consider which self-help strategies might appropriately strengthen self-esteem, and which might risk enhancing the problem patterns.

Giving Interpersonal and Intrapsychic Advice

Advice giving is usually forbidden in therapy, because it can easily violate the principle of enhancing the patient's personal strength; it risks enabling dependency instead. It also may be just plain foolish, since therapists are rarely experts outside their professional field. However, in IRT, advice giving is appropriate in specific interpersonal and intrapsychic contexts—including crisis management, as discussed in Chapter 7. Advice giving in crisis management is precipitated by a very Red plan that needs to be blocked and replaced with concrete alternatives. It is necessary when the patient seems to be in harm's way and is unlikely to take care of him- or herself.

For example, Candy had recently filed for divorce from her violent husband, and he was now threatening to kill her and the children. Candy was overwhelmed and distraught because he was demanding to see the children that night, and she feared for their safety. She said she would comply, however, because she did not want to offend him further. Such self-negating compliance was an old story for Candy. The therapist would probably encourage (advise) her to connect with the police and the battered woman's shelter, with the specific goal of helping her learn about options for assuring her immediate physical safety, as well as about legal methods for protecting herself and the children from harm. The resultant self-care would be consistent with therapy goal activities. The therapist's advice would provide a needed antidote to earlier experiences of neglect by parental figures in face of urgent need. In this plan, Candy's Red pattern of leaving herself in harm's way would be blocked (step 3) by the therapist's suggestion of specific alternative ways to engage in self-care (step 5).

Advice giving in IRT sometimes extends beyond crisis management, but it always conforms to the core algorithm. No matter what the context, advice giving is confined to commentary about interpersonal and intrapsychic patterns.[15] Every effort is made to give advice in a way that enhances the patient's Growth Collaborator (Green). Sometimes advice giving is subtle. For example, if a patient is uncertain about whether to implement his or her own new and sensible solution to a difficult interpersonal situation at step 5 of therapy, the therapist can say, in effect, "Sounds like a good plan to me."

For example, consider Vera, a dependent woman who had been tyrannized by her teenage son. She planned to tell him he could not have the car on Saturday night, because he had not done any of his reasonably assigned tasks around the house that week. Vera knew he would protest, yell, and try to intimidate her, just as her older brother had always done. But she was planning to insist that he do his work before she would allow him to take the car on a weekend. By affirming her intention to set limits and to break her habit of complying in reaction to intimidation, the therapist helped Vera stick to her desired new pattern of assertive, affirming parenting.

If, unlike Vera, a patient does not come up with a Green plan, the therapist may need to mobilize Green and then encourage constructive alternative behaviors. Suppose that Vera had not presented a plan for limit setting, and instead was lamenting her helplessness in relation to her son. A discussion about the origins of her meekness might engage her interest in no longer being trapped in the pattern. If she then decided to stop giving in to and enabling tyranny in her son, she could be encouraged to think of ways to hold her own—ones that would teach him reciprocity and respect for others, as well as provide better protection for herself. A class or book on parent training might help her find specific behaviors that would be helpful in managing this (or a comparable) situation. Therapist role playing would be another way to develop new behaviors.

The distinctive feature of advice giving in IRT is that recommendations focus extensively on interpersonal and intrapsychic process and are consistent with the case formulation (e.g., Vera's son was repeating her brother's tyranny). Such explicit support for Green is often needed and appreciated by the nonresponder population. At the same time, the conventional wisdom to avoid giving advice would be honored in IRT if the patient's Red outweighed the Green by too much. If that had been true for Vera, it might have been too risky for her to try limit setting with her son. Predominant Red might have led her to respond to her son's expected hostile reaction in old ways, followed by certainty that she was hopelessly inept.

Therapists accustomed to working with so-called higher-level patients may feel that such active blocking of a patient's preferred behaviors and development of unfamiliar alternatives demeans the patient. The distinction between Red and Green behaviors is the key to understanding when this activity is helpful and when it is not. Because nonresponders have been so devoted to their old rules and values for so long, their underdeveloped Green needs substantial assistance in getting permission for and help with building personal strength. Higher-level patients already have plenty of Green, so such a degree of therapist activity is not necessary at best and demeaning at worst.

To further develop the unfamiliar idea of interpersonal and intrapsychic advice giving during therapy, additional examples of recommendations that can support new learning are given here. These include advising a patient to call his or her physician for an appointment to treat a physical illness; to seek a second opinion in a difficult medical situation; or to seek a legal opinion. I once "cured" a self-negating woman of debilitating depression in a single session by referring her to a lawyer to check my belief that her errant husband would indeed need to share his retirement fund with her if her were to pursue his threat to divorce her after 50 years of marriage. She called back in a few days, no longer depressed: The lawyer had assured her that although she might have to deal with loneliness, she would not have to live in poverty.[16]

Coaching a Patient through a Current Challenge

Active coaching can help nonresponders develop constructive alternatives. For example, Ronald, a highly placed executive in an insurance company, came to therapy because of an unremitting depression. He effectiveness at work was enhanced by his ability to be nurturant, although he gave help in a patronizing manner. Ronald became depressed when people failed to comply with his suggestions. He also needed to be appreciated and would, for example, feel criticized if somebody offered to help him. He saw an offer to help as a challenge to his honesty and competence. Ronald would become withdrawn and morose when employees and peers failed to appreciate him.

After Ronald had been in IRT for almost a year, a crisis erupted between factions within the company. Ronald was on the side of current management. He felt deeply betrayed by the leader of the "revolution," whom Ronald had previously supported and protected. His close friend, the founder and president of the company, had not yet learned about the revolution. Ronald was trying to decide whether he should let the president know about it. The therapist supported this plan, noting that wise anticipatory discussion with the president about how to handle this problem would probably be a good idea from a strategic point of view. For purposes of therapy, the proactive stance would represent a constructive change from Ronald's more familiar depressive pattern of feeling unappreciated, betrayed, hurt, and victimized.

Ronald then rehearsed the ways he might work with the president to develop a plan for responding to the revolutionaries at an upcoming board meeting. The therapist did not comment on the business details, of course. Instead, the therapist coached the patient on how to maintain a position of active listening and friendly disclosure, instead of scolding and patronizing the colleagues and subordinates at the expected board meeting. This willingness on the therapist's part to take a clear position came from having a clear definition of normal behaviors that had been embraced as a therapy goals by the patient. Explicit focus on a patient's therapy goal behaviors is a major part of step 5 in IRT.

Helping with Children

In therapy sessions, it is common for patients to mention problems they are having with their children. Children matter a lot to most parents, and they also happen to be unusually potent triggers for old patterns and wishes. Nowhere are copy processes more apparent than in parenting behavior. Problems that are likely to be manifested when interacting with children are too much control, too much submission, inattention to their needs, blaming, and (in some cases) outright attack. Nonresponders will quickly see that they are doing to their children what their parents (or other care-takers) did to them. Alternatively, they may be reacting to their children as they reacted to their parents. After the will to change has been engaged, it can be particularly useful to refer such patients to parent training groups and/or the parent training literature. In addition, the IRT therapist can "walk them through" anticipated problem situations with children to get new patterns started, or to supplement the other training.

For example, Dorothy had repeatedly threatened to kill her stepfather, and so the stepfather kicked Dorothy out of the house. He refused to let her come back until she was able to prove she would not talk that way to him again. Melissa, her mother, felt helpless to do anything about it. She could only tell her daughter: "The two of you will have to work it out." Melissa herself had a kindly but entirely overwhelming mother who had decided, for example, what Melissa should wear every day throughout high school. Melissa had dealt with this by just giving in and doing what was expected. However, the submissive solution was not working now. Both her husband and her child had become overbearing. Melissa was intimidated, compliant, resentful, and frightened. Her despair escalated, and she had become nonfunctional for quite some time. Eventually she forced herself to take a new job and decided she needed to try therapy again. After several sessions in IRT, her depression lifted and she began to function better. She learned to speak up with her husband, and sometimes he responded favorably. But Melissa remained upset with him for kicking her daughter out of the house. She wanted to change that situation, but was unsure of how to proceed.

The IRT therapist suggested a role play that involved a future conversation with Dorothy about her relationship with her stepfather. Melissa agreed that saying: "The two of you will just have to work it out," might sound as if she did not care about Dorothy. Here is how the role play went:

MELISSA: (*Role-playing her daughter*) I want to be able to come back to the house.

THERAPIST: (*Role-playing Melissa*) I know. And I want you to come back, too. Let's see if we can figure out a way that will work.

MELISSA: (*As Dorothy*) Like what?

THERAPIST: (*As Melissa*) Well, he says he wants your promise you won't threaten to kill him.

MELISSA: (*As Dorothy*) He is a jerk. I hate him.

THERAPIST: (*As Melissa*) I know you are angry about how bossy he is. But you need to deal with that in a better way. So do I. For my part, I am working hard on learning to express my views so I have equal input to what goes on around here. And I want you home, so I am going to tell him that.

MELISSA: (*As Dorothy*) It's about time.

THERAPIST: (*As Melissa*) Yes, you are right. So let's agree that you will promise not to threaten him again, and that you will keep that promise. I'll be letting him know what I want and need, and that includes having you come home. I suggest we start with an evening or two together, and then, if that goes well, we can try a whole week. After that, if there have been no threats and shouting, then I expect he will agree you can move back in. I would like that very much. For the long term, we'll have to learn to discuss disagreements in a new way. I will try to make sure the rules are fair and agreed on by everybody. Still, it is really important that you do your part by not "losing it." Are you willing to try?

MELISSA: (*As Dorothy*) Maybe.

Here the therapist modeled a new pattern for Melissa. Note that the therapist was descriptive and remained focused on Melissa's way of relating to Dorothy. The therapist did not criticize the husband. For this role play to be successful, it was important that Melissa had already decided to "stop being a wimp," and had become more assertive on several lesser issues. She was a "quick study" and was loving enough that she could assert easily without becoming angry. Melissa began to use her newfound ability to speak up more consistently and was pleased with the results.

Resisting the Wish to Go Back to Old Ways

Helping the Patient Avoid Rejecting the Transplanted Self

The problem of self-sabotage in the face of success, discussed in Chapter 8, can carry over into this last phase of therapy. One patient, a nurse, spoke of herself as rejecting the new, transplanted self. She said, "I went to lunch yesterday, and we talked about how you have to change who you are in therapy. I understand the necessity of that, but it feels self-destructive. I guess it is. (*Cries*) I am killing off the old self."

Such grief over loss of Red hopes and values continues on through step 5, as new patterns clearly take their place in every day life. The IRT therapist is aware of this process, and explains that grief is normal when someone or something so familiar is gone. Normalizing the process in this appropriate way helps the patient sustain change and resist the wish to go back to the old self.

Providing Additional Help with New Learning

Sometimes patients' honesty about the pain of loss is poignant or even funny. The therapist's appreciation and understanding of this unexpected but welcome distress helps sustain the change. It may also be necessary to add helpful structure. Consider the case of June:

JUNE: When I was operating from a hostile position, I was not so troubled. Now my comfortable hostility is gone. I am confused about how to deal with people like my roommate now. And I also had trouble with my dentist this week. Things were so much easier when I could just be pissed off at people.

THERAPIST: You miss the old ways of coping and are unsure of what to do instead.

JUNE: Yes. Absolutely.

June then described the problems with the dentist and the roommate. The therapist listened to and affirmed the story about the dentist, because her behavior there was consistent with therapy goals. However, with the room-mate, June had not yet tried the very first step in dispute resolution—namely, to disclose her feelings in a friendly way. A brief role play set the pattern. Subsequently, June's practice of friendly assertiveness led to a solution of that problem.

Staying Out of the Way When the Problem Is Existential

Toward the end of IRT, increasing numbers of existential problems will arise because of changes that naturally flow from behaving differently. It is important that the therapist recognize these as normative and stay out of the way as the patient struggles to deal with them. The rule is this: So long as decisions are not being driven by the identified problems in the case formulation, and so long as the new behavior patterns are consistent with therapy goals, the IRT therapist "lightens up" and becomes primarily supportive. At this time, the therapist functions mostly as a "secure base" from which the patient ventures into the unknown. The therapist characteristics described so well by Rogers (1951)—empathy, positive regard, and congruence—predominate in this situation. Here is an example:

Susan, who had been very self critical and compliant with others, decided to take a better job in a new city. Even though her daughter, Lynn, was away at college, she did not want her mother to move. Lynn wanted her mother to stay in the city where she had grown up.

SUSAN: Lynn is critical of the idea of my moving. Talking with her, I lapsed into negativism about me. But I was real aware of it. Lynn is ambivalent, really. She does want me to go and be happy. It's just that she likes it here and wants to be able to come back. This has been her only home. This time, while hearing how unhappy she is with me, I was more relaxed, not frantic.

THERAPIST: Lynn likes it that you are taking care of yourself, but she finds it is hard for her personally.

SUSAN: Yes. But I know she will be OK with it.

THERAPIST: So your moving is some kind of marker of change for everybody. It makes it clear there are big life changes now for both of you.

SUSAN: Yes, it really is.

MOVING TOWARD TERMINATION

When Is Reconstruction "Complete"?

Some patients ask, "How will I know when I am done?" The learning speech (Table 2.5) provides a version of a good answer. It really is not possible to say when any learning process is "finished." Because of the expense of therapy, and because IRT is so focused on problem patterns, patients usually do not "hang around" when the problem patterns are no longer an issue. If they do not spontaneously want to terminate, their ambivalence about independence probably needs more work. In addition, it may again be very important to check on *Klute* syndrome practices, discussed in Chapter 8. Ideally, IRT terminates naturally and is not forced by finances, geography, inadequate funding, family politics, and so on. In those cases, the "How will I know?" question can be answered this way:

> "Therapy is like sleeping. When you are tired and you need sleep, it is one of your most important concerns. When you are not tired, you don't want to sleep. So when you are psychologically renewed, you will not be nearly so interested in therapy, and you will be comfortable about stopping."

Given the importance of the therapy relationship in IRT, and given patients' frequent histories of familial neglect and abandonment, it is natural that some nonresponders worry a lot about termination. Many are quite open about this worry. For example, after making tremendous strides during her first year of treatment, Judy said:

JUDY: I am worried about the fact I am so much better. When I have been in therapy before, getting better meant I got kicked out. And I don't feel done at all.

THERAPIST: I agree you still can benefit from therapy, even though you are no longer so desperately depressed, and your voices are quiet. I think therapy is like any other learning process. It is hard to say when you have learned all you need to learn. In fact, I hope you never stop learning! Still, there will come a time when you are really finished with the old ways, and your new social learning is solid enough that you will want to continue it on your own. I agree with you that we are not there yet!

Consolidating Gains

In the later stages of step 5, many IRT patients suggest meeting less frequently. They may ask to switch from once a week to once a month. After a few of those monthly checkups, they become ready to terminate altogether. During these final meetings, the aims are mostly to consolidate gains and mark issues where the patient may need to be especially watchful.

Polly illustrated that process as she tapered her sessions to once a month, following 2 years of IRT. She had been severely abused physically and emotionally by both parents. A part of her treatment had included listening to an extraordinarily cruel tape-recorded family conference that had taken place at the beginning of therapy. The tape provided *in vivo* evidence that Polly was another case of an abused child's becoming the parent of the parents. In the family conference, she ignored their assaults, and expressed her views with clarity and dignity as she tried to reconcile with them on friendly terms.[17] Unfortunately, her parents continued with a long list of accusations. During the therapy that followed, she was able to take their condemnations less literally, and began to take better care of herself. Here is a segment from one of her last checkups before termination.

POLLY: I am not anxious or worried about lapsing or regressing. I am not even anxious about being alone.

THERAPIST: It sounds like you are ready to finish your work here.

POLLY: Yeah. I am. I have been mindful to not do it abruptly. I am still working on the drinking issue. That is the one thing I need to keep watching.[18]

THERAPIST: Would you say a breakthrough with drinking was realizing it was being just like your parents?

POLLY: Absolutely. That was huge. Actually, it goes back several generations. And it's the same thing with the vicious self-criticism.

THERAPIST: You realized that your big problem with self-esteem was based on your parents' critical words?

POLLY: Yes. At a deep level. I see that the way to love my mother was to yell at somebody else the way she yelled at me. I don't do that any more.

Polly understood her case formulation well. With the support of the therapy relationship, she successfully realized the therapy goals.

Green Goodbye When IRT Is Terminated Prematurely by the Therapist

Sometimes IRT is interrupted, especially in institutional settings where therapists rotate through a service and cannot be available for a long-term commitment. Ideally, the patient continues with a new therapist who is familiar with the IRT approach. It is extremely helpful if the patient can have one to three sessions jointly with the old and the new therapists. During the transition meetings, the case formulation and progress to date are reviewed with the new therapist. Current problem issues are marked for immediate attention. Points of vulnerability and methods of coping with them are noted.

To maintain progress, it can be very helpful to agree on a list of "code words" that will remind the patient of connections between particular patterns and IPIRs, and of the countermoves that have been developed as antidotes. For example, suppose a female patient has learned that she gets in big trouble because she scolds her friends just as her mother scolded her for failing to read her mind and meet her needs. The patient can develop key words that help her remember to be more moderate in her expectations and reactions. In turn, this will reduce the likelihood of bitter disappointment, recriminations, alienation, loneliness, and depression. Code words for this scenario might be "Express well rather than expect much." After the task is clearly understood, patients will choose whatever language has deep meaning for them. That language can provide the new therapist and patient with a clear "handle" they can use to connect the new therapy to the previous one as they continue the progress. These efforts to consolidate gains and continue the learning are called a "Green goodbye."

"I Do Like What I Have Become": Patients' Reflections on Termination

During the last step of therapy, patients will spontaneously reflect on their changed condition. Here are examples of things that patients have said as they approach termination of therapy:

- "I do like what I have become."
- "Last night I decided to have fun and please myself, not others. Wow! It was so fun I might make it a regular habit."
- "I am so much less tortured than I was 2 years ago. I see no reason to be tortured now just because he needs me to be. I am a reasonable and good person."
- "I am more detached and yet more accepting of myself. I certainly am less concerned with whether I am liked by everybody. The other day, I let a man know in a nonconfrontational way that I do not like to be ordered around. I reacted very differently in that situation than I would have 2 years ago. I would not have had the needed presence of mind as recently as a year ago. In the last month, some gains are really coming together."

CONCLUSION

With the therapy goals so clearly defined, and the methods of reaching toward them so precisely described, IRT therapists are fully equipped to help nonresponders engage effectively with the challenges they face. Patients sensibly understand and accept that successful IRT does not lead to guaranteed happiness. Rather, it helps people develop the skills to be free of old burdens and to cope with life's challenges in positive, well-modulated ways. Their awareness gives them new choices that can bring them greater comfort and increased satisfaction in love and work.

NOTES

1. This baseline has been defined by the Structural Analysis of Social Behavior (SASB) model and discussed in Chapter 4. See also Chapters 2 and 5.
2. For example, if physically threatened, the patient may choose to try to control the aggressor, escape altogether, or (if necessary) fight back.
3. Described by BLAME in the SASB cluster model, **Condemn** in the parallel affect model, and **Scorn** in the parallel cognitive model.
4. For example, the patient is moving to another city soon.
5. For example, SASB codes of therapy process that establish baseline friendliness and moderate degrees of enmeshment and differentiation.
6. The reader is reminded this sequence is only approximate. Steps overlap, and there often is movement back and forth among them.
7. Mabel was slated for a transfer to a new branch of the company.
8. SASB-coded as AFFIRM. Many patients are very interested to see that these skills are the exact opposite of BLAME, the pattern they know best.
9. Three types of interpersonal focus are defined in Chapter 4.
10. To the contrary, the SASB model classifies ASSERT and **CONTROL** as antitheses.

11. Content coded <u>SEPARATE</u>.
12. Indirect process coded **PROTECT**.
13. Indirect process coded **BLAME**.
14. Readers familiar with the SASB model will recognize how clearly and simply this speech touches on key interpersonal positions.
15. In other words, all components of the advice are SASB-codable. For example, the advice to Candy would help her learn to <u>SEPARATE</u> from oppression, to ask appropriately for help (<u>TRUST</u>), and to *SELF-PROTECT*. It would also be focused on Candy and would not relate to justice or punishment in relation to the husband.
16. In terms of SASB codes, the therapist would be engaging in **PROTECT** in all the examples given in this paragraph. The intended result would be internalization of that behavior as *SELF-PROTECT*.
17. Some readers might object that she should have been encouraged to express her anger, and the parents should have been confronted. Previous discussions of the cathartic and the justice models explain why that was not done here. Instead, there was an honest and benevolent attempt to come to better understanding and to improve family relationships. The parents were unwilling or unable to take advantage of the opportunity. They were more interested in their version of justice (condemning and shaping their child to taste) than in reconciliation and healing.
18. Polly was allowed to continue in IRT despite her drinking problem, because she was very open about it and clearly struggled to curb it. Alcohol was not her preferred coping mechanism. Her collaboration and learning curve were promising enough that it seemed unnecessary to insist on total abstinence. IRT policy about drugs and alcohol was discussed in Chapter 5.

10

Interpersonal Reconstructive Therapy in Clinical and Research Contexts

The main thesis of this book is that so-called nonresponders can become capable of change if the treatment consistently focuses on the underlying motivations for the presenting interpersonal and intrapsychic problems. To explain how to do that, Chapters 1–4 have described the basic principles of Interpersonal Reconstructive Therapy (IRT). Chapters 5–9 have provided detail about how to use these principles when implementing the five recommended therapy steps.

A brief review of the IRT principles appears below, followed by a comparison of IRT to main features of some widely used therapy approaches. The chapter closes with remarks on selected topics, including comments on IRT's potential status as a clinical science and suggestions for how to begin to practice IRT.

A BRIEF SUMMARY OF IRT PRINCIPLES

The Developmental Learning and Loving Theory

The Developmental Learning and Loving (DLL) theory of psychopathology describes the underlying motivations that organize and support the problems to be treated. More specifically, DLL theory proposes that each presenting interpersonal problem is linked to relationships with early caregivers by one or more of three basic copy processes: (1) "Be like him or her" (identification); (2) "Act as if he or she is still there and in control" (recapitulation); and (3) "Treat yourself as he or she treated you" (introjection). The presumed motivation for copy processes is to implement the rules and values of the persons being copied, Important Persons and their Internalized Representations (IPIRs), in order to provide testimony to their beliefs. The hope is that such loyalty will create psychic proximity to and facilitate psychic reconciliation with the IPIRs. Every psychopathology is a gift of love.

Throughout IRT, it is helpful to think of the patient as, in effect, two people. The part that comes to therapy and hopes to function and feel better is called the Growth Collaborator or the Green. The part of the person that wants to remain loyal to old ways is called the Regressive Loyalist, or the Red. The conflict between the Green and the Red is ever present, and is described so clearly that patients understand it at the beginning of treatment. Early in therapy, the Red overshadows the Green. By termination, the Green prevails.

The IRT Goals

The treatment implication of the gift-of-love hypothesis is that the impossible wishes that support the quest for psychic proximity to the IPIRs must be recognized, grieved for, and given up. Then reconstruction of personality can begin. The overall goal of IRT is for a patient to function from a baseline of friendliness with moderate degrees of enmeshment and of differentiation.[1] Hostility and extreme degrees of enmeshment (control or submission) or differentiation (invoking or taking distance) can be observed in normal people in special contexts. However, if present as a baseline, these positions mark psychopathology. The healthy patterns of relationship (friendliness, with moderation in enmeshment and differentiation) are associated with affects that are generally pleasant, and with cognitive styles that are highly functional.[2] These goals are not relativistic, and therefore IRT is inappropriate for use within any culture that advocates baseline function outside of the domain defined as normal by DLL theory. For example, IRT would not be appropriate for members of a culture that gives priority to a lifestyle of revenge over the goals of friendliness and of moderation in enmeshment and differentiation.[3]

The Core Algorithm as the Basis for Every Intervention

Interventions from any and all schools of therapy may be used in IRT. The core algorithm provides the basis for choice of an intervention at any point in time. The core algorithm consists of six rules or guidelines: (1) Accurate empathy should be apparent at all times. (2) An intervention should attempt to support the Growth Collaborator (Green) more than the Regressive Loyalist (Red). (3) Every intervention should clearly relate to the case formulation. (4) The therapy narrative should consistently develop episodes that involve patterns related to the presenting problems, and each discussion of each episode should incorporate concrete detail about input, response, and impact on self. (5) Each episode should be examined in terms of the ABCs (affect, behavior, and cognition). (6) Each intervention should implement one or more of the five therapy steps. These five steps are as follows: (1) collaboration; (2) learning what the patterns are, where they are from, and what they are for; (3) blocking maladaptive patterns; (4) enabling the will to change; and (5) learning new patterns.

Within each therapy step, therapy techniques are classified into two subgroups, depending on whether they facilitate self-discovery or self-management. In general, techniques from client centered and psychodynamic therapies are more likely to encourage self-discovery through experiencing current and uncovered feelings and thoughts about the self and other people. Techniques from behavioral therapies are more likely to invoke self-management techniques through learning and practicing skills such as self-talk or assertiveness. Both self-discovery and self-management activities are needed in IRT.

The Key to Progress: Transformation of the Gift of Love

In its analysis of what needs to be changed, IRT combines fundamental principles from attachment theory with behavior theory. From behavior theory comes the idea that what works is likely to be repeated. Attachment theory provides the definition of what "works" in IRT. Psychic proximity to Important Persons' Internalized Representations (IPIRs) is believed to be the main "reward" for behavior patterns that otherwise seem to be "maladaptive." Hence the key question as to whether there can be progress in reconstruction will center on an assessment of the patient's relationships with the problem IPIRs. Once the loyalty to the IPIRs is transformed, the patient is free to learn new patterns that comprise the therapy goals.

This emphasis on the central role of attachment demotes the role of traditional "drivers" of the psyche, such as anger, rage, power, or superiority. Although these human traits are very much a part of IRT, they are not considered to be the primary targets of intervention. This difference between IRTs and other approaches' views of primary motivators has many treatment implications.[4]

RELATION TO OTHER THERAPY APPROACHES

Although IRT provides that interventions can come from any school of therapy, client-centered, psychodynamic, and behavioral therapies have had the most influence on the IRT approach to nonresponders. IRT's relationship to these three perspectives, as well as others, is described below.

Client-Centered Therapy

Client-centered therapy (Rogers, 1951) emphasizes the need for the thera-pist to show empathy, positive regard, and congruence.[5] Empathy and pos-itive regard are essential to the therapy alliance in IRT and are characteris-tic of most psychotherapies, including those that are psychodynamically oriented. Maintaining empathy is the first component of the core algo-rithm, and keeping collaboration intact is the first of the five IRT steps. Maintaining positive regard for the patient's Green is a constant feature of IRT process. Finally, IRT therapists are relatively active and engage in self-disclosure, provided that it is consistent with the case formulation and the core algorithm. This feature means that therapist congruence is apparent to patients in IRT.

Psychodynamic Therapies

Psychodynamic therapies draw explicitly from principles of psychoanaly-sis. The *American Heritage Talking Dictionary* (1997) provides several definitions for the word "dynamic." The most relevant are these: "1. An interactive system or process, especially one involving competing or con-flicting forces: 'the story of a malign dynamic between white prejudice and black autonomy' (Edmund S. Morgan). 2. A force, especially political, so-cial, or psychological: the main dynamic behind the revolution." The defi-nitions note the presence of conflict and of an underlying force that shapes a process, respectively.

In the original version of psychoanalysis, the basic dynamic forces were said to be the id, the ego, and the superego. According to classical drive theory, conflict among these forces shapes the personality. The under-lying problem motivations are sexuality and/or anger, which are disap-proved of by the superego. The therapy process brings this conflict to awareness (i.e., to the attention of the ego). After "working through" the conflict, the patient becomes a conflict-free, healthy person (e.g., Green-berg & Mitchell, 1983, p. 390). Newer versions of psychoanalysis are less concerned with the conflict among the id, ego, and superego; they focus more on object relations. IRT, also object-relations-oriented, owes most to Sullivan's (1953) interpersonal psychiatry, but it has much in common with the ideas of other important object relations theorists, such as Kernberg (2001).[6]

IRT theory holds that there is conflict between the Regressive Loyalist (Red) and the Growth Collaborator (Green). Figures 1.1 and 9.1 make it clear that this conflict is present at every step in therapy. The treatment approach seeks to resolve this conflict by enhancing the Green and dimin-ishing the Red. Red is diminished primarily by interventions that help reduce the wishes underlying the Red patterns. As the relevant IPIRs are reconsidered, the patient becomes better able to resist the Red side of the conflict, and more reliably choose Green solutions. Green is enhanced primarily by well-known techniques for learning new and more adaptive behaviors.

Because the DLL theory of psychopathology that guides the choice of interventions in IRT addresses the impact of social learning, IRT shares with psychodynamic therapies an interest in talking about the past. In IRT, the main reason for talking about the past is to change motivation. A review of the past that identifies patterns, where they came from, and what they are for can contribute significantly to the task of enabling the will to change. Many of the psychodynamic techniques designed to facilitate recall of the past have been reviewed in Chapter 6. Examples are free association, dream analysis, and simple recall. Gestalt therapy, a derivative of psychoanalysis, has contributed a particularly useful technique for revisiting the past in the light of the Red–Green conflict. In the two-chair technique, a patient "recreates" various members of the family in one chair and reacts to them in another. These activities are most adherent to IRT when the two chairs represent the Red and the Green. By enacting the Red and reacting to it with Green,[7] the patient directly works on better seeing the motivation for presenting problems and on developing constructive alternative behaviors.

Because IRT draws so heavily on the psychodynamic perspective, it may be appropriate to explain how a few illustrative well-known terms from psychoanalysis can be understood within IRT. Menninger (1958) offered a wonderfully succinct summary of basic psychoanalytic therapy principles. More recent, clear, and brief descriptions are available in Greenberg and Mitchell (1983). Useful clinical detail is offered by Thoma and Kachele (1987). Finally, N. E. Miller, Luborsky, Barber, and Docherty (1993) provide important reviews of comparatively credible research studies on basic psychoanalytic therapy concepts.

Transference

According to psychoanalysis, transference refers to the patient's feelings and views about the therapist, which are likely to be distorted because unresolved early conflict has been projected onto the (neutral) therapist. In IRT, the therapist is very active and sometimes self-discloses; therefore, it is not reasonable to suggest that the patient's view of the IRT therapist is necessarily "distorted." In IRT, the patient's view of the therapist will be partly determined by his or her past learning, and partly based on actual experience with the therapist. Hence, in IRT, transference simply refers to the patient's view of the therapy relationship, whether distorted or not. "Transference distortion" specifically means that the patient's view of the therapist is distorted in a way that relates to the case formulation.

Countertransference

Countertransference refers to the therapist's personal feelings about the patient. Early in the history of psychoanalysis, countertransference was supposed to be minimal. If negative, countertransference was an indication that the therapist needed further analysis him- or herself (Fenichel, 1945, p. 580). In contemporary psychoanalysis, a therapist's reaction to the patient, even if hostile, is thought to comprise valuable information about the patient (Greenberg & Mitchell, 1983, pp. 388–389), and therefore can become part of the therapy dialogue. For example, sometimes a therapist using this model tells a patient, "I am feeling angry with you."

In IRT, it does not matter if the therapist's feelings about the patient come from the therapist's history, provided that the impact of those feelings on the therapy process is consistent with the case formulation In fact, if the therapist has recovered from early injuries, he or she may be more rather than less skilled in helping others with those problems. Suppose, for example, that a therapist had to cope with living with a schizophrenic parent. Naturally, there would be injuries from those experiences. However, once the damage has been healed, the skills that enabled survival with the schizophrenic parent can be very handy when the therapist is trying to "read" complicated patients and help them find their way out of their difficulties.

Although a therapist's feelings about the patient are not considered a primary source of data about the patient in IRT, they can provide valuable information simply because of the interactive nature of IRT theory and practice. The connection between the therapist's feelings and the patient him- or herself is likely to be detailed by the predictive principles (especially complementarity) in the SASB model. Hence the therapist's historically based feelings theoretically provide a guide to what is going on if the therapist has been unable to detect it by attending to the therapy process and narrative.[8] Even so, the IRT therapist is unlikely to announce simply that he or she is feeling angry with the patient, and expect the patient to learn from that intervention. In rare situations, the IRT therapist may express anger at the Red, but never simply at "the patient." Too often, a therapist's anger is on behalf of his or her own need to control or to distance from the patient. That should not become the patient's problem. Instead, the IRT therapist does better to appeal to the core algorithm to deal directly with whatever is triggering the anger, and to remain a focused, centered, and consistently friendly advocate for the patient's Green.

In sum, since IRT requires that the focus be primarily on the patient, the therapist's feelings about the patient are not usually considered relevant per se. On the other hand, self-disclosure—which need not, but can include feelings about the patient—is acceptable in IRT so long as it is consistent with the case formulation. Countertransference distortion is defined by instances wherein the therapist's views and feelings interfere with implementation of the core algorithm. An example of countertransference distortion is a therapist's inability or unwillingness to explore a given important concern with a patient because of personal distaste for or fear of the subject that needs to be discussed.

Interpretation

Interpretation in classical psychoanalysis is an effort to help the patient "objectify, visualize and understand the meaning of the place of various bits of his behavior, emotion, memory, fantasy, and experience" (Menninger, 1958, p. 129). It is given rarely and is likely to point to "the existence or possible existence of connections and implications and meanings which tend to elude the patient. He [the analyst] reminds the patient of forgotten statements or he confronts him with a discrepancy or self-contradiction, a misrepresentation, an obvious but unrecognized omission" (Menninger, 1958, p. 128). The object relations versions of psychoanalysis also propose that an interpretation conveys information of this sort, but they add the dimension of therapy process: "A correct interpretation implies a deep and empathic form of relatedness. A deep and empathic engagement of the patient by the analyst communicates information—about the patient, about the analyst, or about their interaction" (Greenberg & Mitchell, 1983, p. 392).

An IRT therapist engages in interpretation if he or she collaboratively introduces the case formulation into a discussion of a current problem pattern. That pattern may be anchored in past, present, or future; in experienced reality or fantasy; and/or in therapy narrative or process. Both insight (Chapter 6) and the therapist–patient relationship (Chapter 5) are central to interpretations and other interventions in IRT.

Resistance

"Resistance as it is used in psychoanalytic theory may be defined as the trend of forces within the patient which oppose the process of ameliorative change. It is not the analyst who is being resisted; it is the process within the patient which the analyst is encouraging" (Menninger, 1958, p. 104). Object relations analysts think of resistance in diverse ways. The view that is closest to IRT comes from Fairbairn, who viewed resistance in terms of devotion to "bad objects." IPIRs are the "bad objects" in IRT, although it would be more accurate consistently to call them "good–bad objects." Red is an IRT code word for the constellation of problem attachments to IPIRs and the associated problem behaviors. Fairbairn provided a clear description of this proposed basis of resistance:

The actual overcoming of repression as such would, accordingly, appear to constitute if anything a less formidable part of the analyst's difficult task than the overcoming of the patient's devotion to his repressed objects—a devotion which is all the more difficult to overcome because these objects are bad and he is afraid of their release from the unconscious. (Fairbairn, 1943/1996, p. 73)

In IRT, resistance reflects domination of the therapy by the Red. It is manifested when a patient who has already agreed with and understood the case formulation objects to a collaborative attempt to apply the formulation to a current problem. Resistance is treated with the procedures summarized in Figure 3.3, and discussed in detail in Chapter 7.

Regression

Regression is at the core of psychoanalytic treatment. Menninger (1958) notes that psychoanalysis induces regression by a process that leads

to the denudation of the original wish to be cured and its replacement with more primitive, buried wishes and the employment of techniques that once applied to expectations of other kinds from other persons for whom the therapist is substituted. With this regressive trend go fluctuations and variations in the "I" concept, or self estimate, including body image and ego-ideal. This regression proceeds in waves and cycles of alternating attitudes, with frequent "surfacing" and realigning. By maintaining a steady position of no reaction and an optimum degree of frustration, the therapist assists the process of self visualization, objectification, and stabilization which represent aspects of the self knowledge enabling an abandonment of the regressive position and progressive return to "health." (pp. 43–44)

In other words, with all social rules suspended, the patient lets go and talks about early feelings and views. As these are stirred up and the analyst says nothing to "get in the way," the patient is likely to project those early feelings and views onto the analyst (transference projection). He or she then behaves in a regressive (i.e., more appropriate to earlier times) manner. As the analysis proceeds, the patient "works through" these uncovered feelings and views, and eventually lets go of them and returns to health. An IRT perspective on this view would be that the patient projects Red expectations onto the blank screen therapist, making the therapist resemble an IPIR. Given that the therapist is nothing like the IPIR, the patient discovers his or her distortions and reconsiders his or her responses. This learning generalizes to other situations.

The expected process of immersing oneself in earlier ways of being is probably the basis of the popular warnings given in many psychodynamically oriented therapies: "Things will get worse before they get better."[9] Object relations psychoanalysts, who disagree with each other as well as with classical psychoanalysts, have varying views of regression. Their explanations tend to be technical and to draw heavily on underlying assumptions that are difficult to test. Winnicott, for example, suggested that regression "is not a return to points of libidinal fixation or specific erotogenic zones. Regression represents a return to the point at which the environment has failed the child" (Greenberg & Mitchell, 1983, p. 200).

In IRT, regression is defined relative to the patient's highest level of functioning in the preceding year, which is a moving target. If, for example, a patient improves early in therapy relative to the year preceding therapy, and then goes back to old ways a year after therapy starts, the patient is considered regressed even if he or she is no worse than when therapy started. Regression is identified when problem patterns appears in a situation wherein the patient has previously demonstrated the ability to behave in a more adaptive manner; in other words, it reflects increased salience of Red in the given situation. It is treated with procedures summarized in Figures 3.2, 3.3, and 3.4, and discussed in detail in Chapter 7. If an individual has never progressed beyond a developmental level appropriate to early childhood, he or she is not considered "regressed," because there has been no retreat from an earlier higher level. If labels are needed, such a person may be labeled developmentally arrested.

Behavioral and Cognitive-Behavioral Therapies

Thorndike (see Boring, 1950, pp. 562–563), who studied trial-and-error learning in cats, focused particularly on the effects of success, which "stamps in" the movements that were the cause of it. He noted that if the sequence a cat used to solve a laboratory problem occurred repeatedly ("was exercised"), it would occur more readily thereafter. Skinner incorporated this fundamental principle of learning in his model for operant conditioning, and it is central to modern-day behavior therapy. The main idea is this: What works is likely to be repeated. The technical way of saying it is that a positive reinforcer increases the probability of the behaviors that led to it. For example, if a laboratory monkey gets a grape when it picks a triangle instead of a square in a learning task, the monkey is more likely to pick triangles. The grape therefore is a positive reinforcer. Many writers with a behavioral orientation have applied this idea to clinical process. A contemporary review of the history of behaviorism, and a useful discussion of its current clinical applications, appears in Goldfried and Davison (1994).

Reinforcement and the Operant Model

The IRT version of the fundamental principle of learning begins with the DLL proposal that the perceived (implied) approval of an IPIR serves as positive reinforcement for problem behaviors, affects, and cognitions. As therapy progresses, the internalizations of the therapist and other helpful persons in the patient's world provide positive reinforcement for the desired new goal behaviors. These versions of positive reinforcement invoke a "mental" version[10] of Skinner's operant or instrumental conditioning model of behavior therapy (Delprato & Midgley, 1992).

The operant model also specifies that a negative reinforcement decreases the frequency of responses leading to it. For example, the IRT therapist reliably discourages chronic crisis behaviors by meeting them with diminished, rather than intensified, therapy work. Hospitalization does not yield more comfortable time with the therapist. Instead, it sends the patient into the world of symptom management (see Figure 3.4 and Chapter 7).

Likewise, crisis behaviors are negatively reinforced in IRT outpatient work. If a patient has engaged in self-cutting, the entire episode has to be reviewed in great detail and linked to a problem IPIR. This therapy activity tends to decrease the incidence of such behaviors, because the type of attention it elicits is not supportive of the original motivation—namely, providing testimony to and enjoying the psychic proximity of the abusing IPIR. The IRT therapist and current significant others do not ignore such serious behaviors; at the same time, they do not get drawn into the implicit invitation to "replace" the IPIR and/or to do battle with the IPIR over "possession" of the patient. In IRT, the actual impact of the self-cutting action is not at all as typically planned and reflected in such movies as *Sunset Boulevard* (1950) or *Fatal Attraction* (1987; see also Benjamin, 1996a, Ch. 5). In each film, the woman who cuts herself takes center stage, and her (abandoning) nurturer/protector is brought to heel.[11]

Negative reinforcement is not the same as punishment. There is controversy within the behavioral literature over what actually defines punishment, and whether it is ever appropriate (Griffin, Paisey, Stark, & Emerson, 1988). Given that retributive justice is not consistent with rehabilitative efforts in IRT, there is no further discussion of punishment here.

The Pavlovian or Classical Conditioning Model

An alternative learning model, the Pavlovian or classical conditioning model, is also used by behavioral therapists for such procedures as desensitization, hierarchical conditioning, and so on (Wolpe & Plaud, 1997). Those procedures are also imported to IRT when they are consistent with the case formulation.

For example, suppose a patient has public speaking anxiety. The IRT therapist does not hesitate to treat such a clearly defined presenting complaint with the brief and sometimes effective desensitization procedures so well described by Wolpe and others. However, many nonresponders have already had no success with such symptom-oriented short-term approaches.

If that is the case, then interventions may be better chosen in relation to the DLL case formulation. Perhaps the IRT therapist will discover that the patient imagines the audience is packed with replicas of his or her critical and violent stepfather. Appreciating the connection between anxiety and the imagined words of the IPIR can quickly help the patient become more responsive to the desensitization procedure. Alternatively, the patient's dread may be relieved if he or she constructs a role play giving the speech, but in the therapy fantasy, digresses to tell the stepfather that he was just a coward who picked on little kids to make his own inadequacies seem smaller. The patient is sick of being intimidated by that, and so the stepfather can "take a hike to you know where."[12] This sort of exercise creates different self-talk that can counter the anxiety the patient feels when actually giving a speech.

Whether or not these short-term techniques are used to try to get immediate relief from the specific symptom of public speaking anxiety, the lengthier process of coming to terms (Figure 3.2) with the problem IPIRs (Chapter 8) will provide relief even if there has not been any particular technical focus on the anxiety. The anxiety disappears because after the patient has come to terms, the IPIR can no longer reward the problem behavior.

Extinction

Extinction refers to the weakening of the association between the positive (or negative) reinforcer and the response in question. When a response has been extinguished, it no longer is displayed in the original context.

Suppose a female patient has road rage whenever a female driver in a fine car and fancy hairdo causes her to slow down or wait. In IRT, it is likely that the patient will discover a link to an IPIR such as the following: The patient's mother was devoted to and compliant with the role of wife and parent, and was completely miserable in it. Nonetheless, the mother demanded that the patient, her oldest daughter, pursue the same destiny. Now the patient knows that the women who elicit her road rage mean more to her than just "offensive" politics and lifestyle. These drivers activate memories of her mother's misery and her apparent insistence that the patient share her mother's dismal destiny. The patient's rage when such women move slowly in traffic ahead of her now is understood as an effort to distance herself from all that they remind her of. Once the patient has come to terms with her relationship with her mother, the road rage will have extinguished. When she is in a state of friendly differentiation from and perhaps even feeling compassion for her mother, the patient will no longer have to deal with the conflict between her attachment to her mother and her terror of becoming like her.

Stimulus Generalization

Learning theorists note that connections learned in one situation are likely to spread to another. Transference of views and feelings about parents or influential others to the therapist is a frequently occurring example of stimulus generalization. For example, the learning may have been this: "People in authority will try to control every single minute of your day, and most of their plans for you do not take your perspective into account. The best way to deal with this is to say yes when you mean no" (see Benjamin, 1996a, Ch. 11, for further detail on this pattern). The generalization to therapy is this: "The therapist will try to take over your life with a lot of dumb and probably harmful suggestions. Agree to the therapy plan, but die before you carry it out."

Stimulus Discrimination

Most definitions of learning provide that in addition to developing new links between a specific stimulus and a specific response, inappropriate generalization is minimized. In therapy, the patient learns about links between early experience and current problems, and also learns how to tell the difference between the current people (e.g., the therapist) and earlier important figures. The therapist avoids acting like problem IPIRs and tries to facilitate corrective learning. For example, if the IPIRs were very bossy, the therapist is cautious about engaging in any behaviors suggestive of control. By contrast, if IPIRs were neglectful, the IRT therapist is more likely to provide helpful structure, and this is a form of moderate control. If the IPIRs adored the patient and expected incredible feats, the IRT therapist is likely to provide remarks that relieve the patient of the burden of having to be admirable—for example,

> "What you are saying is truly impressive, but I have the feeling that today you are working hard on affecting what I think about you. I do think you have a lot of wonderful abilities, but I also don't see how telling me about it is helping you become more comfortable in your own skin. To do that, can we work more on what you feel about yourself in [here the therapist mentions a current issue that has probably set off this pattern]?"

In short, the therapist encourages stimulus discrimination as he or she implements the core algorithm in whatever way is appropriate at the moment. There are many different ways to implement the core algorithm successfully at any point in therapy. In the example just given, the therapist might instead ask the patient to say how he or she is feeling about his or her relationship with the therapist today, and then track back to the pattern with the early IPIR and how that felt. Probably the first version, with emphasis on self-definition, would come later in therapy (step 3, 4, or 5), whereas this second version would come earlier to facilitate learning about patterns (step 2).

Family, Couple, and Systems Therapies

Conferences with the Family of Origin

Addressing IPIRs is central to IRT. Because important others are typically family members, family therapy can be an important resource. In this book, discussion of the contribution of family therapy is restricted to the use of the occasional conference for two clearly defined purposes:

1. *Establishing new rules of relating to IPIRs that are consistent with the goals of IRT.* This purpose is rarely achieved, but not impossible. One barrier to this kind of success, mentioned earlier, is that even if the actual person has changed, the internalized representation may not have changed. If and when the family conference actually can change a driving internalization in the desired direction, the therapy can be very brief.

2. *Approaching the family in a collaborative way, and tape-recording what unfolds from there.* This procedure will produce an *in vivo* sample of the patterns and purposes confronted by the patient. Later review of the tape typically provides a powerful boost to step 2 (learning about patterns, where they are from, and what they are for). It can also enhance progress in step 4 (enabling the will to change). This particular use of a family intervention, discussed in Chapter 8, is often powerful even if the replay of the "same old, same old" seems discouraging during the conference itself.

Fantasy Family Conferences

A related alternative is to make a videotape of the patient role-playing the various family members, taking a different chair for each. The patient views and discusses the tape with the therapist in subsequent sessions. Acting out the templates for the IPIRs, and then discussing them with the support of the therapist, can be amazingly effective. Exposition of these procedures (plus the range of many other possibilities for family therapy) is deferred for elsewhere.

Couple Therapy

The couple forum can also be helpful in IRT. If a loving partner is willing to come and work toward the two-circle model of relationship presented in Figure 4.4, IRT can be accelerated. Complementarity theory usually correctly predicts that the patient will have selected a partner who matches and enables his or her own problem patterns. If a loved one stops offering behaviors that complement or otherwise enable problem patterns, their likelihood diminishes. Moreover, mutual commitment in couple therapy to friendly baselines with moderate enmeshment and moderate differentiation can help participants become more willing to learn new ways of relating.

If the partner is relatively stable and does not need much focus on his or her own problem patterns and motivations, the IRT therapist can see the identified patient intensively in individual therapy, and the couple occasionally. More often than not, however, the partner has his or her own entrenched problem patterns and IPIRs. When each partner is significantly damaged, it is better to have separate individual therapists for each partner, and both therapists for couple sessions. IRT-adherent therapists will be able to resist the inevitable behavioral invitations to do battle for "their" individual patients. Instead, they will consistently model, and help patients work toward, the general therapy goal of friendliness with moderate degrees of enmeshment and differentiation.

Extended Family and System Conferences

Extended family conferences, or even system conferences with the neighbors or other affected persons, can be part of IRT as well. This approach can be good in crisis management, as discussed below and in Chapter 7, but is not usually necessary for reconstructive work. Extended family conferences can even create problems, because when the whole family gets together around an identified patient, old alliances and battles sometimes emerge. Family systems are not easily engaged in the task of challenging these habits and myths, even if it is almost always simple to see how the problem patterns are bouncing through the generations and repeatedly reflecting the same damages.

For example, if the patient's mother is treating her father just as she saw the grandmother treat the grandfather, the recognition initially serves to "justify" the mother and the patient in their ways of being. Giving up the underlying fantasies about what it costs to keep the grandmother alive in this way is—as the reader of this book will probably realize by now—not a simple matter. Everyone has to come to terms with his or her own IPIRs and, at the same time, learn to develop more appropriate relationships with the "real deals." Use of individual IRT principles in IRT-based family therapy is like changing from playing a simple keyboard to trying to master a cathedral organ. So much is going on at once that it is uncommonly difficult to bring it all together.

Large system meetings can be very helpful, however, if somebody is out of control with suicidality or homicidality. This intervention, if implemented carefully, can help the concerned parties collaboratively work out ways to support the patient's Green. It can provide a coordinated forum for working out plans to monitor and transport the patient as needed. It can involve minimizing the patient's exposure to high-risk situations and maximizing whatever is supportive to him or her. It can involve collaboration to manage doses of medications, or collaboratively correcting family members' fantasies about what the health care system can and cannot do.

Everyone in the system needs to understand that measures worked out in a meeting devoted to blocking dangerous symptoms do not constitute reconstructive treatment. Their purpose is only to try to preserve the option for the patient to pursue reconstruction later.

Group Therapy

Group therapy is an underdeveloped but potentially vital part of IRT. It can provide compelling opportunity to develop multiple collaborations that support Green (step 1); learn about one's patterns (step 2); learn new and better rules and values that can inhibit problem patterns (step 3); develop, through the eyes of others, a broader perspective on one's own history and thereby enable the will to change (step 4); and learn new and better patterns (step 5). These possibilities can be realized best if the therapist controls the group process so that it remains truly collaborative and devoted to IRT goals.[13] It is important to establish these goals in the earliest group meetings. Just letting a group evolve as it will, without definition of goals or methods, is likely to lead to iatrogenic events. For example, problem patterns can be enabled through joining of Regressive Loyalists. Contagion is one of many hazards in uncontrolled group therapy. Effective group therapy requires quite a bit more than "assemble patients and stir."

The IRT group therapist develops a case formulation for each person before the group starts. The patient is oriented to the learning model and to the ways the group can contribute to this learning. Each patient considers his or her own specific areas of needed learning, and commits to the goal of working on each of the five steps. Once the group meets and agrees on the process and goals, each intervention attempts to implement the core algorithm for as many participants as possible. Ideally, group members quickly learn to help each other identify interactive patterns in the group; discuss their roots; participate actively in discussion of different perspectives on early and current scenarios; and provide clear structure for learning goal patterns of interaction—first within the group, and later in their lives at large.

The group therapist blocks problem behaviors early in therapy. Later on, group members may take over any blocking that is still needed. For example, if the group begins to scapegoat an individual, the IRT therapist blocks that pattern by helping the attacker explore what his or her anger is supposed to accomplish, and how that relates to his or her own internalizations. The scapegoat's views are also elicited. Both attacker and scape-goat are supported in efforts to address their own vulnerabilities. Then other group members are encouraged to discuss feelings about the process, describe their personal associations to it, and establish whether they wish to continue in attack mode or learn to understand and communicate in new ways. The original agreement to help each other implement the five steps and work toward therapy goal behaviors is reaffirmed and increasingly implemented by group members. The therapist consistently supports Green interactions among members, and calls the group's attention to Red process only if and when the group allows Red to escalate.

MacKenzie (1990, 1997) has described his principles of stages of group therapy, supplemented by SASB concepts, to construct and conduct groups effectively. Elsewhere (Benjamin, 2000a), I have provided a data-based illustration of how principles of IRT and the SASB technology can enhance group therapy.

Organizational Psychology

Consultants to companies with problems with managers may recognize the fact that referral of key figures for IRT can effectively relieve difficult system problems. One example, the cases of Ronald and Mabel, has been discussed in Chapter 9.

Brief Therapies

It is highly desirable for treatments to be brief rather than not brief. By definition, IRT seeks reconstruction or "cure," not merely symptom relief. This book has been about the use of IRT with nonresponders. The successfully reconstructed IRT case of this type should be without major symptoms, off most medications, and unlikely to need to return to treatment (barring extraordinary new circumstances). Effectiveness of a personality-changing long-term therapy like IRT should be assessed in terms of long-term total system costs. These could include the usual measures of symptom relief, as well as other factors of concern (number and length of rehospitalizations, medical visits, medications, therapy sessions, days lost at work, and so on). Assessments should be longer-term in nature. For example, system costs for the year preceding treatment might be compared to system costs in the years during and following IRT. The context and reasons for this recommendation to apply broader and longer-term measurements to assess treatment effectiveness for patients with personality disorders are discussed elsewhere (Benjamin, 1997).

If a patient can respond quickly and stably to a brief therapy, he or she probably should have the brief therapy. IRT will be employed if and when a referral source has found that there are no effective shortcuts for the person in question. Although it is not brief, IRT presumes to be accelerated compared to other approaches to the nonresponder population. That said, there have been some rather amazing brief courses of IRT with nonresponders (e.g., Martha, described in Chapter 6). Unfortunately, brevity is not the norm.

ASSESSMENTS OF VALIDITY
OF IRT THEORY AND PRACTICE

Testimonials from Former Trainees

Just about any therapist using any approach can produce testimonials from former patients as to effectiveness. That fact makes a listing of such testimonials relatively meaningless. Still, the nature (and number) of IRT testimonials from ex-patients is encouraging, because they almost universally include two features: (1) "This therapy has been very helpful," and (2) "I have tried many other approaches before that were not helpful." It is particularly noteworthy when testimonials come from supervisees who report significant change in the progress within their caseloads after switching to IRT. Here are examples:

> "The self-mutilating and manipulative [patient with Borderline Personality Disorder] I had hoped to get while you were supervising me finally arrived 3 months ago while [I was] working at my new placement. When she started treatment, she was cutting deeply into her arms, chest, and legs, and burning words like 'blood,' into her flesh with hot matches. The first step to a good alliance, I believe, came when she began by telling me how five previous therapists had failed her, and that she hoped I'd be the one to help her. I had sense enough to respond with, 'Well, I just may be your next disappointing therapist,' which quickly engaged her. Also, when she requested more frequent sessions, I was able to orchestrate the agreement of doing so on an experimental basis, with the expectation of seeing clear progress if it was to continue. We then proceeded with the IRT model, and she was able to make a commitment to growth, to exploring new ways of being, and so on. She has demonstrated remarkable progress in totally ending self-mutilation, making sense of her copy process patterns, and doing a great job at reevaluating and changing them. It's wonderful to be a part of such an amazing transformation, and, even more, to have a valuable framework (i.e., IRT) from which to facilitate her transformation!"

IRT students discussing their internship experience seem especially to appreciate having a clear method to develop a case formulation and knowing how to use that to proceed effectively in therapy. Their competence is noted by their peers, who may complain of feeling "lost." Here is an excerpt from a representative letter[14] sent by a student a few years after he completed postdoctoral training:

> "[When we meet] I will tell you of the many good things that your practicum sequence did for me on my pre-doc internship, and how different my experience was when compared to the other interns. In fact, I think that it probably got me my current job."

Research Studies to Date

For the past 3 years, my psychology practicum class has constituted a pilot program wherein IRT trainee therapists provide brief inpatient therapy for clearly defined nonresponders after I developed the case formulation. To date, there have been over 50 such brief inpatient treatments. Each discharge report included a consultative report and a summary of the brief inpatient treatment. Many of these patients were enthusiastic about following the IRT plan in their further work. Sometimes they requested that copies of videotapes of their consultative interviews be sent to their outpatient therapists for further discussion.[15]

Recently, cases that did not have other placements have been transferred to outpatient follow-up by IRT psychology practicum student therapists for periods ranging from 4 months to 2½ years. To date, there have been five such outpatient treatments by students following discharge. None of these patients has committed suicide. Only one attempted suicide; she was rehospitalized twice after two attempts that occurred within 3 weeks of discharge. Following an IRT-based family conference during the second rehospitalization, the treatment of this desperately suicidal person resumed with full support of the family and of the primary physician. Subsequent progress was dramatic and has been long-lasting. No other patients in the practicum were rehospitalized, despite long records of many previous hospitalizations and multiple suicide attempts. Three of these erstwhile nonresponders with IRT student therapists filled out measures of symptoms before and after treatment. Data show that all three returned to full functioning that matched or exceeded levels prior to their first hospitalization. All three patients no longer felt a need for medications.[16]

When the three empirically documented student cases were combined with five patients from my private practice who also elected to complete forms on their symptoms before and after treatment, a Wilcoxon signed-ranks nonparametric test of differences between "before" and "after" scores revealed significant improvement ($p < .01$) on the following measures from the Symptom Checklist 90—Revised (Derogatis, 1977): the General Symptom Index; the Positive Distress Level; and individual scales for Somatization, Interpersonal Sensitivity, Anxiety, and Phobic Anxiety.

Significant changes were also found on individual Wisconsin Personality Inventory (Klein et al., 1993) scales for Narcissism, Borderline, Avoidant, and Dependent Personality Disorders.

In addition, about 20 students to date have provided outpatient IRT to "ordinary" cases from the hospital outpatient clinic's waiting list. These treatments did not begin with IRT inpatient work; the patients were assessed and treated by the IRT students, and many showed clear progress during their semester-long treatments. None made a suicide attempt or needed hospitalization.

Finally, there have been six more IRT supervisions of students from another university. Their severely disordered cases had been handed down over the years from therapist to therapist. Although some of these patients were suicidal and two were homicidal, none made any attempts, and none was hospitalized. Most made obvious constructive changes.

This list of results—some of which are properly based on objective, symptom-oriented data gathered before and after treatment hardly constitutes a formal clinical trial. But the data are a step above the "testimonial" or isolated "case report" methods of validation.

Research Studies in the Future

Clearly, formal clinical trials are needed next. The plan is to do more than simply demonstrate improvement in patients who receive IRT versus a contrast condition. The goal is also to assess the validity and relevance of the DLL hypotheses, and the effect of adherence to the core algorithm in relation to outcome. This will test the conceptual validity of the IRT model, as well as provide formal overall evidence as to whether it is effective.

The SASB model will be central in tests of DLL theory, adherence to the therapy model and interpersonal as well as intrapsychic impacts of treatment. SASB codes of the therapy narrative and patient ratings on SASB questionnaires can systematically survey and quantify the patient's interactive patterns and internal representations. Assessments are highly reliable (Benjamin, 2000b). The ability of SASB to make social cognitions amenable to the rules of science has been acknowledged by other investigators and theoreticians,[17] including important figures within mainstream behavioral psychology (e.g., Goldfried & Davison, 1994, pp. 296–297).

RESPONSES TO MAJOR CRITICISMS OF PSYCHODYNAMIC THERAPIES USING IRT

IRT is responsive to the seriously challenging criticisms of psychodynamically oriented therapies offered by Walter Mischel in 1973. Mischel's paper helped marginalize psychoanalysis and psychodynamic psychotherapy within the scientific community. The present movements toward empirically validated therapies (EVTs) and empirically supported therapies (ESTs), mentioned in Chapter 1, are wholly consistent with Mischel's suggestion that preferred treatments be based on clearly specified methods and well-documented effects. As noted in Chapter 1, selected behavioral, interpersonal, and medication approaches have met that standard, and therefore predominate in current practices. However, these approaches, by definition, have not been effective with the nonresponder population. IRT claims to be effective with many erstwhile nonresponders, and also to be amenable to the EST standards. IRT includes psychodynamic as well as interpersonal and behavioral methods. Even though it includes discussions of the past, consistent focus on conflict, and an emphasis on motivation, IRT is responsive to Mischel's criticisms of psychodynamic approaches. A review of Mischel's main points and the IRT responses to them follows. Clinical examples are drawn from the case of Marie, introduced in Chapter 1 and discussed in subsequent chapters.

1. *There is a large gap between symptoms and presumed motive.* With this comment, Mischel questioned the relevance of psychoanalytic theory to the problems that brought the patients to therapy in the first place. His arguments are not reviewed here. As has been said many times before, the DLL case formulation method requires explicit links between the presenting problems and the values and rules associated with key figures or IPIRs. For example, Marie's "ultimate fear" was linked directly to her internalized relationship with her father.

2. *Psychoanalysis is ineffective.* Mischel declared, "Clients often may have remained crippled by their disadvantageous behaviors while waiting (how long?) for insight based relief from psychodynamic treatments" (1973, p. 337). IRT assumes full responsibility for taking measures before, during, and after treatment. Although there has not yet been a formal clinical trial of IRT, clinical results are very encouraging, as are the preliminary research results mentioned above.

3. *Behavioral approaches focus on behavior–condition relations.* Here, in effect, Mischel required that the treatment approach define and address the "reasons" for the presenting problems. He cited the behavioral model, wherein there is an "analysis of behavior patterns in relation to the conditions that evoke, maintain, and modify those patterns" (1973, p. 338).

Similarly, the functional analysis according to IRT proposes that the wish for psychic proximity to and reconciliation with an IPIR is the motivator of the problem patterns. That wish has to change before there can be behavior change. For example, Marie's lingering attachment to the internalization of her abusive father kept her locked in her need to find someone to protect from danger. She recapitulated her patterns with him, presumably because of an unconscious hope that "next time," she would manage things so well that he would become more loving. Then everyone, including Marie, would truly be safe. Since neither the reality nor the internalization was likely to change in that way, the only resolution was for Marie to decide that her father's internalization was no longer centrally important to her. Her anger at him could then be redirected to help her separate (differentiate) from his representation, rather than to continue psychic enmeshment via ongoing blaming for sexual abuse. After letting the anger help her separate, she would regain the greatest control of her psyche as she decided simply that she could let her father "rest in peace."

This functional analysis of Marie's anxiety is not based on environmentally observable antecedent and consequent conditions, as would be required by Skinner (and probably also by Mischel). Nonetheless, the approach implements the idea of trying to extinguish the connections that maintain the problem responses. As mentioned earlier, SASB measures of the IPIRs, and the use of predictive principles to link them to problem patterns, does enhance the objectivity of the theory and treatment approach. Research studies (Benjamin, 1996c) have repeatedly shown strong associations between SASB measures of internalizations and DSM-relevant symptoms.

4. *The approach should acknowledge that people create situations.* Here, Mischel elaborated upon his idea that it is a mistake to think of people simply as a collection of dispositions or traits. People behave differently, depending on the situations they are in. Moreover, they seek and create situations. A functional analysis is incomplete without considering the person's role in choosing or creating as well as reacting to the context.

In DLL theory, links between persons and their social situations are detailed by the three copy processes and can be codified via the SASB model's predictive principles. The "reward" or "function" of the person × situation interaction is to implement the rules and values of the key figure or IPIR in order to achieve psychic proximity. For example, Marie remained married to a very cruel man for many years. An IRT-based functional analysis of this problem situation would suggest that she was recapitulating her pattern with her father. Her marriage allowed her to carry on her father's tradition. Even after the separation had continued for many years, she still had the role of protecting their adult children from her husband and other dangers. As suggested in the discussion of Mischel's third criticism, the purpose of recapitulation would be to try for "one more chance" to achieve loving psychic proximity to the internalization of her father. The analysis "explains" why Marie remained so long in an abusive marital relationship.[18] IRT is wholly compatible with Mischel's point about persons and situations.[19]

5. *Memory of childhood is distorted.* Mischel worried that psychodynamic psychotherapy concentrates on stories from the past, and that there is often no way of checking their validity. Mischel might therefore ask this

question: How can one possibly implement cure while working on "bad information"?

DLL theory, the basis of the case formulation, depends on the belief that how the person sees things directs his or her behavior, cognition, and affect. Reality is not important in explaining "why" people do what they do. If a delusional man believes that the FBI is after him, his behavior reflects his belief, not the reality. Murray (1938) called the connection between the perception and action the beta press. Case formulation in IRT invokes beta press.

By contrast, treatment planning in IRT requires careful attention to current reality. It makes no sense to ignore the patient's actual situation in efforts to encourage new and more adaptive behaviors. For example, it would be vital to compare Marie's labeling of her husband as cruel to her concrete (SASB-codable) descriptions of interactions with him. To gather these data, the therapist inquires: "What did he say, do? What did you say, do, feel, think?" If the codes of her narrative suggested that he was overcontrolling, but not attacking, any such discrepancy between the supporting detail and her conclusion would be important.[20] No discrepancies were noted for Marie, since the concrete descriptions of the words from her husband and father documented that each was physically and verbally attacking.

6. *Interventions must generalize outside the therapist's office.* Mischel referred to the belief that patients and their analysts typically have wonderful relationships, but nothing in the patients' lives seems to change. Without assessing the validity of the accusation, and instead embracing the need to address the issue, I emphasize that IRT does consistently focus on current patterns. Stories of ongoing relationships are likely to reflect the problem patterns early in treatment, and then offer opportunities for new social learning later on. If the therapist is enabling problem patterns, then codes of therapy process will be Red, and the therapy will not be IRT-adherent. Properly implemented IRT includes substantial efforts to enhance awareness of current patterns and motives and to try to change them. Reports by the patient of interactions with family, friends, and associates should reflect progression toward the therapy goals of normative behaviors, affects, and cognitions described in detail in Chapter 9.

Information about progress in interactions with current people is easily available in nearly any session of ongoing IRT. My colleagues and I have not found that patients give specific narratives about interactions with others during therapy that conflict with the judgments of their significant others about the patients' progress. In a context of collaboration and specificity in therapy, there is excellent accuracy. Patient ratings on the Retrospective Assessment of the Therapy Experience (RATE; Strupp, Fox, & Lessler, 1968) indicate that improvement is apparent in varying degrees to spouses/partners, friends, and colleagues. Nonetheless, it will be vital eventually to obtain objective ratings of patients by significant others, both be-fore and after treatment. This plan to use informants should perhaps also be included in the EVT and EST standards.

7. *Assessment and prediction must be based directly on the model.* Mischel noted that in psychoanalytic theory, the connections between the theoretically underlying drives and structures have little to do with the therapy model. Again, the validity of Mischel's point here might fall some-what short of "granted," in the eyes of analysts. Nonetheless, the goal marked by Mischel is worthy, whether or not analysis achieves it. In IRT, assessment, case formulation, treatment planning, choice of interventions, and measurement of outcome are all closely related. The therapy consis-tently focuses on the attachments to IPIRs that organize the problem be-haviors.

For example, therapy with Marie would consistently attend to her anxi-ety and its relationship to her internal struggle with her father IPIR. Anxiety would be assessed with traditional symptom measures. Her relationship to her father IPIR could be assessed with the SASB Intrex questionnaires, as well as with clinician or observer SASB codes of her narratives. The prediction would be that when she differentiated[21] from that IPIR, her anxiety would diminish. In sum, IRT offers highly specific descriptions of mechanisms of pathology and the directly related treatment model. Assessment methods re-late directly to the theories of etiology and treatment.

In conclusion, IRT provides reasonable responses to each of Mischel's criticisms of psychodynamic psychotherapies.

FUTURE DEVELOPMENTS IN THE NEAR TERM

In addition to pursuing research study of the validity of the models and ef-fectiveness of the approach, systematic ways of teaching IRT need to be de-veloped. Presently, the University of Utah Neuropsychiatric Institute (UNI) is supporting a clinic that specializes in using IRT to treat nonresponders. Emphasis on service, training, and research is evenly distributed. A re-search protocol to document effectiveness is under way.

PRELIMINARY REMARKS ON HOW TO LEARN IRT

Among the planned work products from the IRT clinic at UNI, just de-scribed, will be training manuals that will supplement the present book in helping clinicians learn this approach efficiently. In the meantime, miscella-neous recommendations for clinicians who wish to learn to use IRT are as follows:

- Read an earlier book (Benjamin, 1996a) for background in using interpersonal patterns to identify and better understand individuals with DSM-IV Axis II personality disorders.
- Study the present book on IRT carefully (and perhaps repeatedly).
- Select one or two cases that have been difficult, and develop case formulations according to Figures 2.1, 2.2, and 2.3.
- Be sure that the therapy dialogue is always concrete enough to provide valid data. For example, elicit "He said, 'I am sorry I have to go back to work tonight, but I will be home by 11,' " rather than "My husband doesn't love me any more." Accomplish this by frequently asking if needed, "Can you give me an example of _____?", "Help me understand how you know _____," and "What did he say or do that makes you feel _____?"
- Frequently be empathic by providing accurate and compassionate reflections of what the patient is saying. This facilitates collaboration by letting the patient know that you understand what is being said.
- Frequently attend to therapy process (what is happening between the patient and you), as well as to content (what the patient is talking about). If therapy process becomes negative, address the situation rapidly.
- Once you have a clear case formulation and are empathically facilitating collaborative discussions of concrete interpersonal narratives, begin to add other elements of the core algorithm. (See the summary of the core algorithm provided at the beginning of this chapter.)
- Audiotape a few sessions (or make exact notes) and review them. Ask yourself whether and how you have used the core algorithm.
- Create session notes as suggested in Figure 3.5 or in a comparable data base. This process forces adherence to the IRT model. You need not have an entry for every line in the table, but be sure to include a complete SOAP (subjective patient report, objective data, analysis, plans) summary of each session (see Chapter 3).
- Learn to use the SASB model. Constant SASB coding helps keep the therapy dialogue concrete and clarifies patterns and links. For example, SASB coding enables you to be clear about complex messages even when the narrative "bends your mind." The predictive principles help focus your intuition about antecedents and consequences.
- Participate regularly in a peer group that is trying to learn the IRT approach. In that group, share results of the preceding exercises (with requisite permissions from the patients). Think more about the therapy process in relation to each patient's presenting problems and less about the "nature" of the patient. Such statements as "She did something sooo borderline last week" are not IRT-adherent.
- Obtain supervision from a certified IRT trainer.
- Try to remember that the therapy is about the patient, not the thera-

pist. The outcome of the treatment does not define the therapist. Rather, the outcome of treatment defines the patient!

EPILOGUE

Thanks to my readers for continuing on to the end of this dense book. It summarizes over 30 years of practice, teaching, and research, and is not an "easy read." However, I believe the book is worth the energy and time it demands, and I have several wishes for its impact. The first is that its ideas and materials will enable clinicians to approach the nonresponder population with good cheer and increased effectiveness. The second is that its ideas and materials will facilitate further research documentation of the belief that psychotherapy can be extremely helpful to severely disordered individuals, as well as to the "worried well." The third is that its ideas and materials will help the many readers who still have palpable Red parts themselves to progress further in their personal struggle toward Green. The fourth, and most grandiose, is that its ideas and materials will eventually contribute to ongoing efforts to increase societal investments (financial, emotional, social, and conceptual) in more benign and effective ways to raise children.

NOTES

1. According to the Structural Analysis of Social Behavior (SASB) model.
2. According to the parallel affect and cognitive models presented in Appendix 4.1.
3. This statement applies to a lifestyle that has revenge as its baseline. Isolated, contextually appropriate episodes of revenge taking or administration of punishment can be accommodated within IRT. Please see the discussion of the justice model, Chapter 8.
4. For example, anger is not an energy that must be expressed one way or another (see the discussion of the cathartic model in Chapter 8). As another example, an apparent need to control may be a defense against abandonment rather than an end in itself. Alternatively, it may be a strategy that evolved to attempt to keep a volatile parent from explosive episodes. Still other reasons for a pathological need to control can be identified by study of patterns learned in relation to an important person and his or her internalization.
5. Klein, Kolden, Michels, and Chrisholm-Stockard (2002) describe congruence in terms of two facets. The first is the

> therapist's personal integration in the relationship, that "he is freely and deeply himself, with his actual experience accurately represented by his awareness of himself" (Rogers, 1967, p. 97). By placing the emphasis on the relationship Rogers does not require the therapist to be well-integrated in all aspects of his life, but at least be "accurately himself in this hour of this relationship . . . in this moment of time" (p. 97).

The second facet of congruence characterizes the therapist's capacity to communicate his personhood *to* the client, as appropriate. (p. 396)

6. See Benjamin (2001) for a brief description of major degrees of overlap between Kernberg's view of treatment for severe personality disorders and IRT.

7. Of course, the two-chair technique can be used for other purposes. It can, for example, simply clarify patterns when the patient acts out two different family members in the respective chairs.

8. SASB coding typically increases a therapist's ability to read therapy process and content correctly.

9. The reader is reminded that a regressive attitude is discouraged in IRT. If the patient cannot confine his or her regressive behaviors to the therapy sessions, the procedure changes (see Figures 3.2, 3.3, and 3.4) until he or she can.

10. It should be noted that Skinner disliked attempts to study unobservables and therefore disapproved of cognitive-behavioral therapies (Skinner, 1990), which are concerned with mental events. He preferred to consider the "behaving organism" as a black box, and held that "prediction and control" of behavior require only a clear knowledge of antecedent and consequent conditions. It can therefore be inferred that Skinner would not approve of the IRT adaptation of his basic operant model, which considers fantasies about relations with IPIRs as reinforcements.

11. Recognition of this possibility does not suggest that the target caregiver should therefore ignore the gesture; unfortunately, that will yield escalation. The challenge is to respond by supporting Green and blocking Red, using principles discussed in Chapter 7.

12. Naturally, the content of this fantasied counterattack will vary, depending on the evidence about the nature of the stepfather's attacks on the patient. Even though attack is not a goal of IRT, fantasy attacks and other in-therapy expressions of anger are often necessary and important interim steps in the process of escaping the influence of a destructive IPIR.

13. And not, for example, to goals that might be consistent with a justice model. Hostile confrontation of a patient, even if he or she has been physically or sexually abusive, is not likely to be consistent with the IRT core algorithm and collaborative orientation. Individuals who have abused others often have dreadful histories themselves, and therapist replication of the same patterns is unlikely to inspire anything new on a long-term basis.

14. There have been dozens of such letters, phone messages, conversations, and e-mails over the years.

15. After patients have given written permission to release these tapes, they have been sent to the patients' current health care providers.

16. The patient who made the overdose attempts immediately after discharge did not provide "after" data, but continued in treatment with an expert object relations therapist after the IRT student left for his internship. She reportedly also has returned to full functioning and is "doing extremely well."

17. A list of publications based on the SASB model is available on request at Intrex@Psych.utah.edu.

18. It could also explain why she separated from her husband when her children left home.

19. The accompanying SASB model assesses within a trait × state × situation perspective (Benjamin, 2000b).

20. One might note that each patient is still the data source, and therefore might wonder how one can test "reality" this way. The answer is that unless the patient is deliberately lying, the SASB-coded details in the narrative will describe actual behaviors. The clinician who elicits and codes the concrete detail emerging from the input–response algorithm is rarely surprised when the person described appears for a family session. However, the ultimate test of DLL theory would be to SASB-code family interactions at critical times and situations during development, follow children across the years, and then compare the early assessments of subjects with normal outcomes to those with pathological destinies.

21. Her SASB Intrex ratings should show better circumplex order centering on the point SEPARATE.

References

American Heritage talking dictionary. (1997). Novato, CA: The Learning Company.

American Psychiatric Association. (1994). *Diagnostic and statistical manual of mental disorders* (4th ed.). Washington, DC: Author.

American Psychological Association (APA). (2002, April). *Ethical principles of psychologists and code of conduct* (Draft 7) [Online]. Available: http://www.apa. org/ethics/code.html [2002, June 12].

Aschen, S. R. (1997). Assertion training therapy in psychiatric milieus. *Archives of Psychiatric Nursing, 11,* 46–51.

Barlow, S. H., & Bergin, A. E. (2001). *The phenomenon of spirit in a secular psychotherapy.* Thousand Oaks, CA: Sage.

Beck, A. T. (1997). The past and future of cognitive therapy. *Journal of Psychotherapy Practice and Research, 6,* 276–284.

Beck, A. T. (1999). Cognitive aspects of personality disorders and their relation to syndromal disorders: A psychoevolutionary approach. In C. R. Cloninger (Ed.), *Personality and psychopathology.* Washington, DC: American Psychiatric Press.

Beck, A. T., Brown, G., & Steer, R. A. (1989). Prediction of eventual suicide in psychiatric inpatients by clinical ratings of hopelessness. *Journal of Consulting and Clinical Psychology, 57,* 309–310.

Beck, A. T., Rush, A. J., Shaw, B. E., & Emery, G. (1979). *Cognitive therapy of depression.* New York: Guilford Press.

Benjamin, L. S. (1974). Structural Analysis of Social Behavior. *Psychological Review, 81,* 392–425.

Benjamin, L. S. (1978). Structural analysis of differentiation failure. *Psychiatry: Journal for the Study of Interpersonal Processes, 42,* 1–23.

Benjamin, L. S. (1984). Principles of prediction using Structural Analysis of Social Behavior. In R. A. Zucker, J. Aronoff, & A. J. Rabin (Eds.), *Personality and the prediction of behavior.* New York: Academic Press.

Benjamin, L. S. (1986). Using SASB to add social parameters to Axis I of DSM-III. In T. Millon & G. L. Klerman (Eds.), *Contemporary directions in psychopathology.* New York: Guilford Press.

Benjamin, L. S. (1989). Is chronicity related to the quality of the relationship with the hallucination? *Schizophrenia Bulletin, 15,* 291–310.

Benjamin, L. S. (1993). Every psychopathology is a gift of love. *Psychotherapy Research, 3,* 1–24.

Benjamin, L. S. (1994). SASB: A bridge between personality theory and clinical psychology. *Psychological Inquiry, 5,* 273–316.

Benjamin, L. S. (1995). Good defenses make good neighbors. In H. R. Conte & R. Plutchik (Eds.), *Ego defenses: Theory and measurement.* New York: Wiley.

Benjamin, L. S. (1996a). *Interpersonal diagnosis and treatment of personality disorders* (2nd ed.). New York: Guilford Press.

Benjamin, L. S. (1996b). An interpersonal theory of personality disorders. In J. F. Clarkin (Ed.), *Major theories of personality disorder.* New York: Guilford Press.

Benjamin, L. S. (1996c). Introduction to the special section on Structural Analysis of Social Behavior (SASB). *Journal of Consulting and Clinical Psychology, 64,* 1203–1212.

Benjamin, L. S. (1996d). A clinician-friendly version of the interpersonal circumplex: Structural Analysis of Social Behavior (SASB). *Journal of Personality Assessment, 66,* 248–266.

Benjamin, L. S. (1997). Personality disorders: Models for treatment and strategies for treatment development. *Journal of Personality Disorders, 11,* 307–324.

Benjamin, L. S. (2000a). Interpersonal diagnosis and treatment in group therapy. In A. Beck & C. Lewis (Eds.), *The process of group psychotherapy: Systems for analyzing change.* Washington, DC: American Psychological Association.

Benjamin, L. S. (2000b). *Intrex user's manual.* Salt Lake City: University of Utah.

Benjamin, L. S. (2000c). Scientific discipline can enhance clinical effectiveness. In S. Soldz & L. McCullough (Eds.), *Reconciling empirical knowledge and clinical experience: The art and science of psychotherapy.* Washington, DC: American Psychological Association.

Benjamin, L. S. (2001). Commentary on Kernberg's "The suicidal risk in severe personality disorders: Differential diagnosis and treatment." *Journal of Personality Disorders, 15,* 209–211.

Benjamin, L. S. (in preparation). *Personality guided Interpersonal Reconstructive Therapy for anxiety, anger, and anhedonia.*

Benjamin, L. S., & Cushing, G. (2000). *Manual for coding social interactions in terms of Structural Analysis of Social Behavior.* Salt Lake City: University of Utah.

Benjamin, L. S., & Friedrich, F. (1991). Contributions of SASB to the bridge between cognitive science and object relations psychotherapy. In M. Horowitz (Ed.), *Person schemas and maladaptive interpersonal patterns.* Chicago: University of Chicago Press.

Benjamin, L. S., & Karpiac, C. (2001). Personality disorders. *Psychotherapy Theory/Research/Practice/Training, 38,* 487–494.

Benjamin, L. S., & Karpiac, C. (2002). Personality disorders. In J. C. Norcross (Ed.), *Psychotherapy relationships that work: Therapists' relational contributions to effective psychotherapy.* New York: Oxford University Press.

Bergin, A. E. (1991). Values and religious issues in psychotherapy and mental health. *American Psychologist, 46,* 394–403.

Bergin, A. E., & Lambert, M. J. (1978). The evalution of therapeutic outcomes. In S. L. Garfield & A. E. Bergin (Eds.), *Handbook of psychotherapy and behavior change: An empirical analysis* (2nd ed.). New York: Wiley.

Blatt, S. J., & Behrends, R. S. (1987). Internalization: Separation–individuation and the nature of therapeutic action. *International Journal of Psycho-Analysis, 68,* 279–297.

Bonner, D., & Howard, R. (1995). Treatment-resistant depression in the elderly. *International Psychogeriatrics, 7*(Suppl.), 83–94.

Boring, E. G. (1950). *A history of experimental psychology* (2nd ed.). New York: Appleton-Century-Crofts.

Blatt, S. J. (1998). Contributions of psychoanalysis to the understanding and treatment of depression. *Journal of the American Psychoanalytic Association, 46,* 723–752.

Bowlby, J. (1969). *Attachment and loss: Vol. 1. Attachment.* New York: Basic Books.

Bowlby, J. (1977). The making and breaking of affectional bonds. *British Journal of Psychiatry, 130,* 201–210.

Braswell, L., & Kendall, P. C. (1987). Treating impulsive children via cognitive-behavioral therapy. In N. S. Jacobson (Ed.), *Psychotherapists in clinical practice: Cognitive and behavioral perspectives*. New York: Guilford Press.

Breggin, P. (1994). *Toxic psychiatry*. New York: St. Martin's Press.

Buckley, P. F., Wiggins, L. D., Sebastian, S., & Singer, B. (2001). Treatment-refractory schizophrenia. *Current Psychiatry Reports, 3*, 393–400.

Carson, R. C. (1969). *Interaction concepts of personality*. Chicago: Aldine.

Carter, J. C., & Fairburn, C. G. (1998). Cognitive-behavioral self-help for binge eating disorder: A controlled effectiveness study. *Journal of Consulting and Clinical Psychology, 66*, 616–623.

Cassidy, J. R. (1999). The nature of the child's ties. In J. R. Cassidy & P. E. Shaver (Eds.), *Handbook of attachment: Theory, research, and clinical applications*. New York: Guilford Press.

Chambless, D. L., & Hollon, S. D. (1998). Defining empirically supported therapies. *Journal of Consulting and Clinical Psychology, 66*, 7–18.

Connolly, M. B., Crits-Christoph, P., Demorest, A., Azarian, K., Muenz, L., & Chittams, J. (1996). Varieties of transference patterns in psychotherapy. *Journal of Consulting and Clinical Psychology, 64*, 1213–1221.

Connolly, M. B., Crits-Christoph, P., Shelton, R.C., Hollon, S., Kurtz, J., Barber, J. P., Butler, S. F., Baker, S., & Thase, M. E. (1999). The reliability and validity of a measure of self-understanding of interpersonal patterns. *Journal of Counseling Psychology, 46*, 472–482.

Constantino, M. J. (2000). Interpersonal process in psychotherapy through the lens of the Structural Analysis of Social Behavior. *Applied and Preventive Psychology: Current Scientific Perspectives, 9*, 153–172.

Cousens, P., & Nunn, K. P. (1997). Is "self-regulation" a more helpful construct than "attention"? *Clinical Child Psychology and Psychiatry, 2*, 27–43.

Crits-Christoph, P., Cooper, A., & Luborsky, L. (1988). The accuracy of therapists' interpretations and the outcome of dynamic psychotherapy. *Journal of Consulting and Clinical Psychology, 56*, 490–495.

Darwin, C. (1952). The descent of man. In R. M. Hutchins (Ed.), *Great books of the Western world*. Chicago: Encyclopedia Britannica. (Original work published 1871)

Davison, G. C. (2000). Stepped care: Doing more with less? *Journal of Consulting and Clinical Psychology, 68*, 580–585.

DeLay, T. (2000). Fighting for children. *American Psychologist, 55*, 1054–1055.

Delprato, D. J., & Midgley, B. D. (1992). Some fundamentals of B. F. Skinner's behaviorism. *American Psychologist, 47*, 1507–1520.

Dench, S., & Bennett, G. (2000). The impact of brief motivational intervention at the start of an outpatient day programme for alcohol dependence. *Behavioural and Cognitive Psychotherapy, 28*, 121–130.

Derogatis, L. R. (1977). *SCL-90 administration, scoring and procedures manuals for the revised version*. Baltimore: Author.

Downey, L., Rosengren, D. B., & Donovan, D. M. (2000). To thine own self be true: Self-concept and motivation for abstinence among substance abusers. *Addictive Behavior, 5*, 743–757.

Dunkle, J. H., & Friedlander, M. L. (1996). Contribution of therapist experience and personal characteristics to the working alliance. *Journal of Counseling Psychology, 43*, 456–460.

Elkin, I., Gibbons, R. D., Shea, M. T., Sotsky, S. M., Watkins, J. T., Pilkonis, P. A., & Hedeker, D. (1995). Initial severity and differential treatment outcome in the National Institute of Mental Health Treatment of Depression Collaborative Research Program. *Journal of Consulting and Clinical Psychology, 63*, 841–847.

Elkin, I., Shea, M. T., Watkins, J. T., Imber, S. D., Sotsky, S. M., Collins, J. F., Glass, D. R., Pilkonis, P. A., Leber, W. R., Docherty, J. P., Fiester, S. J., & Parloff, M. B. (1989). NIMH Treatment of Depression Collaborative Research Program: General effectiveness of treatments. *Archives of General Psychiatry, 46*, 971–982.

Elliott, R., Shapiro, D. A., Firth-Cozens, J., Stiles, W. B., Hardy, G. E., Llewelyn, S. P., & Margison, F. R. (1994). Comprehensive process analysis of insight events in cognitive behavioral and psychodynamic–interpersonal psychotherapies. *Journal of Counseling Psychology, 41,* 449–463.

Ellis, A. (1973). *Humanistic psychotherapy: The rational–emotive approach.* New York: Julian Press.

Eronen, M. (1995). Mental disorders and homicidal behavior in female subjects. *American Journal of Psychiatry, 152,* 1216–1218.

Fairbairn, W. R. D. (1996). The repression and the return of Bad Objects (with special reference to the "war neuroses." In *Psychoanalytic studies of the personality.* London: Routledge. (Original work published 1943)

Feeney, M. C., & Davidson, J. A. (1996). Bridging the gap between the practical and the theoretical: An evaluation of a conflict resolution model. *Peace and Conflict: Journal of Peace Psychology, 2,* 255–269.

Fenichel, O. (1945). *The psychoanalytic theory of neurosis.* New York: Norton.

Finkelhor, D., & Dziuba-Leatherman, J. (1994). Determinants of violence in the family: Towards a theoretical integration. *American Psychologist, 49,* 173–183.

First, M. B., Spitzer, R. L, Gibbon, M., Williams, J. B. W., & Benjamin, L. S. (1997). *Structured clinical interview for DSM-IV Axis II personality disorders (SCID-II).* Washington, DC: American Psychiatric Press.

Forman, D. R., & Kochanska, G. (2001). Viewing imitation as child responsiveness: A link between teaching and discipline domains of socialization. *Developmental Psychology, 37,* 198–206.

Frank, E., Kupfer, D. J., Wagner, E. F., McEachran, A., & Cornes, C. (1991). Efficacy of interpersonal psychotherapy as maintenance treatment for recurrent depression: Contributing factors. *Archives of General Psychiatry, 48,* 1053–1059.

Frank, J. D., & Frank, J. B. (1993). *Persuasion and healing: A comparative study of psychotherapy* (3rd ed.). Baltimore: Johns Hopkins University Press

Freedman, S. R., & Enright, R. D. (1996). Forgiveness as an intervention goal with incest survivors. *Journal of Consulting and Clinical Psychology, 64,* 983–992.

Freud, S. (1959a). Hysterical phantasies and their relation to bisexuality. In E. Jones (Ed.), *Sigmund Freud: Collected papers* (Vol. 2). New York: Basic Books. (Original work published 1908)

Freud, S. (1959b). Psycho-analytic notes upon an autobiographical account of a case of paranoia (dementia paranoides). In E. Jones (Ed.), *Sigmund Freud: Collected papers* (Vol. 3). New York: Basic Books. (Original work published 1911)

Fromm-Reichmann, F. (1959). *Psychoanalysis and psychotherapy: Selected papers of Frieda Fromm-Reichmann* (D. M. Bullard, Ed.). Chicago: University of Chicago Press.

Gabbard, G. O., Lazar, S. G., Hornberger, J., & Spiegel, D. (1997). The economic impact of psychotherapy: A review. *American Journal of Psychiatry, 154,* 147–155.

Garfield, S. L., & Bergin, A. E. (Eds.). (1986). *Handbook of psychotherapy and behavior change* (3rd ed.). New York: Wiley.

Garland, A. F., & Zigler, E. (1993). Adolescent suicide prevention: Current research and social policy implications. *American Psychologist, 48,* 169–182.

Gelder, M. (1997). The future of behavior therapy. *Journal of Psychotherapy Practice and Research, 6,* 285–293.

Gidycz, C. A., Layman, M. J., Rich, C. L., Crothers, M., Gylys, J., Matorin, A., Jacobs, C. D. (2001). An evaluation of an acquaintance rape prevention program: Impact on attitudes, sexual aggression, and sexual victimization. *Journal of Interpersonal Violence, 16,* 1120–1138.

Goldbeck, R., Myatt, P., & Aitchison, T. (1997). End-of-treatment self-efficacy: A predictor of abstinence. *Addiction, 92,* 313–324.

Golden, O. (2000). The federal response to child abuse and neglect. *American Psychologist, 55,* 1050–1053.

Goldfried, M. R., & Davison, G. C. (1994). *Clinical behavior therapy.* New York: Wiley.

Gordon, T. (1970). *P.E.T. Parent effectiveness training.* New York: Wyden.

Graham, D. T., Lundy, R. M., Benjamin, L. S., Kabler, J. D., Lewis, W. C., Kunish, N. W., & Graham, F. K. (1962). Specific attitudes in initial interviews with patients having different 'psychosomatic' diseases. *Psychosomatic Medicine, 25,* 260–266.

Greenberg, J. R., & Mitchell, S. A. (1983). *Object relations in psychoanalytic theory.* Cambridge, MA: Harvard University Press.

Greenberg, L. S., & Foerster, F. S. (1996). Task analysis exemplified: The process of resolving unfinished business. *Journal of Consulting and Clinical Psychology, 64,* 439–446.

Greenberg, L. S., Rice, L. N., & Elliott, R. (1993). *Facilitating emotional change.* New York: Guilford Press.

Greenberg, M. A., Wortman, C. B., & Stone, A. A. (1996). Emotional expression and physical health: Revising traumatic memories or fostering self-regulation? *Journal of Personality and Social Psychology, 71,* 588–602.

Griffin, G. A., & Harlow, H. F. (1966). Effects of three months of total social deprivation on social adjustment and learning in the rhesus monkey. *Child Development, 37,* 533–547.

Griffin, J. C., Paisey, T. J., Stark, M. T., & Emerson, J. H. (1988). B. F. Skinner's position on aversive treatment. *American Journal on Mental Retardation, 93,* 104–105.

Grissom, R. J. (1996). The magical number .7 + .2: Meta-meta-analysis of the probability of superior outcome in comparisons involving therapy, placebo, and control. *Journal of Consulting and Clinical Psychology, 64,* 973–982.

Gurtman, M. (2000). Interpersonal complementarity: Integrating interpersonal measurement with interpersonal models. *Journal of Counseling Psychology, 48,* 97–110.

Hamberger, L. K. (1997). Cognitive behavioral treatment of men who batter their partners. *Cognitive and Behavioral Practice, 4,* 147–169.

Harlow, H. F., & Harlow, M. K. (1967, January). The young monkeys. *Psychology Today,* pp. 40–47.

Harlow, H. F., Harlow, M. K., Dodsworth, R. O., & Arling, G. L. (1966). Maternal behavior of rhesus monkeys deprived of mothering and peer associations in infancy. *Proceedings of the American Philosophical Society, 110,* 58–66.

Harlow, H. F., & Suomi, S. J. (1974). Induced depression in monkeys. *Behavioral Biology, 12,* 273–296.

Hatcher, R. L., & Barends, A. W. (1996). Patients' view of the alliance in psychotherapy: Exploratory factor analysis of three alliance measures. *Journal of Consulting and Clinical Psychology, 64,* 1326–1336.

Hazelwood, R. R., & Warren, J. I. (2000). The sexually violent offender: Impulsive or ritualistic? *Aggression and Violent Behavior, 5,* 267–279.

Hazen, C., & Shaver, P. R. (1994). Deeper into attachment theory. *Psychological Inquiry, 5,* 68–79.

Heavey, C. L., Layne, C., & Christensen, A. (1993). Gender and conflict structure in marital interaction: A replication and extension. *Journal of Consulting and Clinical Psychology, 61,* 16–27.

Hellerstein, D. J., Rosenthal, R. N., Pinsker, H., Samstag, L. W., Muran, J. C., & Winston, A. (1997). A randomized prospective study comparing supportive and dynamic therapies: Outcome and alliance. *Journal of Psychotherapy Practice and Research, 7,* 261–271.

Henry, W. P. (1996). Structural Analysis of Social Behavior as a common meteric for programmatic psychopathology and psychotherapy research. *Journal of Consulting and Clinical Psychology, 64,* 1263–1275.

Henry, W. P., Schacht, T. E., & Strupp, H. H. (1992). Structural Analysis of Social Behavior: Application to a study of interpersonal process in differential psychotherapeutic outcome. In A. E. Kazdin (Ed.), *Methodological issues and strategies in clinical research.* Washington, DC: American Psychological Association.

Hesse, E. (1999). The Adult Attachment Interview: Historical and current perspectives. In J.

Cassidy & P. R. Shaver (Eds.), *Handbook of attachment: Theory, research, and clinical applications.* New York: Guilford Press.

Hoglend, P. (1996). Motivation for brief dynamic psychotherapy. *Psychotherapy and Psychosomatics, 65,* 209–215.

Horowitz, M. J., Merluzzi, T., Ewert, M., Ghannam J., Hartley, D., & Stinson, C. H. (1991). Role-relationship models configuration. In M. J. Horowitz (Ed.), *Person schemas and maladaptive interpersonal patterns.* Chicago: University of Chicago Press.

Horvath, A. O. (1994a). Research on the alliance. In A. O. Horvath & L. S. Greenberg (Eds.), *The working alliance: Theory, research, and practice.* New York: Wiley.

Horvath, A. O. (1994b). Empirical validation of Bordin's pantheoretical model of the alliance: The Working Alliance Inventory perspective. In A. O. Horvath & L. S. Greenberg (Eds.), *The working alliance: Theory, research, and practice.* New York: Wiley.

Horvath, A. O., & Symonds, B. D. (1991). Relation between working alliance and outcome in psychotherapy: A meta-analysis. *Journal of Counseling Psychology, 38,* 139–149.

Humes, D. L., & Humphrey, L. L. (1994). A multimethod analysis of families with a polydrug-dependent or normal adolescent daughter. *Journal of Abnormal Psychology, 103,* 676–685.

Humphrey, L. L., & Benjamin, L. S. (1986). Using Structural Analysis of Social Behavior to assess critical but elusive family processes: A new solution to an old problem. *American Psychologist, 41,* 979–989.

Humphreys, K., & Moos, R. (2001). Can encouraging substance abuse patients to participate in self-help groups reduce demand for health care?: A quasi-experimental study. *Alcoholism: Clinical and Experimental Research, 25,* 711–716.

Iacoboni, M., Woods, R. P., Brass, M., Bekkering, H., Mazziotta, J. C., & Rizzolatti, G. (1999). Cortical mechanisms of human imitation. *Science, 286,* 2526–2528.

Jacobson, N. S., & Christensen, A. (1996). *Integrative couple therapy: Promoting acceptance and change.* New York: Norton.

Janicak, P. G., Davis, J. M., Preskorn, S. H., & Ayd, F. J. (1997). *Principles and practice of psychopharmacotherapy* (2nd ed.). Baltimore: Williams & Wilkins.

Jobes, D. A., & Berman, D. L. (1993). Suicide and malpractice liability: Assessing and revising policies, procedures, and practice in outpatient settings. *Professional Psychology: Research and Practice, 30,* 83–87.

Johnson, D. W. (1972). *Reaching out: Interpersonal effectiveness and self-actualization.,* Englewood Cliffs, NJ: Prentice-Hall.

Johnson, D. W., & Matross, R. (1977). Interpersonal influence in psychotherapy: A social psychological view. In A. S. Gurman & A. M. Razin (Eds.), *Effective psychotherapy: A handbook of research.* Oxford: Pergamon Press.

Johnson, J. G., Rabkin, J. G., Williams, J. B. W., Reiman, R. H., & Gorman, J. M. (2000). Difficulties in interpersonal relationships associated with personality disorder and Axis I disorders: A longitudinal community-based investigation. *Journal of Personality Disorders, 14,* 42–56.

Johnson, M. E., Popp, C., Schacht, T. E., Mellon, J., & Strupp, H. H. (1989) Converging evidence for identification of recurrent relationship themes: Comparison of two methods. *Psychiatry, 52,* 275–288.

Joiner, T. E., Walker, R. L., Rudd, M. D., & Jobes, D. A. (1999). Scientizing and routinizing the assessment of suicidality in outpatient practice. *Professional Psychology: Research and Practice, 30,* 447–453.

Julien, R. M. (1995). *A primer of drug action: A concise, nontechnical guide to the actions, uses, and side effects of psychoactive drugs* (7th ed.). New York: Freeman.

Kagan, J. (1994). *Galen's prophecy: Temperament in human nature.* New York: Basic Books.

Kaslow, N., Thompson, M. P., Meadows, L. A., Jacobs, D., Chance, S., Gibb, B., Bornstein, H., Hollins, L., Rashid, A., & Phillips, K. (1998). Factors that mediate and moderate the link between partner abuse and suicidal behavior in African American women. *Journal of Consulting and Clinical Psychology, 66,* 533–544.

Kernberg, O. F. (2001). The suicidal risk in severe personality disorders: Differential diagnosis and treatment. *Journal of Personality Disorders, 15,* 195–208.

Kiesler, D. J. (1983). The 1982 interpersonal circle: A taxonomy for complementarity in human transactions. *Psychological Review, 90,* 185–214.

Kivlighan, D. M., Multon, K. D., & Patton, M. J. (2000). Insight and symptom reduction in time-limited psychoanalytic counseling. *Journal of Counseling Psychology, 47,* 50–58.

Kleespies, P. M., Deleppo, J. D., Gallagher, P. L., & Niles, B. L. (1999). Managing suicidal emergencies: Recommendations for the practitioner. *Professional Psychology: Research and Practice, 30,* 454–463.

Klein, D. F. (1996). Preventing hung juries about therapy studies. *Journal of Consulting and Clinical Psychology, 64,* 81–87.

Klein, M. H., Benjamin, L. S., Rosenfeld, R., Treece, C., Husted, J., & Greist, J. H. (1993). The Wisconsin Personality Disorders Inventory: I. Development, reliability, and validity. *Journal of Personality Disorders, 7,* 285–303.

Klein, M. H., Kolden, G. G., Michels, J., & Chrisholm-Stockard, S. (2002). Effective elements of the therapy relationship: Congruence/genuineness. In J. C. Norcross (Ed.), *Psychotherapy relationships that work: Therapists' relational contributions to effective psychotherapy.* New York: Oxford University Press.

Kolb, B., & Whishaw, I. (1998). Brain plasticity and behavior. *Annual Review of Psychology, 49,* 43–64.

Kosmicki, F. X., & Glickauf-Hughes, C. (1997). Catharsis in psychotherapy. *Psychotherapy, 34,* 154–159.

Kroll, J. (2000). Use of no-suicide contracts by psychiatrists in Minnesota. *American Journal of Psychiatry, 157,* 1684–1686.

Krupnik, J. L., Sotsky, S. M., Simmens, S., Moyer, J., Elkin, I., Watkins, J., & Pilkonis, P. A. (1996). The role of the therapeutic alliance in psychotherapy pharmacotherapy outcome. *Journal of Consulting and Clinical Psychology, 64,* 532–539.

Lambert, M. J., & Bergin, A. E. (1994). The effectiveness of psychotherapy. In A. E. Bergin & S. L. Garfield (Eds.), *Handbook of psychotherapy and behavior change* (4th ed.). New York: Wiley.

Lambert, M. J., Hawkins, E .J., & Hatfield, D. R. (2002). Empirishe forschung uber negative effekte in der psychotherapie: Befunde und ihre bedeutung fur praxis und forschung. In M. Martens & H. Petzold (Eds.), *Therapieschaden: Risiken und nebenwirkungen von psychotherapie.* Mainz, Germany: Matthias-Grunewald-Verlag.

Leary, T. (1957). *Interpersonal diagnosis of personality: A functional theory and methodology for personality evaluation.* New York: Ronald Press.

Lecomte, T., Liberman, R. P., & Wallace, C. J. (2000). Identifying and using reinforcers to enhance the treatment of persons with serious mental illness. *Psychiatric Services, 51,* 1312–1314.

Lee, R., & Coccaro, E. (2001). The neuropsychopharmacology of criminality and aggression. *Canadian Journal of Psychiatry, 46,* 24–25.

Leitenberg, H., & Henning, K. (1995). Sexual fantasy. *Psychological Bulletin, 117,* 469–496.

Levendosky, A. A., & Graham-Bermann, S. A. (2000). Behavioral observations of parenting in battered women. *Journal of Family Psychology, 14,* 80–94.

Lewinsohn, P. M., Rohde, P. E., & Seeley, J. R. (1994). Psychosocial risk factors for future adolescent suicide attempts. *Journal of Consulting and Clinical Psychology, 62,* 297–304.

Linehan, M. M. (1993). *Cognitive-behavioral treatment of borderline personality disorder.* New York: Guilford Press.

Linneberg, D. M. (1999). Moral education and choice theory/reality therapy: An initial examination. *International Journal of Reality Therapy, 19,* 52–55.

Loftus, E. F., Garry, M., & Feldman, J. (1994). Forgetting sexual trauma: What does it mean when 38% forget? *Journal of Consulting and Clinical Psychology, 62,* 1177–1181.

Lowenstein, L. F. (1997). Research into causes and manifestations of aggression in car driving. *Police Journal, 70,* 263–270.

Luborsky, L. (1984). *Principles of psychoanalytic psychotherapy: A manual for supportive-expressive treatment.* New York: Basic Books.

Luborsky, L., Barber, J. P., & Crits-Christoph, P. (1990). Theory-based research for understanding the process of dynamic psychotherapy. *Journal of Consulting and Clinical Psychology, 58,* 281–287.

Luborsky, L., Singer, B., & Luborsky, L. (1975). Comparative studies of psychotherapies: Is it true that "everyone has won and all must have prizes"? *Archives of General Psychiatry, 32,* 995–1008.

Luborsky, L., Popp, C., Luborsky, E., & Mark, D. (1994). The core conflictual relationship theme. *Psychotherapy Research, 4,* 172–183.

Lunnen, K. M., & Ogles, B. M. (1998). A multiperspective, multivariable evaluation of reliable change. *Journal of Consulting and Clinical Psychology, 66,* 400–410.

Lynch, K. (2000). The long road back. *Journal of Clinical Psychology, 56,* 1427–1432.

MacKenzie, K. R. (1990). *Introduction to time-limited group psychotherapy.* Washington, DC: American Psychiatric Press.

MacKenzie, K. R. (1997). *Time-managed group psychotherapy. Effective clinical applications.* Washington D.C.: American Psychiatric Press.

Malan, D. H. (1976). *The frontier of brief psychotherapy.* New York: Plenum Press.

Martin, D. J., Garske, J. P., & Davis, M. K. (2000). Relation of the therapeutic alliance with outcome and other variables. A meta-analytic review. *Journal of Consulting and Clinical Psychology, 68,* 438–450.

McEwen, T. (1997). Communication training in corporate settings: Lessons and opportunities for the academe. *Mid-American Journal of Business, 12,* 49–58.

Menninger, K. (1958). *Theory of psychoanalytic technique.* New York: Basic Books.

Michaud, S. G., & Aynesworth, H. (1989). *Ted Bundy: Conversations with a killer.* New York: New American Library.

Miller, N. E., Luborsky, L., Barber, J. P., & Docherty, J. P. (Eds.). (1993). *Psychodynamic treatment research: A handbook for clinical practice.* New York: Basic Books.

Miller, T. Q., Smith, T. W., Turner, C. W., Guijarro, M. L., & Hallet, A. J. (1996). A meta-analytic review of research on hostility and physical health. *Psychological Bulletin, 119,* 322–348.

Miller, W. (2000). Motivational interviewing: IV. Some parallels with horse whispering. *Behavioural and Cognitive Psychotherapy, 28,* 285–292.

Miller, W. R. (1985). Motivation for treatment: A review with special emphasis on alcoholism. *Psychological Bulletin, 98,* 84–107.

Miller, W. R., Benefield, R. G., & Tonigan, J. S. (1993). Enhancing motivation for change in problem drinking: A controlled comparison of two therapist styles. *Journal of Consulting and Clinical Psychology, 61,* 455–461.

Miller, W. R., Meyers, R. J., & Tonigan, J. S. (1999). Engaging the unmotivated in treatment for alcohol problems: A comparison of three strategies for intervention through family. *Journal of Consulting and Clinical Psychology, 67,* 688–697.

Mischel, W. (1973). On the empirical dilemmas of psychodynamic approaches: Issues and alternatives. *Journal of Abnormal Psychology, 82,* 335–344.

Morrison, L. L., & Downey, D. L. (2000). Racial differences in self-disclosure of suicidal ideation and reasons for living. *Cultural Diversity and Ethnic Minority Psychology, 6,* 374–386.

Murphy, C. M., & Baxter, V. A. (1997). Motivating batterers to change in the treatment context. *Journal of Interpersonal Violence, 12,* 607–619.

Murray, H. A. (1938). *Explorations in personality.* New York: Oxford University Press.

Neale, M. S., & Rosenheck, R. A. (2000). Therapeutic limit setting in an assertive community treatment program. *Psychiatric Services, 5,* 499–505.

Nerdrum, P. (1997). Maintenance of the effect of training in communication skills: A controlled follow-up study of level of communicated empathy. *British Journal of Social Work, 27,* 705–722.

Newman, L. S., Duff, K. J., & Bandmaster, R. F. (1997). A new look at defensive projection. Thought suppression, accessibility, and biased person perception. *Journal of Personality and Social Psychology, 72,* 980–1001.

Norcross, J. C. (2000). Here comes the self-help revolution in mental heath. *Psychotherapy: Theory, Research, Practice, Training, 37,* 370–377.

Norcross, J. C. (Ed.). (2002). *Psychotherapy relationships that work: Therapists' relational contributions to effective psychotherapy.* New York: Oxford University Press.

Ogles, B. M., Lambert, M. J., & Sawyer, J. D. (1995). Clinical significance of the National Institute of Mental Health Treatment of Depression Collaborative Research Program data. *Journal of Consulting and Clinical Psychology, 63,* 321–326.

Ouimette, P. C., Finney, J. W., & Moos, R. H. (1997). Twelve-Step and cognitive-behavioral treatment for substance abuse: A comparison of treatment effectiveness. *Journal of Consulting and Clinical Psychology, 65,* 230–240.

OPD Task Force. (Ed.) *OPD: Operationalized psychodynamic diagnostics. Foundations and manual.* Toronto: Hogrefe & Huber.

Overholser, J. C. (1997). Treatment of excessive interpersonal dependency: A cognitive-behavioral model. *Journal of Contemporary Psychotherapy, 27,* 283–301.

Paivio, S. C., & Greenberg, L. (1995). Resolving "unfinished business": Efficacy of experiential therapy using empty-chair dialogue. *Journal of Consulting and Clinical Psychology, 63,* 419–425.

Pam, A. (1994). Limit setting: Theory, techniques, and risks. *American Journal of Psychotherapy, 48,* 432–440.

Pavio, S. C., & Bahr, L. M. (1998). Interpersonal problems, working alliance, and outcome in short-term experiential therapy. *Psychotherapy Research, 8,* 392–407.

Perry, J. C., Banon, E., & Ianni, F. (1999). Effectiveness of psychotherapy for personality disorders. *American Journal of Psychiatry, 156,* 1312–1321.

Peruzzi, N., & Bongar, B. (1999). Assessing risk for completed suicide in patients with major depression: Psychologists' views of critical factors. *Professional Psychology: Research and Practice, 30,* 576–580.

Pincus, A., & Benjamin, L. S. (in preparation). *Structural Analysis of Social Behavior: A method for the scientific study of psychopathology and psychotherapy.* Washington, DC: American Psychological Association.

Piper, W. E., Rosie, J. S., Joyce, A. S., & Azim, H. F. A. (1996). *Time-limited day treatment for personality disorders: Integration of research and practice in a group program.* Washington, DC: American Psychological Association.

Poincaré, H. (1947). Science and hypothesis. In D. J. Bronstein, Y. H. Krikorian, & P. P. Wiener (Eds.), *Basic problems of philosophy.* New York: Prentice-Hall. (Original work published 1905)

Prentky, R. A., Burgess, A. W., Rokous, F., Lee, A., Hartman, C., Ressler, R., & Douglas, J. (1989). The presumptive role of fantasy in serial sexual homicide. *American Journal of Psychiatry, 146,* 887–891.

Prochaska, J. O., DiClemente, C. C., & Norcross, J. C. (1992). In search of how people change: Applications to addictive behaviors. *American Psychologist, 47,* 1102–1114.

Prochaska, J. O., Velicer, W. F., Rossi, J. S., Goldstein, M. G., Marcus, B. H., Rakowski, W., Fiore, C., Harlow, L. L., Redding, C. A., Rosenbloom, D., & Rossi, S. R. (1994). Stages of change and decisional balance for 12 problem behaviors. *Health Psychology, 13*, 39–46.

Pugh, C. (1999). *Impact of therapist affirmation on the process and outcome of psychotherapy.* Unpublished doctoral dissertation, University of Utah.

Rawls, J. (1963). The sense of justice. *Philosophical Review, 72*, 281–305.

Reid, W. H. (1989). Treatment of violent patients: Concerns for the psychiatrist. In A. Tasman, R. E. Hales, & A. J. Frances (Eds.), *American Psychiatric Press review of psychiatry* (Vol. 8). Washington, DC: American Psychiatric Press.

Reik, T. (1949). *The inner experience of a psychoanalyst.* London: George Allen and Unwin, Ltd.

Reiss, D., Plomin, R., & Hetherington, E. M. (1991). Genetics and psychiatry: An unheralded window on the environment. *American Journal of Psychiatry, 148*, 283–291.

Rogers, C. R. (1951). *Client-centered therapy.* Cambridge MA: The Riverside Press.

Rose, R. J. (1995). Genes and human behavior. *Annual Review of Psychology, 46*, 625–654.

Rosenbaum, M., & Bennett, B. (1986). Homicide and depression. *American Journal of Psychiatry, 143*, 367–370.

Rosenberg, J. I. (1999). Suicide prevention: An integrated training model using affective and action-based interventions. *Professional Psychology: Research and Practice, 30*, 83–87.

Rudd, M. D., Joiner, T. E., Jobes, D. A., & King, C. A. (1999). The outpatient treatment of suicidality: An integration of science and recognition of its limitations. *Professional Psychology: Research and Practice, 30*, 437–446.

Rudd, M. D., Joiner, T. E., & Rajab, M. H. (1995). Help negation after acute suicidal crisis. *Journal of Consulting and Clinical Psychology, 63*, 499–503.

Safran, J. D., & Muran, J. C. (1996). The resolution of ruptures in the therapeutic alliance. *Journal of Consulting and Clinical Psychology, 64*, 447–458.

Santrock, J. W., Minnett, A. M., & Campbell, B. D. (1994). *The authoritative guide to self-help books.* New York: Guilford Press.

Schulberg, H. C., Pilkonis, P. A., & Houck, P. (1998). *The severity of major depression and choice of treatment in primary care practice.* Unpublished manuscript, Department of Psychiatry, University of Pittsburgh School of Medicine.

Seligman, M. (1975). *Helplessness: On depression, development and death.* San Francisco: Freeman.

Seligman, M. (1995). The effectiveness of psychotherapy: The *Consumer Reports* study. *American Psychologist, 50*, 965–974.

Shea, M. T. (1993). Psychosocial treatment of personality disorders. *Journal of Personality Disorders, 7*(Suppl.), 167–180.

Sifneos, P. E. (1979). *Short-term dynamic psychotherapy: Evaluation and technique.* New York: Plenum Press.

Simon, L. M. J. (1995). A therapeutic jurisprudence approach to the legal processing of domestic violence cases. *Psychology, Public Policy, and Law, 1*, 43–79.

Skinner, B. F. (1990). Can psychology be a science of mind? *American Psychologist, 45*, 1206–1210.

Soloff, P. (1997). Psychobiologic perspectives on treatment of personality disorders. *Journal of Personality Disorders, 11*, 336–344.

Strupp, H. H., & Binder, J. L. (1984). *Psychotherapy in a new key.* New York: Basic Books.

Strupp, H. H., Fox, R. E., & Lessler, K. (1964). *Patients view their psychotherapy.* Baltimore: Johns Hopkins University Press.

Suddendorf, T., & Whiten, A. (2001). Mental evolution and development: Evidence for secondary representation in children, great apes, and other animals. *Psychological Bulletin, 127*, 629–650.

Sullivan, H. S. (1953). *The interpersonal theory of psychiatry.* New York: Norton.

Sullivan, H. S. (1954). *The psychiatric interview* (H. S. Perry & M. L. Gawel, Eds.). New York: Norton.

Suomi, S. (1999). Attachment in rhesus monkeys. In J. Cassidy & P. R. Shaver (Eds.), *Handbook of attachment: Theory, research, and clinical applications.* New York: Guilford Press.

Sykes, C. M., & Marks, D. F. (2001). Effectiveness of a cognitive behaviour therapy self-help programme for smokers in London. *Health Promotion International, 16,* 255–260.

Task Force on Promotion and Dissemination of Psychological Procedures. (1995). Training in and dissemination of empirically-validated psychological treatments. *The Clinical Psychologist, 48,* 3–23.

Teyber, E. (1997). *Interpersonal process in psychotherapy: A relational approach* (3rd ed.). Pacific Grove, CA: Brooks/Cole.

Thase, M. E., Friedman, E. S., & Howland, R. H. (2001). Management of treatment-resistant depression: Psychotherapeutic perspectives. *Journal of Clinical Psychiatry, 62*(Suppl. 18), 18–24.

Thoma, H., & Kachele, H. (1987). *Psychoanalytic practice: Vol. 1. Principles.* New York: Springer-Verlag.

Tiihonen, J., & Hakola, P. (1994). Psychiatric disorders and homicide recidivism. *American Journal of Psychiatry, 151,* 436–438.

Tiihonen, J., Kuikka, J., Bergstrom, K., Lepola, U., Koponen, H., & Leinonen, E. (1997). Dopamine reuptake site densities in patients with social phobia. *American Journal of Psychiatry, 154,* 239–242.

Valenstein, E. S. (1998). *Blaming the brain: The truth about drugs and mental health.* New York: Free Press.

VandenBos, G. R. (1996). Outcome assessment of psychotherapy. *American Psychologist, 51,* 1005–1006.

van Doom, C., Kasl, S. V., Beery, L. C., Jacobs, S. C., & Prigerson, H. G. (1998). The influence of marital quality and attachment styles on traumatic grief and depressive symptoms. *Journal of Nervous and Mental Disease, 186,* 566–573.

Watzlawick, P., Beavin, J. H., & Jackson, D. D. (1967). *Pragmatics of human communication.* New York: Norton.

Weissman, M. M., Markowitz, J. C., & Klerman, G. L. (2000). *Comprehensive guide to interpersonal psychotherapy.* New York: Basic Books.

White, J. (1995). Stresspac: A controlled trial of a self-help package for the anxiety disorders. *Behavioural and Cognitive Psychotherapy, 23,* 89–107.

Wiggins, J. S. (1982). Circumplex models of interpersonal behavior in clinical psychology. In P. C. Kendall & J. N. Butcher (Eds.), *Handbook of research methods in clinical psychology.* New York: Wiley.

Williams, L. M. (1994). Recall of childhood trauma: Women's memories of child sexual abuse. *Journal of Consulting and Clinical Psychology, 62,* 1167–1176.

Witt, P. H., Rambus, E., & Bosley, T. (1996). Current developments in psychotherapy for child molesters. *Sexual and Marital Therapy, 11,* 173–185.

Wolpe, J., & Plaud, J. J. (1997). Pavlov's contributions to behavior therapy: The obvious and the not so obvious. *American Psychologist, 52,* 966–972.

Woodsie, R., Blake, D., Kaplan, A. S., Olmsted, M. P., & Carter, J. C. (2001). Pretreatment motivational enhancement therapy for eating disorders: A pilot study. *International Journal of Eating Disorders, 29,* 393–400.

Worthington, E. L., & Rachal, K. C. (1997). Interpersonal forgiving in close relationships. *Journal of Consulting and Clinical Psychology, 64,* 983–992.

Yahne, C. E., & Miller, W. R., (1999). Enhancing motivation for treatment and change. In B. S. McCrady & E. E. Epstein (Eds.), *Addictions: A comprehensive guidebook.* New York: Oxford University Press.

Yeomans, F. E., Selzer, M. A., & Clarkin, J. F. (1992). *Treating the borderline patient: A contract-based approach.* New York: Basic Books.

Zimmerman, M., Mattia, J. I., & Posternak, M. A. (2002). Are subjects in pharmacological treatment trials of depression representative of patients in routine clinical practice? *American Journal of Psychiatry, 159,* 469–473.

Zinbarg, R. E., Barlow, D. H., Brown, T. A., & Hertz, R. M. (1992). Cognitive-behavioral approaches to the nature and treatment of anxiety disorders. *Annual Review of Psychology, 43,* 235–267.

Index

ABC domains
  in case formulation, 45, 46
  internalized representations link, 45, 46
  in IRT core algorithm, 24, 25
  operationalization, 85
  SASB model, 135, 147–152, 153n11
    predictive principles, 151, 152
Abreaction, 262, 263
Active love code, 143n4
Adherence, 108, 109
Administrative issues, 109–114, 256, 257
Advice giving, 314–316
  case formulation context, 315
  in crisis management, 314
Affective domain
  in case formulation, 45, 46
  Growth Collaborator pattern, 77
  internalized representations link, 45, 46
  in IRT core algorithm, 24, 25
  in normal interpersonal behaviors, 300, 301
  Regressive Loyalist pattern, 77
  SASB model, 135, 147–152, 153n11
    predictive principles, 151, 152
Affiliation dimension, SASB model, 123–128
Aggression
  management of, 233, 242–250
  toward therapist, 258
Alcohol abuse
  and consent to treatment form, 119
  IRT policy, 106, 107
  symptom-focused management, 106, 107
Algorithm (see Core algorithm)
All-or-nothing thinking, 243, 301

Anger
  and countertransference reaction, 186, 187
  in differentiation process, 276–278
  mobilization of, 94
  toward therapist, 257, 258
Antithesis concept
  and copy processes, 134, 135
  SASB-based analysis, 132, 134, 135
Anxiety, and internalized representations, 40
Assertiveness
  case examples, 308, 309, 317, 318
  role play, 317, 318
  SASB model in teaching of, 311, 312
Assessment
  in case formulation, 55–58
  of IRT theory and practice, 341–343
  traditional methods, 57, 58, 111
Associative method, 205, 206
Attachment
  Bowlby's theory, 64–67
  and case formulation, 43–45
  change process link, 199–201
  definitions, 157, 158
  Developmental Learning and Loving Theory basis, 63–68
  and dependent–independent behavior, 66, 67
  inborn propensity toward, 203
  IRT link, 157–161, 327
  neurochemical correlates, 66
  primate model, 65–67
  in psychopathology development, 9, 10
  and self-discovery, change process, 266–269

to therapist, 159–161, 200
and therapy goals, 136–138, 327
therapy outcome role, 160, 161
Attendance issues, 109, 110, 118, 257
Attention-seeking behavior, 264
Audiotape, of family conference, 211, 212
"Auto mechanic" model, 270, 271
Awareness
  mindfulness in, 306, 307
  therapy goal, 301, 306, 307
Axis I–Axis III symptoms (*see* DSM symptoms)

Beck Depression Inventory, 57, 111
Behavioral therapies, 333–337
  empirical validation, 5
  IRT relationship, 333–337
  in learning new patterns, 309, 310
  model of, 344, 345
  self-management emphasis, 89
  therapy alliance–outcome link, 155, 156
Billing issues, 110, 111, 118
Bisexuality, 176, 177
"Black box" concept, 116*n*17
Blame seeking (*see* Self-blame)
"Blocking silence," 172, 173
Bonding, 66, 157, 158
Borderline personality disorder
  case formulation, 41
  and couple relationship, 294, 295
  internalized representations link, 41
  stabilization phase, 255, 256
Bowlby's attachment theory, 64–67
Brief psychotherapy, 340, 341
  collaboration precondition, 303, 304
  indications for, 340, 341
  long–term therapy comparison, 27

Case formulation, 31–71
  and adherence facilitation, 108
  in crisis management, 234–238, 251
  development of, 35–53
  Developmental Learning and Loving theory in, 9, 10, 32–63
    scientific basis, 58–63
  essential components, 32–34
  inpatient consultation, 36, 37
  intervention link, 81, 82
  in IRT core algorithm, 23

outpatient consultation, 37, 38
report writing component, 55–57
specificity importance, 82–84
theory role in, 31, 32
and treatment planning, 53–55
Case report, 55–57
"Cat therapy," 115*n*11
Catharsis
  as change model, 262, 263, 270, 271
  misuse potential, 270, 271
Causal-factors assumption
  in Developmental Learning and Loving theory, 58, 59
  direct tests of, 58, 59
  internalized representations–symptom link, 60–63
  treatment implications, 62
Change process (*see also* Will to change)
  and attachment security, 200, 201
  collaboration as precondition, 269, 270
  and copy process recognition, 267–269
  fear of, 101, 305
  and goal setting, 285, 286
  insight relationship, 199, 200
  maintenance of, 290, 296
  motivation for, 262, 266
  models, 263, 264
  precontemplation stage, 264, 266–273
  resistance to, 318, 319
  self-discovery role, 266–269, 273–279, 281–285
  self-management approach, 279–281
  stages, 263, 264
  tests of, 58, 59
  therapy models, 270–273
  transtheoretical approach, 263, 264, 296*n*3
Child abuse
  case formulation specificity, 83, 84
  correlates, 231, 232
  reporting requirements, 115*n*14
"Childlike" behaviors, 124
  and copy processes, 135
  SASB analysis, 124, 135
Children, and parenting behavior, 317, 318
Choice behavior
  mindfulness in, 306, 307
  self-management approach, 308, 309
  and therapy goals, 301, 306–309
Classical conditioning model, 334, 335
Client-centered therapy, 328
Clinical trials standard, 5
Cluster model, overview, 128–130
Coaching, 316

Cognitive-behavioral therapy, 333–337
  definition, 28n2
  empirical validation, 5
  IRT relationship, 333–337
  self-management emphasis of, 89
  therapy alliance–outcome link, 155,
    156
Cognitive domain
  in case formulation, 45, 46
  and Growth Collaborator, 77
  internalized representations link, 45,
    46
  in IRT core algorithm, 24, 25
  in normal interpersonal behavior, 300,
    301
  and Regressive Loyalist, 77
  SASB model, 135, 147–152, 153n11
    predictive principles, 151, 152
Collaboration, 154–192
  brief therapy precondition, 303, 304
  as change precondition, 269, 270
  confrontation approach contrast, 168
  dilemmas in, 171–180
  in group therapy, 339
  intervention hierarchy, 86, 87
  in IRT core algorithm, 21, 24
  and therapy goals achievement, 161–
    185
  and therapy tasks, 88
Coming to terms
  flow chart, 89–97
  and motivational change, 262, 296n1
Commitment to hospital, 228, 229, 246,
    247
Common-factors effect, 155, 156
Complementarity
  and couple therapy, 337, 338
  recognition in therapy process, 204
  SASB model, 130–133
  and self-management, 96
Complex coding, 144, 145, 152
Confidentiality, 117, 118
Conflict engagement
  in IRT core algorithm, 22–24
  psychodynamic theory, 328, 329
Confrontation approach, 168
Congruence, 328, 349n5
Consent to treatment form, 109, 117–
    119, 198, 222n9
Consumer Reports article, 28n3
Control code, definition, 142n2
Copy process speech, 46, 47
Copy processes
  causal assumption, 58–63
  in current problem review, 91
  dangerous behavior link, 238–240
  depression link, 40
  genetics compatibility, 63

gift-of-love link, 197, 198
  identification of, 206, 207
  motivation for change link, 266–269
  normality of, 67
  in parenting, 317, 318
  presentation to patient, 46–49, 69n13
  in psychopathology development, 9,
    10, 325, 326
  SASB-based analysis, 134, 135
  in social development, 67
  and suicidality, 234, 236, 238–240
  theory of, 49
  in treatment planning, 54, 55
Core algorithm, 22–25, 73–89, 326, 327
Core Conflict Relational Themes method
  components, 195
  insight-related outcome application,
    195, 196
Cost-effectiveness, psychotherapy, 27
Countertransference, 185–188
  interpretation of, 187, 330
    IRT perspective, 330, 331
  manifestations, 186, 187, 330
Couple therapy (*see* Marital/couple
    relationship)
"Courtroom" model (*see* "Justice"
    model)
Crisis management, 228–256
  advice giving, 314
  anticipatory interventions, 251
  and case formulation, 234–238, 251
  copy process review in, 234–236
  family conferences, 338, 339
  flow chart, 238–245
  follow-up, 250
  and homicidality, 231–233, 242–250
  hospitalization, 228, 229, 246, 247
  IRT perspective, 233–256
  medication in, 242, 243
  problem-solving approach, 243, 244
  stabilization expectation, 255, 256
  suicidality, 229–231
  telephone handling of, 247–249
Cultural values, and therapy goals, 137
Cyclical Maladaptive Pattern analysis,
    222n1

Dangerous behavior, 228–256
  copy process links, 238–240
  hospitalization, 228, 229
  IRT approach, 233–256
    flow chart, 238–245
  no-harm contracts, 244–246
Darwinian theory, 8, 29n13,n14
Decision making, 308, 309

Defenses, 213–217
  adaptive aspects, 215
  experimental data, 213, 214
  functions, 214, 215
  recognition of, 213–217
  relevance, 214
  SASB-based analysis, 135
Denial, in therapist, 219
Dependency
  attachment theory, 66, 67
  and therapy relationship, 200
Depression
  case formulation–intervention link, 81, 82
  internalized representations link, 40, 60
Desensitization procedure, 334, 335
Detached behavior, 136
Deterioration problem, 7, 29n7
Developmental Learning and Loving theory
  attachment theory relationship, 63–68
  and case formulation, 9, 10, 20, 26, 27, 32–63
    scientific basis, 58–63
  causal factors interpretation, 61–63, 345
  limits of applicability, 34, 35
  overview, 9, 10, 325, 326
  predictive aspects, 133
  treatment implications, 33, 34, 53–55
Dialectical behavior therapy, 309
Differentiation (see Enmeshment–differentiation)
Disaffiliative behavior, 136
Disclosure
  and countertransference, 330, 331
  therapist's use of, 174–177, 330, 331
Domestic violence, 231, 232, 242–250
Dream analysis, 207–209
  and insight development, 207–209
  SASB coding, 209, 224n31
  will to change facilitation, 209
Drive theory, 328
Drug abuse
  on consent to treatment form, 119
  IRT approach, 106, 107, 119
  symptom-focused approach, 106, 107
DSM symptoms
  in case assessment, 35, 36
  internalized representations connection, 40–42
Duty to warn, 246, 247

E-mail contact, 110
Effectiveness of psychotherapy
  definition, 6, 29n10
  overstatement of, 6, 7

Efficacy of psychotherapy, 6, 29n9
Efficiency of psychotherapy, 6
Ego, and Growth Collaborator, 78
Eligibility, for IRT, 107, 108
Emergencies (see also Crisis management)
  hospitalization, 228, 229
  telephone contact, 118, 119
Empathic listening, 309
Empathy
  in case formulation interview, 39
  in core algorithm, 22, 74
  and IRT adherence, 220
  phrasing of, 74–76
Empirically supported therapies
  definition, 5, 6
  long-term therapy comparison, 27
  overstated effectiveness of, 6, 7
  side effects, 6, 7
Empirically validated therapies, 5, 6
Empowerment, 281
Enmeshment–differentiation
  and couple therapy, 338
  and IRT goals, 136–138, 142n2, 299–301, 326
  relativistic nature of, 326
  role plays in, 312, 313
  SASB model in teaching of, 311, 312
Eroticized homicide, 232 (see also Klute syndrome)
Eroticized pain, 289, 290
Ethics, APA code, 114
Evolutionary factors, 8, 29n13,n14, 137, 138
Existential problems, 319, 320
Extended family, conferences, 338, 339
Externalizing patients, responsibility taking, 286, 287
Extinction, learning theory, 335

"False memories," 217, 218
Family conference
  fantasy format, 337
  in new pattern learning, 207, 208, 337–339
  tape of, 211, 212
Family violence, 231, 232 (see also Violence, management of)
Fantasy (see also Important Persons and their Internalized Representations)
  in Klute syndrome, 289, 290
  reconstruction "shortcut," 92, 93
  relinquishing of, 287, 288
  about therapist, and suicidality, 253, 254
Fear of change, 101, 305

Fear of therapy, 180, 181
Fees, 110, 111, 118
Forgiving, 97, 116n19, 283
Free association, 211
Frequency of sessions, 111
Friendliness, therapy goal, 136–138, 299–302, 326

Generalization of results, 346
Genetics, and copy processes, 63
Gestalt therapy, 329
Gift of love
  blame-seeking function, 217
  causal assumption, 58, 59
  confronting of, in change process, 266–273, 327
  explanation to patient, 49–51
  identification of, 197, 198
  treatment implication, 326
Gift-of-love speech, 48–51
Goals
  in change process, 285, 286
  and collaboration, 161–185
  in IRT final stage, 299–302
  rationale, 137, 138
  SASB utilization, 135–138
"Goals" speech, 162, 163
The Green, 154–192
  in case formulation, 33
  ego comparison, 78
  empathy enhancement of, 75, 76, 79, 80
  and "goals speech," 162
  internalized representations link, 78, 79
  in IRT core algorithm, 22–24
  maximization of, 165–171
  in problem pattern identification, 196, 197
  Red conflict, resolution of, 89–97
  and psychodynamic theory, 328, 329
  and self-management, 94–97
Green empathy, 75, 76, 79, 80, 128
Green goodbye, 322
Green grief, 281
Grief and lost internalizations, 93, 281, 282, 318, 319
  and self-discovery, 281, 282
Group therapy, 95, 339, 340
Growth Collaborator (*see* The Green)

Habits, and copy processes, 64
Homicidality, 231–233, 242–250
Homosexuality, 176, 177

Hope factor, 156, 189n9
Hospitalization
  crisis management, 228, 229, 246, 247
  in symptom management, 105

Id, 77, 328
Identification
  and gift-of-love message, 197, 198
  SASB-based analysis, 134
Important Persons and their Internalized Representations (IPIRs)
  attachment theory, 64, 65
  and case formulation, 13, 14, 16, 20, 33, 49
  causal factors assumption, 58–63
  compassion for, 284, 285
  constructive anger toward, 276–278
  differentiation from, 275–278
  forgiveness, 283
  functional analysis, 344, 345
  in gift-of-love speech, 49
  loss of, grief work, 93
  in psychopathology development, 10, 326
  SASB assessments, 120–122, 134, 135
  in self-discovery process, 91–93
  symptoms link, 40–42, 46, 47, 59
Impression management, 82
Independence
  attachment theory, 66, 67
  IRT goal, 299
  SASB definition, 142n1
Informants, in case formulation, 218
Informed consent, 117
Inpatient consultation, 36, 37
Insight, 193–225
  definitions, 194–198
  and dream analysis, 207, 208
  facilitation of, 202–218
  markers of, 199
  outcome connection, 195, 196
  psychoanalytic view, 194
  will to change facilitation, 198–201
Instrumental conditioning, 334
Insurance companies, disclosure, 118
Internal working models
  Bowlby's hypothesis, 49, 64, 65
  in psychopathology development, 9, 10
Internalization (*see also* Important Persons and their Internalized Representations)
  of new figures, 283, 284
  of therapist, 159, 284

Internalizing patients, responsibility taking, 286, 287
Interpersonal psychotherapy
empirical validation, 5
and self-management, 89
therapy alliance–outcome link, 155, 156
Interpretation
and collaboration, 331
insight facilitation function, 209–211
method, 48, 69*n*14, 331
psychoanalytic approach, 331
Interpretive reflection, 209
Interviews
case report basis, 55–57
inpatients, 36, 37
methods, 37–46
outpatients, 37, 38
Intrex questionnaire (*see* SASB Intrex)
Introjection
copy processes, 134
and gift-of-love message, 197, 198
predictive aspects, 131
SASB-based analysis, 123, 124, 126, 134
in self-system formation, 124, 139*n*8
of therapist, 161
Isolation defense, 254, 255

"Justice" model
clinical judgment in use of, 301, 302
problematic aspects, 271, 272, 301
of therapy, 270–272, 297*n*8, 301, 302

Klute syndrome, 101, 102, 259, 288–290

Learning speech, 51–53
breaking an impasse function, 102
intervention integration, 85–87
presentation to patient, 51–53
in therapy termination, 320
Legal disputes, therapist's participation, 180
Letting go, 282, 283
Limit setting, therapy behaviors, 257–259
Long-term therapy, 27
Loss (*see* Grief)
Love (*see* Gift of love)

Maintenance of change, 291–296
Manualization of therapy, 5
Marital/couple relationship
and complementarity, 337, 338
IRT goals, 135–138, 293–295, 337, 338
two-circle model, 294, 337
Medication, in crisis management, 242, 243
Memorabilia, 211
Memories
accuracy of, 217, 218
changes during therapy, 217
and psychodynamic theory validity, 345, 346
Mirroring, 48, 69*n*14
Missed appointments, 109, 110, 118, 257
Modeling
role-play use, 312, 313
therapy relationship in, 310–313
Moral choice technique, 265
Mother–infant bond, 65, 66
Motivation
abreaction effects on, 262, 263
for change, 262–266, 273–279
internalized representations role, 60–63
and IRT eligibility, 107
self-discovery link, 226, 227, 273–279
Motivational enhancement therapy, 264

Negative reinforcement, 334
No-harm contracts, 244–246, 249–250
Nonresponders
definition, 6, 28*n*4
evaluation, 2–4
Normality, SASB definition, 135–138

Object relations theory, 328
Operant conditioning, 74, 75, 333, 334
Opposites
and copy processes, 134, 135
SASB-based analysis, 131, 134, 135
Organizational psychology, 340
Outcome (*see* Therapy outcome)
Outpatient consultation, 37, 38
"Outpatient hospitalizations," 247
"Overdetermined" behavior, 94, 115*n*17

Paradoxical technique, 54
Paraphilias, 232
Parenting behavior
  copy processes in, 317
  and role play, 317, 318
"Parentlike" behaviors
  and copy processes, 135
  SASB analysis, 123, 124
Participant observer concept, 186
Passive–aggressive personality disorder
  brief therapy contraindication, 304
  case formulation, 41, 81
    intervention link, 81, 115n11
    internalized representations link, 41
  limit setting, 257
  and therapy relationship monitoring, 253
Pavlovian model, 334, 335
Payment issues, 110, 111, 118
Peer group support, 313
Performance model, 59, 60
"Peripatetic empathy," 38
Personality disorders
  case formulation, 41
  internalized representations, 41
  nonresponse to treatment, 3, 4
  therapy relationship monitoring, 253
Personality theory, 8, 9
Placebo effect, psychotherapy outcome, 156
"Pointing out," 108
Pornography, and eroticized violence, 232
Positive reinforcement, 333, 334
Presenting problems, 55–57, 59
Primate model, attachment relationship, 65–67
Problem solving approach, 243, 244
Projection
  experimental data, 213, 214
  relevance of, 214
Psychic proximity
  causal assumption, 58, 59, 327, 344
  functional analysis, 344, 345
  in gift-of-love speech, 49
  normality of, 67
  in social development, 67
Psychodynamic therapy, 328, 329
  criticisms, 343–347
  insight role in, 194
  IRT link, 328, 329
  self-discovery emphasis, 89
Psychosomatic symptoms, 41, 42
Public relations orientation, 82
Punishment, 334

Quadrant model, 122–128
  coding, 125–128
  dimensions, 122–125
  overview, 128, 129
QUAINT coding system, 222n2

Rapprochement, 33
"Real-time coding," 121
Reality therapy, 265
Recapitulation
  and gift-of-love message, 197, 198
  SASB-based analysis, 134
Record keeping, 111–113
The Red
  and blockers to progress, 97–100
  in case formulation, 33, 34
  Green conflict, resolution of, 89–97
  id comparison, 77
  internalized representations in, 78, 79
  intervention, 76–79, 89–97, 165–171
    flow chart, 89–97
  in IRT core algorithm, 22–24
  minimization of, 165–171
  psychodynamic theory, 328, 329
  and therapy goals, 163
Red empathy
  and adherence facilitation, 108
  examples, 79, 80
  SASB-based analysis, 128
Regression (*see also* The Red)
  IRT approach, 333
  psychoanalytic theory, 323, 333
Regressive Loyalist (*see* The Red)
Reinforcement
  and change motivation, 265
  and IRT, 333–337
Religion, of therapist, 176
"Remember it" model, 270
Repression
  experimental data, 213, 214
  function, 214, 215
  relevance of, 214
Rescuer role, 10–13
Research, IRT outcome, 342, 343
Resistance, 331, 332
  IRT perspective, 332
  psychoanalytic perspective, 331, 332
Responsibility issue, 184, 185, 286, 287
Retrospective Assessment of the Therapy
    Experience, 111, 346
Role playing
  insight facilitation, 212, 213
  in new learning new patterns, 312, 313
  parenting behavior, 317, 318
Role Relationship Models method, 222n1

Safety contracts, 244–246, 249, 250
SASB Intrex, 311
 availability, 116*n*24
 goals and method, 58, 121, 122
 transference assessment, 121
Secondary reinforcement, 265
Secure base
 as change requirement, 199–201
 therapist's role in existential problems, 319
Self-blame, 215–217
 and "courtroom" therapy model, 272
 motivation, 215–217
 and responsibility taking, 287
Self-care, 143*n*5
Self-concept
 development of, 124, 139*n*8
 interview exploration, 39, 40
 intervention approach, 82–84
Self-disclosure (*see* Disclosure)
Self-discovery
 activities in, 166–168, 199
 in change process, 266–269, 273–279, 281–285
 and Green grieving, 281, 282
 and internalized representations, 91–94
 in learning new patterns, 304–308
 letting go process, 282, 283
 in maintenance of change, 291–293
 markers, 199
 motivation link, 226, 227
 in psychodynamic therapy, 89
 "shortcuts" to, 92–94
 therapeutic tasks, 87–89
 unconscious role in, 166
Self-help groups, 313
Self-help literature, 313, 314
Self-management
 in change process, 269–273, 279–281, 285–290
 collaborative approach to, 168, 269, 270
 coming to terms function, 94–97
 and complementary theory, 96
 implicit training, 168, 169
 in maintenance of change, 293–296
 in new pattern learning, 308–320
 self-discovery in, 226–228
 and short-term therapies, 89
 shortcuts, 96, 97
 therapeutic tasks in, 87–89, 168–171
Self-talk, 227, 228, 310
Self-Understanding of Interpersonal Patterns, 195, 196
Session summary form, 113
Sexual abuse
 repression of, 213, 214
 therapeutic approach, 275, 276, 297*n*11

Sexual fantasies, and *Klute* syndrome, 289, 290
Sexual orientation, therapist's attitude, 176
Sexuality, therapist's beliefs, 176, 177
Short-term therapy (*see* Brief psychotherapy)
Signs, definition, 70*n*27
Silences, 171–173
SOAP algorithm, 112, 303
Social deprivation, consequences, 67
Social skills training, 243
Social support, 242, 243
Specificity
 in problem pattern identification, 202, 203
 in therapy process channeling, 82–85
Spirituality, 176, 242
Stalking, 258, 259
"Stepped care" policy, 6
Stimulus discrimination, 336, 337
Stimulus generalization, 336
Structural Analysis of Affective Behavior, 148–152, 153*n*11
Structural Analysis of Cognitive Behavior, 148–152, 153*n*11
Structural Analysis of Social Behavior (SASB), 120–153
 assessment instruments, 120, 121
 cluster model, 128–130
 coding, 125–128, 144, 145
 full model, 145–147
 in interpersonal skills teaching, 311, 312
 normality definition, 135–138
 parallel models, 135, 147–152
 predictive principles, 129–135
 quadrant model, 122–128
 software, 121
 in therapy goals definition, 135–138
 underlying dimensions, 20, 21, 122–128
Structured Clinical Interview for DSM-IV Axis II, 111
Substance dependence, 106, 107, 119
Suicidality
 anticipatory interventions, 251
 copy process links, 238–240
 and fantasies about therapist, 253, 254
 and hospitalization, 228, 229, 246, 247
 impact, 230, 231
 IRT approach, 233–256
 medication role, 242, 243
 no-harm contract, 244–246
 perceived "benefits," 240
 risk factors, 229, 230

Suicidality (*continued*)
    social support mobilization, 242, 243
    telephone management, 247–249
    and threat management, 230, 238–245
"*Sunset Boulevard* syndrome," 274, 275,
    287, 304
Symptom Checklist 90—Revised, 57, 111
Symptom management
    flow chart, 103–107
    IRT results, 342, 343
    switch to, 103–106
    and therapy adherence, 108
    treatment as usual approach, 4, 5
Symptoms
    definition, 59, 70n27
    internalized representations link, 40,
        42, 59, 62, 63
    psychoanalytic explanations criticism,
        344

Telephone contact, 110, 118, 119, 247–
    249
"Telling" error
    exceptions, 105, 234
    in interpretation, 46–48, 220, 221, 268
    predictable response to, 268
Termination issues, 111, 320–323
Testimonials, IRT trainees, 341, 342
Theory
    case formulation role, 7, 8, 31, 32,
        58–63
    function of, 31, 32
Therapist (*see also* Countertransference)
    attachment to, 159–161, 200
    denial in, 219, 220
    internalization of, 159, 283, 284
    limit setting by, 257–259
    negative feelings toward, 181–183
    self-disclosure, 174–177
    as "substitute fantasy figure," 200
    and suicide fantasies, 253, 254
    threatening behavior toward, 258, 259
Therapy goals (*see* Goals)
Therapy outcome
    attachment role in, 160, 161
    empirically validated therapies, 6, 7
    insight connection, 195, 196
    IRT research findings, 342, 343
    specificity link, 202, 203
    therapy alliance link, 155, 156
Therapy relationship
    in crisis-prone cases, 246, 310, 311
    love relationship distinction, 158, 159
    in modeling new patterns, 310–311
    outcome link, 155, 156

"Thought experiment,", 92, 93
Traits, SASB coding, 133, 134
Trainees, IRT testimonials, 341, 342
Transference
    distortions in, 181–184, 329
    and negative feelings toward therapist,
        101
    psychoanalytic theory, 329
Transtheoretical model, of change, 263,
    264, 296n3
Trauma, catharsis benefits, 262, 263
Treatment as usual, 4–8
Treatment plan, formulation of, 53–
    55
Treatment recommendations, in case
    report, 55–57
Twelve-step programs, 106
Two-chair technique, 212, 213, 329

Unconditional acceptance approach,
    165, 166, 184, 328
Unconscious, therapist's use of, 209

Validation, IRT effectiveness, 341–343
Violence, management of, 233, 242–
    250
Voluntary hospitalization, 229

Will to change, 8, 9, 262–298
    attachment security link, 199–201
    collaboration in facilitation of, 269,
        270
    enabling of, 262–298
    and goal setting, 285, 286
    insight role in, 198–200
    and intervention hierarchy, 86
    models, 263, 264
    self-discovery role, 266–269, 273–
        279, 281–285
    stages of, 263–265
Wisconsin Personality Inventory,
    111
"Working silence," 172
"Working through" process, 262

Zero tolerance policy, 107, 119